Pediatric Demyelinating Disease and its Mimics

Editor

MANOHAR SHROFF

NEUROIMAGING CLINICS OF NORTH AMERICA

www.neuroimaging.theclinics.com

Consulting Editor
SURESH K. MUKHERJI

May 2013 • Volume 23 • Number 2

ELSEVIER

1600 John F. Kennedy Boulevard • Suite 1800 • Philadelphia, Pennsylvania, 19103-2899

http://www.theclinics.com

NEUROIMAGING CLINICS OF NORTH AMERICA Volume 23, Number 2
May 2013 ISSN 1052-5149, ISBN 13: 978-1-4557-7120-2

Editor: Pamela M. Hetherington
Developmental Editor: Teia Stone

Neuroimaging Clinics of North America (ISSN 1052-5149) is published quarterly by Elsevier Inc., 360 Park Avenue South, New York, NY 10010-1710. Months of issue are February, May, August, and November. Business and editorial offices: 1600 John F. Kennedy Blvd., Suite 1800, Philadelphia, PA 19103-2899. Business and editorial offices: 6277 Sea Harbor Drive, Orlando, FL 32887-4800. Periodicals postage paid at New York, NY, and additional mailing offices. Subscription prices are USD 342 per year for US individuals, USD 489 per year for US institutions, USD 172 per year for US students and residents, USD 396 per year for Canadian individuals, USD 612 per year for Canadian institutions, USD 502 per year for international individuals, USD 612 per year for international institutions and USD 246 per year for Canadian and foreign students and residents. To receive student/resident rate, orders must be accompanied by name of affiliated institution, date of term, and the *signature* of program/residency coordinator on institution letterhead. Orders will be billed at individual rate until proof of status is received. Foreign air speed delivery is included in all *Clinics* subscription prices. All prices are subject to change without notice. POSTMASTER: Send address changes to *Neuroimaging Clinics of North America*, Elsevier Health Sciences Division, Subscription Customer Service, 3251 Riverport Lane, Maryland Heights, MO 63043. Telephone: 1-800-654-2452 (U.S. and Canada); 314-447-8871 (outside U.S. and Canada). Fax: 314-447-8029. E-mail: journalscustomerservice-usa@elsevier.com (for print support); journalsonlinesupport-usa@elsevier.com (for online support).

Reprints. For copies of 100 or more of articles in this publication, please contact the Commercial Reprints Department, Elsevier Inc., 360 Park Avenue South, New York, NY 10010-1710. Tel.: 212-633-3812; Fax: 212-462-1935; E-mail: reprints@elsevier.com.

Neuroimaging Clinics of North America is covered by *Excerpta Medica/EMBASE,* the RSNA Index of Imaging Literature, *MEDLINE/PubMed (Index Medicus),* MEDLINE/MEDLARS, SciSearch, Research Alert, and Neuroscience Citation Index.

Printed and bound by CPI Group (UK) Ltd, Croydon, CR0 4YY
Transferred to Digital Printing, 2013

PROGRAM OBJECTIVE

The goal of *Neuroimaging Clinics of North America* is to keep practicing radiologists and radiology residents up to date with current clinical practice in radiology by providing timely articles reviewing the state of the art in patient care.

TARGET AUDIENCE

Practicing radiologists, radiology residents, and other healthcare professionals who utilize neuroimaging findings to provide patient care.

LEARNING OBJECTIVES

Upon completion of this activity, participants will be able to:
1. Recognize childhood transverse myelitis and its mimics.
2. Discuss standardized MRI acquisition and reporting as well as advanced MRI imaging in pediatric multiple sclerosis.
3. Review childhood central nervous system vasculitis.

ACCREDITATION

The Elsevier Office of Continuing Medical Education (EOCME) is accredited by the Accreditation Council for Continuing Medical Education (ACCME) to provide continuing medical education for physicians.

The EOCME designates this journal-based CME activity for a maximum of 11 *AMA PRA Category 1 Credit*(s)™. Physicians should claim only the credit commensurate with the extent of their participation in the activity.

All other health care professionals completing continuing education credit for this activity will be issued a certificate of participation.

DISCLOSURE OF CONFLICTS OF INTEREST

The EOCME assesses conflict of interest with its instructors, faculty, planners, and other individuals who are in a position to control the content of CME activities. All relevant conflicts of interest that are identified are thoroughly vetted by EOCME for fair balance, scientific objectivity, and patient care recommendations. EOCME is committed to providing its learners with CME activities that promote improvements or quality in healthcare and not a specific proprietary business or a commercial interest.

The planning committee, staff, authors and editors listed below have identified no financial relationships or relationships to products or devices they or their spouse/life partner have with commercial interest related to the content of this CME activity:

Brenda Banwell, MD, FRCPC; Susanne M. Benseler, MD, PhD; Sandra Bigi, MD; Helen M. Branson, BSc, MBBS, FRACR; David J.A. Callen, MD, PhD, FRCPC; Nicole Congleton; Pamela Hetherington; Kevin Charles Jones, MD; Sandy Lavery; Wayne Lee, MSc; Samantha E. Marin, MD; Jill McNair; Mahendranath Moharir, MD, MSc, FRACP; Suresh K. Mukherji, MD, FACR; Sridar Narayanan, PhD; Julia O'Mahony, BSc; Manohar Shroff, MD, DABR, FRCPC; John G. Sled, PhD; Karthikeyan Subramaniam; Sniya Sudhakar, MBBS, DNB, MD; Terrence Thomas, MD, MRCPCH; Leonard H. Verhey, PhD; and Victor Wycoco, MBBS, FRANZCR.

The planning committee, staff, authors and editors listed below have identified financial relationships or relationships to products or devices they or their spouse/life partner have with commercial interest related to the content of this CME activity:

Naila Makhani, MD, MPH, FRCPC is on the speaker's burea for EMD Serono and Teva Neurosciences, Inc.

UNAPPROVED/OFF-LABEL USE DISCLOSURE

The EOCME requires CME faculty to disclose to the participants:
1. When products or procedures being discussed are off-label, unlabelled, experimental, and/or investigational (not US Food and Drug Administration (FDA)) approved; and
2. Any limitations on the information presented, such as data that are preliminary or that represent ongoing research, interim analyses, and/or unsupported opinions. Faculty may discuss information about pharmaceutical agents that is outside of FDA-approved labelling. This information is intended solely for CME and is not intended to promote off-label use of these medications. If you have any questions, contact the medical affairs department of the manufacturer for the most recent prescribing information.

TO ENROLL

To enroll in the *Neuroimaging Clinics of North America* Continuing Medical Education program, call customer service at 1-800-654-2452 or sign up online at http://www.theclinics.com/home/cme. The CME program is available to subscribers for an additional annual fee of $212 USD.

METHOD OF PARTICIPATION

In order to claim credit, participants must complete the following:
1. Complete enrolment as indicated above.
2. Read the activity.
3. Complete the CME Test and Evaluation. Participants must achieve a score of 70% on the test. All CME Tests and Evaluations must be completed online.

CME INQUIRIES/SPECIAL NEEDS

For all CME inquiries or special needs, please contact elsevierCME@elsevier.com.

NEUROIMAGING CLINICS OF NORTH AMERICA

FORTHCOMING ISSUES

August 2013
Modern Imaging of the Brain, Body and Spine
Lara Brandao, MD, *Editor*

November 2013
Endovascular Management of Neurovascular Pathology in Adults and Children
Neeraj Chaudhary, MD, and
Joseph Gemmete, MD, *Editors*

RECENT ISSUES

February 2013
Head and Neck Cancer
Patricia A. Hudgins, and Amit M. Saindane, *Editors*

November 2012
Central Nervous System Infections
Gaurang V. Shah, MD, *Editor*

August 2012
Socioeconomics of Neuroimaging
David M. Yousem, MD, MBA, *Editor*

RELATED INTEREST

Neuroimaging, Vol. 21, No. 3, August 2011
Congenital Anomalies of the Brain, Spine, and Neck
Hemant A. Parmar, and Mohannad Ibrahim, *Editors*

Contributors

CONSULTING EDITOR

SURESH K. MUKHERJI, MD, FACR
Department of Radiology, University of
Michigan Health System, Ann Arbor, Michigan

EDITOR

MANOHAR SHROFF, MD, DABR, FRCPC
Professor of Radiology, Radiologist in Chief,
Ontasian Chair of Pediatric Imaging and Staff
Neuroradiologist, Division of Neuroradiology,
Department of Diagnostic Imaging, The
Hospital for Sick Children, University of
Toronto, Toronto, Ontario, Canada

AUTHORS

BRENDA BANWELL, MD, FRCPC
Professor of Pediatrics (Neurology) and Senior
Associate Scientist, Division of Neurology,
Department of Pediatrics, Research Institute,
The Hospital for Sick Children, University of
Toronto, Toronto, Ontario, Canada

SUSANNE M. BENSELER, MD, PhD
Division of Rheumatology, Department of
Pediatrics, The Hospital for Sick Children,
University of Toronto, Toronto, Ontario,
Canada

SANDRA BIGI, MD
Clinical Research Fellow, Division of
Neurology, Department of Pediatrics, Hospital
for Sick Children, University of Toronto,
Toronto, Ontario, Canada

HELEN M. BRANSON, BSc, MBBS, FRACR
Pediatric Neuroradiologist, Department of
Medical Imaging, The Hospital for Sick
Children, University of Toronto, Toronto,
Ontario, Canada

DAVID J.A. CALLEN, MD, PhD, FRCP(C)
Division of Pediatric Neurology, Department
of Pediatrics, McMaster Children's Hospital,
Hamilton, Ontario, Canada

KEVIN CHARLES JONES, MD
Division of Neurology, Department of
Pediatrics, The Hospital for Sick Children,
Toronto, Ontario, Canada

WAYNE LEE, MSc
Division of Neuroradiology, Department of
Diagnostic Imaging, The Hospital for Sick
Children, Toronto, Ontario, Canada

NAILA MAKHANI, MD, MPH, FRCPC
Clinical Research Fellow, Division of
Neurology, Department of Pediatrics, Hospital
for Sick Children, University of Toronto,
Toronto, Ontario, Canada

SAMANTHA E. MARIN, MD
Division of Pediatric Neurology, Department
of Pediatrics, McMaster Children's Hospital,
Hamilton, Ontario, Canada

MAHENDRANATH MOHARIR, MD, MSc, FRACP
Division of Neurology, Department of Pediatrics, The Hospital for Sick Children, University of Toronto, Toronto, Ontario, Canada

SRIDAR NARAYANAN, PhD
Faculty Lecturer, Department of Neurology and Neurosurgery, Montreal Neurological Institute, McConnell Brain Imaging Centre, McGill University, Quebec, Canada

JULIA O'MAHONY, BSc
Division of Neurology, Department of Pediatrics, Research Institute, The Hospital for Sick Children, Toronto, Ontario, Canada

MANOHAR SHROFF, MD, DABR, FRCPC
Professor of Radiology, Radiologist in Chief, Ontasian Chair of Pediatric Imaging and Staff Neuroradiologist, Division of Neuroradiology, Department of Diagnostic Imaging, The Hospital for Sick Children, University of Toronto, Toronto, Ontario, Canada

JOHN G. SLED, PhD
Associate Professor and Senior Scientist, Program in Physiology and Experimental Medicine, The Hospital for Sick Children, Toronto Centre for Phenogenomics, Mouse Imaging Centre; Department of Medical Biophysics, Ontario Cancer Institute, Princess Margaret Hospital, University of Toronto, Toronto, Ontario, Canada

SNIYA SUDHAKAR, MBBS, DNB, MD
Department of Radiology, Christian Medical College, Vellore, Tamil Nadu, India

TERRENCE THOMAS, MD, MRCPCH
Neurology Service, Department of Paediatrics, KK Women's and Children's Hospital, Singapore, Singapore

LEONARD H. VERHEY, PhD
Post-Doctoral Research Fellow, Pediatric Demyelinating Disease Program, Program in Neuroscience and Mental Health, The Hospital for Sick Children; Institute of Medical Science, University of Toronto, Toronto, Ontario, Canada

VICTOR WYCOCO, MBBS(Hons), FRANZCR
Division of Neuroradiology, Department of Diagnostic Imaging, The Hospital for Sick Children, Toronto, Ontario, Canada

Contents

Foreword   xi

Suresh K. Mukherji

Preface   xiii

Manohar Shroff

Normal Myelination: A Practical Pictorial Review   183

Helen M. Branson

> MRI is currently the best imaging modality to assess myelin maturation in the human brain. Myelin is the insulator for nerves and is present in both the peripheral nervous system and the central nervous system (CNS). In the CNS, it is a modified extension of the oligodendrocyte cell and is made up of multiple sheaths of protein-lipid-protein-lipid-protein. Standard T1-weighted and T2-weighted sequences can be performed on any MR imaging platform and with knowledge of normal age-related myelin maturation, myelin delay can be detected. Myelination progresses in a constant predetermined pattern from bottom to top, central to peripheral and back to front.

White Matter Anatomy: What the Radiologist Needs to Know   197

Victor Wycoco, Manohar Shroff, Sniya Sudhakar, and Wayne Lee

> Diffusion tensor imaging (DTI) has allowed in vivo demonstration of axonal architecture and connectivity. This technique has set the stage for numerous studies on normal and abnormal connectivity and their role in developmental and acquired disorders. Referencing established white matter anatomy, DTI atlases, and neuroanatomical descriptions, this article summarizes the major white matter anatomy and related structures relevant to the clinical neuroradiologist in daily practice.

Standardized Magnetic Resonance Imaging Acquisition and Reporting in Pediatric
Multiple Sclerosis   217

Leonard H. Verhey, Sridar Narayanan, and Brenda Banwell

> Magnetic resonance (MR) imaging is one of the most important paraclinical tools for the diagnosis of multiple sclerosis (MS), and monitoring of disease progression and treatment response. This article provides clinicians and neuroradiologists caring for children with demyelinating disorders with a suggested standard MR imaging acquisition and reporting protocol, and defines a standard lexicon for lesion features typical of MS in children. As there is considerable overlap between the MR imaging features of pediatric- and adult-onset MS, the recommendations provided herein may be of relevance to radiologists and clinicians caring for adults with multiple sclerosis.

Pediatric Multiple Sclerosis: Pathobiological, Clinical, and Magnetic Resonance Imaging
Features   227

Leonard H. Verhey, Manohar Shroff, and Brenda Banwell

> In this article, the pathobiological, clinical, and treatment aspects of pediatric-onset multiple sclerosis (MS) are summarized, and the conventional magnetic resonance

(MR) imaging (ie, T1-weighted, proton-density, and T2-weighted imaging) features of MS in children are discussed, as well as the application of MR imaging in the diagnosis of pediatric-onset MS and in prediction of MS in children with an incident central nervous system demyelination. Insights gained from studies comparing MR imaging features of pediatric-onset and adult-onset MS are presented.

The Magnetic Resonance Imaging Appearance of Monophasic Acute Disseminated Encephalomyelitis: An Update Post Application of the 2007 Consensus Criteria   245

Samantha E. Marin and David J.A. Callen

Acute disseminated encephalomyelitis (ADEM) is an immunologically mediated inflammatory disease of the central nervous system that typically occurs after a viral infection or recent vaccination, and is most commonly seen in the pediatric population. In 2007 the International Pediatric Multiple Sclerosis Study Group proposed a consensus definition for ADEM for application in research and clinical settings. This article gives an overview of ADEM in children, focusing on differences that have emerged since the consensus definition was established. Although the focus is on neuroimaging in these patients, a synopsis of the clinical features, immunopathogenesis, treatment, and prognosis of ADEM is provided.

Childhood Transverse Myelitis and Its Mimics   267

Terrence Thomas and Helen M. Branson

Childhood transverse myelitis is an acute inflammatory disorder of the spinal cord with a risk of permanent disability. A timely and accurate diagnosis is imperative, and the radiologist needs to discern between a variety of extra-axial and spinal cord abnormalities that produce similar symptoms but require vastly differing treatments. This article presents the range of imaging characteristics seen in childhood transverse myelitis and the differentiation from its mimics.

Diagnosing Neuromyelitis Optica   279

Naila Makhani, Sandra Bigi, Brenda Banwell, and Manohar Shroff

Neuromyelitis optica (NMO) is a severe inflammatory demyelinating disorder typically characterized by attacks of recurrent optic neuritis and transverse myelitis. Advances in magnetic resonance imaging techniques and the discovery of the relatively specific NMO IgG biomarker have led to improved diagnostic accuracy and greater recognition of the broad clinical spectrum of aquaporin 4–related autoimmunity. Brain lesions in NMO typically follow the distribution of aquaporin 4 expression and may be symptomatic. Prompt diagnosis of NMO and NMO spectrum disorders has important therapeutic implications given the high risk of recurrent attacks and consequent severe disability, especially in childhood-onset disease.

Childhood Central Nervous System Vasculitis   293

Mahendranath Moharir, Manohar Shroff, and Susanne M. Benseler

Inflammatory brain diseases in childhood are underrecognized and lead to devastating yet potentially reversible deficits. New-onset neurologic or psychiatric deficits in previously healthy children mandate an evaluation for an underlying inflammatory brain disease. Distinct disease entities, such as central nervous system (CNS) vasculitis, are now being increasingly reported in children. Clinical symptoms, initial laboratory test, and neuroimaging studies help to differentiate between different causes; however, more invasive tests, such as lumbar puncture, conventional angiography, and/or brain biopsy, are usually necessary before the start of treatment. This article focuses on childhood CNS vasculitis.

Anti–NMDA Receptor Encephalitis

309

Kevin Charles Jones, Susanne M. Benseler, and Mahendranath Moharir

Anti–N-methyl-D-aspartate (NMDA) receptor encephalitis is a severe but potentially reversible neurologic disorder that is clinically recognizable in children and adolescents. Prompt diagnosis and treatment are essential to facilitate recovery. Treatment consists of corticosteroids, intravenous immunoglobulin, or plasma exchange as first-line therapy followed by cyclophosphamide or rituximab, if necessary, as second-line immunotherapy. Patients with tumor-associated encephalitis benefit from tumor resection. More than 75% of patients make a substantial recovery, which occurs in the reverse order of symptom presentation associated with a decline in antibody titers.

Mimics and Rare Presentations of Pediatric Demyelination

321

Julia O'Mahony, Manohar Shroff, and Brenda Banwell

This article reviews the features that should prompt consideration of diseases that mimic acquired demyelinating syndromes and multiple sclerosis using vignettes to highlight unusual clinical and radiologic features. Cases of transverse myelitis, spinal infarction, acute disseminated encephalomyelitis, fever-induced refractory epileptic encephalopathy in school-aged children, small-vessel vasculitis, Griscelli syndrome type 2, cysticercosis, vitamin B12 deficiency, and chronic relapsing inflammatory optic neuropathy are presented.

Advanced Magnetic Resonance Imaging in Pediatric Multiple Sclerosis

337

Leonard H. Verhey and John G. Sled

This review summarizes results from studies that have applied advanced magnetic resonance (MR) imaging techniques to patients with pediatric-onset multiple sclerosis (MS), and includes a discussion of cortical imaging techniques, volumetry, magnetization transfer and diffusion tensor imaging, proton magnetic resonance spectroscopy, and functional MR imaging. Multicenter studies on the sensitivity of these techniques to natural history of disease and treatment response are required before their implementation into clinical practice.

Index

355

Foreword

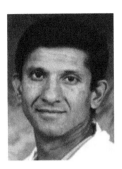

Suresh K. Mukherji, MD, FACR
Consulting Editor

White matter disorders and demyelinating processes are very challenging in the adult, but near impossible in children!! With this in mind, we embarked on creating an issue of *Neuroimaging Clinics* dedicated to this topic. Manu Shroff is Radiologist-in-Chief and Ontasian Chair of Pediatric Imaging at the Hospital for Sick Kids. We are extremely privileged and honored to have him guest edit this very special edition of *Neuroimaging Clinics* on Pediatric Demyelinating Disorders.

This is a state-of-the-art issue devoted to pediatric demyelinating disorders that is both comprehensive and practical. There are several articles dedicated to pediatric multiple sclerosis and its mimics. The authors are world-renowned experts in their chosen topics and I thank them for their extraordinary contributions. I especially want to mention the articles entitled, "Standardized MR Protocols for Pediatric Multiple Sclerosis, Structured Reporting, and Lexicon for Lesion Location and Distribution" and "White Matter Anatomy on MRI: What the Radiologist Needs to Know." These articles are very important for many of us that interpret pediatric neuroimaging but have not had a dedicated pediatric neuroradiology fellowship. These articles will help standardize our technique and ensure we understand the normal myelination pattern of the brain so that abnormal studies are easier to detect.

I have had the distinct privilege to have known Dr Shroff for nearly 20 years and have seen his career progress. The only thing more remarkable than his congeniality and academic accomplishments is his humility. He has already accomplished more in his career than many of us (myself included!) will accomplish in our careers. However, many of you may not be aware of his numerous achievements because of his very understated personality. He never talks about himself and always finds time for his many friends and colleagues. It is truly an honor both to have Dr Shroff guest edit this issue of *Neuroimaging clinics* and, most importantly, to call him my "friend."

Suresh K. Mukherji, MD, FACR
Department of Radiology
University of Michigan Health System
1500 East Medical Center
Ann Arbor, MI 48109-0030, USA

E-mail address:
mukherji@med.umich.edu

Neuroimag Clin N Am 23 (2013) xi
http://dx.doi.org/10.1016/j.nic.2013.02.001
1052-5149/13/$ – see front matter © 2013 Published by Elsevier Inc.

neuroimaging.theclinics.com

1932-2275/13/\$ – see front matter © 2013 Published by Elsevier Inc.
vetquip.theclinics.com   http://dx.doi.org/10.1016/j.cvsm.2013.03.001

Preface

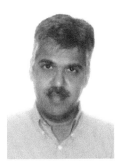

Manohar Shroff, MD, DABR, FRCPC
Editor

It is a privilege to be guest editing this issue, and I am grateful to Dr Suresh Mukherjee for this opportunity. Pediatric demyelinating diseases can often be difficult for clinicians and radiologists to correctly distinguish and diagnose. With 2.7% to 10% of multiple sclerosis (MS) diagnoses occurring in children under the age of 18, and an increased prevalence of demyelination diseases in North America,[1-3] it is important for radiologists and clinicians to be aware of how neuroimaging can facilitate the correct diagnosis of these diseases. This issue of the *Neuroimaging Clinics* offers insight in improving the understanding of demyelinating diseases in children and in distinguishing the various differential diagnoses and mimics of these diseases through the use of MR techniques.

This issue begins with providing an overview of normal myelination and a guide to understanding white matter anatomy on MR imaging. This is followed by a discussion of standardized MR protocols and standardized reporting nomenclature in MS. This article is particularly useful for radiologists, given that even in pediatric MS, MR is an important surrogate clinical tool in the evaluation and follow-up of the diverse clinical representations of MS. Subsequent articles focus on a discussion of other white matter diseases including acute demyelinating encephalomyelitis, childhood transverse myelitis, neuromyelitis optica, childhood central nervous system vasculitis, and anti-NMDA receptor-mediated encephalitis. Further discussion regarding differential diagnoses of MS is provided in later sections, enabling clinicians to correctly distinguish MS from its mimics, allowing for more accurate diagnoses of the disease. This issue culminates in an article surrounding the use of diffusion tensor imaging, magnetic transfer ratio, and MR spectroscopy as complementary measures to conventional MR techniques in understanding the various nuances of pediatric MS.

Every author in this issue is a strong subject matter expert on the topics that they have contributed to. Each of them is passionate about this subject and it is my privilege to know them personally and be able to learn from them. I sincerely thank them for their contributions and insights. I would like to specially thank 2 people who contributed to multiple articles: (1) Leonard Verhey, MSc, PhD—Len is an exceptionally gifted individual who worked long and hard hours on pediatric MS, analyzing in detail a few hundred MR studies for his PhD thesis; and (2) Brenda Banwell, MD, FAAP, FRCPC, who until recently was the director of the Pediatric Demyelinating Disease Program at the Hospital for Sick Children. Brenda is a fantastic physician who excels both as a clinician and a researcher. She has and I am sure will continue to provide valuable dynamic leadership, insight, clinical expertise, and research on pediatric demyelination.

Manohar Shroff, MD, DABR, FRCPC
Department of Diagnostic Imaging
Hospital for Sick Children
University of Toronto
555 University Avenue
Toronto, Ontario M5G 1X8, Canada

E-mail address:
manohar.shroff@sickkids.ca

1052-5149/13/$ – see front matter © 2013 Published by Elsevier Inc.

neuroimaging.theclinics.com

REFERENCES

1. Marin SE, Banwell BB, Till C. Cognitive trajectories in 4 patients with pediatric-onset multiple sclerosis: serial evaluation over a decade. J Child Neurol 2012. http://dx.doi.org/10.1177/0883073812465010. [Epub ahead of print].

2. Popescu BF, Lucchinetti CF. Pathology of demyelinating diseases. Annu Rev Pathol Mech Dis 2012;7:185–217.

3. Ascherio A, Munger KL. Epidemiology of Multiple Sclerosis: Environmental Factors. In: Lucchinetti CF, Hohlfeld R, editors. Multiple sclerosis. 3rd edition. Philadelphia: Saunders Elsevier; 2010. p. 57–82.

Normal Myelination
A Practical Pictorial Review

Helen M. Branson, BSc, MBBS, FRACR

KEYWORDS

• Myelin • Myelination • T1 • T2 • MR • Diffusion

KEY POINTS

- MR imaging is the best noninvasive modality to assess myelin maturation in the human brain.
- A combination of conventional T1-weighted and T2-weighted sequences is all that is required for basic assessment of myelination in the central nervous system (CNS).
- It is vital to have an understanding of the normal progression of myelination on MR imaging to enable the diagnosis of childhood diseases including leukodystrophies as well as hypomyelinating disorders, delayed myelination, and acquired demyelinating disease.

INTRODUCTION

Assessment of the progression of myelin and myelination has been revolutionized in the era of MR imaging. Earlier imaging modalities such as ultrasonography and computed tomography have no current role or ability to contribute to the assessment of myelin maturation or abnormalities of myelin. The degree of brain myelination can be used as a marker of maturation.

The authors discuss

1. Myelin function and structure
2. The MR imaging appearance of myelin
3. The normal progression of myelination on conventional MR imaging
4. Terminal zones of myelination

DISCUSSION
Myelin Function and Structure

To discuss normal myelination in the human brain, knowledge of the purpose and function of myelin and its role in the human nervous system is needed.

Myelin is present in both the CNS and the peripheral nervous system. In the CNS, it is primarily found in white matter (although small amounts are also found in gray matter) and thus is responsible for its color.[1] Myelin acts as an electrical insulator for neurons.[1] Myelin plays a role in increasing the speed of an action potential by 10–100 times that of an unmyelinated axon[1] and also helps in speedy axonal transport.[2] Edgar and Garbern[3] (2004) demonstrated that the absence of a major myelin protein (PLP/DM20) from the oligodendrocyte resulted in major impairments in axonal transport in a mouse model of hereditary spastic paraplegia. It has also been well established that axonal integrity depends on the myelinating cell body for support. Myelin also likely has a role in the regulation of both ion composition and fluid volume around the axon.[4]

Myelination is the formation of a myelin lipid bilayer around an axon.[4,5] Myelination allows rapid transfer of information needed for cognitive

The author has nothing to disclose.
Department of Medical Imaging, The Hospital for Sick Children, University of Toronto, 555 University Avenue, Toronto, Ontario, M5G 1X8, Canada
E-mail address: helen.branson@sickkids.ca

Neuroimag Clin N Am 23 (2013) 183–195
http://dx.doi.org/10.1016/j.nic.2012.12.001
1052-5149/13/$ – see front matter

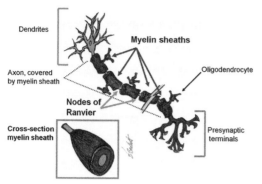

Fig. 1. Schematic of a neuron demonstrating the myelin sheaths wrapped around the axon and the separating nodes of Ranvier. (*Courtesy of* Dr E. Bartlett, Princess Margaret Cancer Centre, Joint Department of Medical imaging, University of Toronto, Toronto, Canada.)

functioning as well as emotional and behavioral functioning and decision making.[5] Myelination begins during fetal life[6,7] and continues after birth.

Myelin is a modified extension of an oligodendroglial cell process.[6,8] An oligodendroglial cell is the key cell in myelination of the CNS and is the predominant type of neuroglia in white matter.[9] Myelin sheaths are composed of multiple

segments of myelin, which are then wrapped around an axon.[6,8] This sheath is instrumental in containing an electrical current around an axon and increasing the action potential of an axon because of the nodes of Ranvier, which are sodium channels in between the myelin sheaths that increase the traveling speed of an electric current down an axon (**Fig. 1**). Thus, myelin is thought to make impulses travel faster by increasing the speed of travel of a current. Myelin is also thought to be symbiotic with the axon.[10] Myelin is metabolically active and involved in the turnover of its own components[11] and contains a large number of myelin-intrinsic enzymes.[12] Myelin also has a role in ion transport, which contributes to its own maintenance, and in the buffering of ions around the axon.[11,12]

A single oligodendrocyte may be responsible for the production and maintenance of up to 40 fibers.[9] Myelin has a high lipid content, having approximately 70% lipid and 20 to 30% protein.[8,9,11] The main proteins that play a part in myelin structure are myelin basic protein (30%), proteolipid protein (50%), and cyclic nucleotide phosphodiesterase (4%).[1] Other proteins involved include myelin-associated glycol protein and myelin oligodendrocyte protein. Lipids that contribute to myelin ultrastructure include cholesterol, phospholipids, and glycosphingolipids.[1,9]

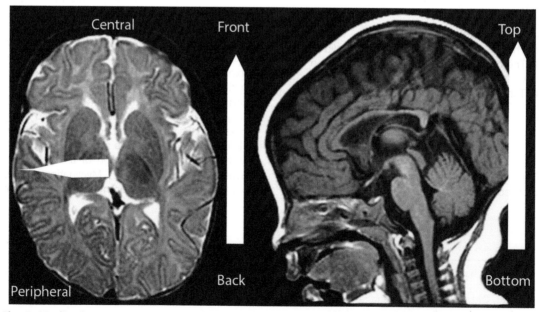

Fig. 2. Myelination progresses in a predictable manner from bottom to top (caudocranial), back to front (posterior to anterior), and central to peripheral (deep to superficial).

A

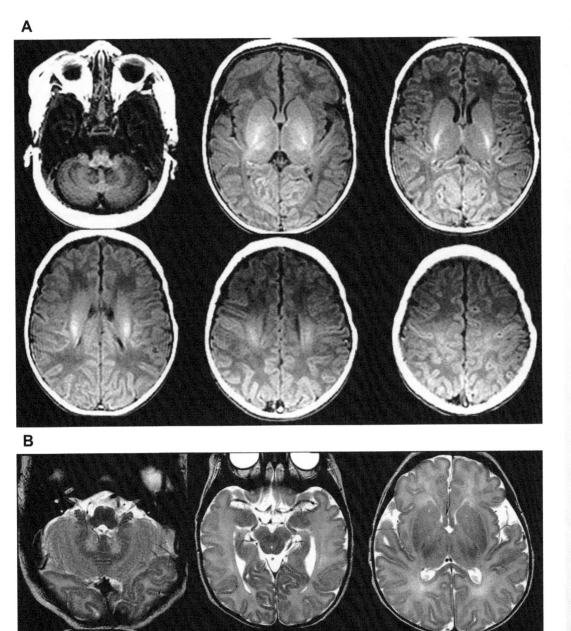

B

Fig. 3. Imaging of myelination. (A) Normal myelination for a term infant on T1. Structures myelinated at birth include the T1 dorsal brainstem, lateral thalami, posterior limbs of the internal capsule, central coronal radiata, and rolandic and perirolandic gyri. (B) Normal myelination for a term infant on T2. On T2, there is expected myelination in the dorsal brainstem, lateral thalami, posterior limbs of the internal capsule, and central corona radiata.

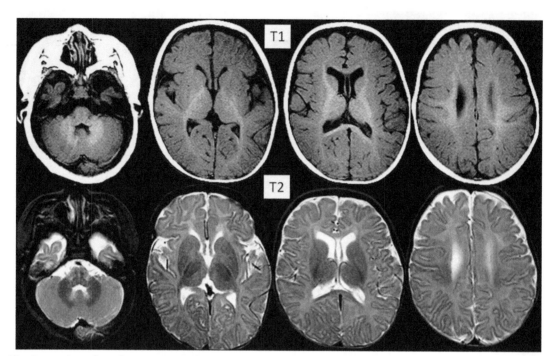

Fig. 4. Imaging of myelination. By 4 months, myelination on T1 in the anterior limbs of the internal capsule as well as thickening of those areas previously described especially central corona radiata and centrum semiovale should be seen. In addition, there should be evolving myelination in the splenium of the corpus callosum. Myelin is not yet well seen in the anterior limb of the internal capsule on T2.

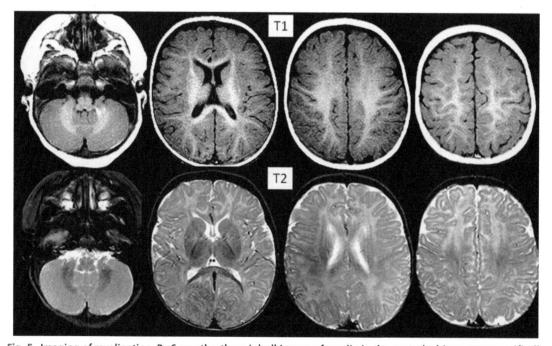

Fig. 5. Imaging of myelination. By 6 months, there is bulking up of myelin in the central white matter specifically in the centrum semiovale and corona radiata as well as the areas previously discussed. This bulking is most evident on T1 and lags on T2 where there is just a faint T2 hypointensity in the anterior limbs of the internal capsule as well as thickening of the myelin in the corpus callosum.

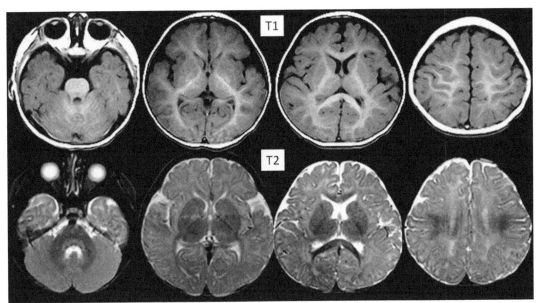

Fig. 6. Imaging of myelination. By 9 months, there is progressive darkening on T2 as well as further bulking up of the myelinated white matter on T1. Myelin should now be seen in the anterior limb of the internal capsule on T2.

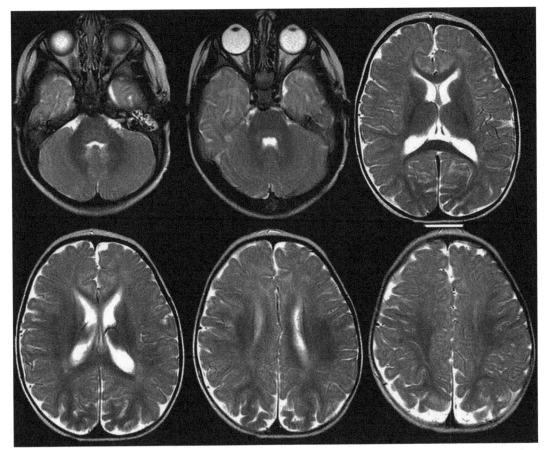

Fig. 7. Imaging of myelination. By 12 months, myelination on T1 is complete and there has been further myelination in the centrum semiovale and coronal radiata as well as the corpus callosum and internal capsule on T2. There is still a fairly large amount of unmyelinated white matter, in particular in the frontal and temporal lobes.

Electron microscopy has demonstrated that myelin is composed of multiple sheaths wrapped around the axon and that the sheaths are made up of a "protein-lipid-protein-lipid-protein" structure. Compaction of these sheaths or processes gives rise to apposition of extracellular and cytoplasmic surfaces, which represents alternating extracellular and intracellular spaces.[12] The lipid bilayer is composed of phospholipids, glycolipids, and cholesterol. Most of the glycolipids (sulfatide and cerebroside) and cholesterol are in the outer layer and exposed to the extracellular space, whereas the phospholipids (plasmalogen) are in the inner layer and are hydrophobic.[6] The formation of compact myelin is required for the growth and maturation of the axon.[10]

The MR Imaging Appearance of Myelin

There is no technique that has been developed to view the myelin lipid bilayer directly with imaging. Myelin is assessed qualitatively. The commonly used MR techniques include conventional anatomic imaging, that is, T1-weighted and T2-weighted sequences as well as MR spectroscopy and diffusion tensor imaging (DTI). Other techniques that have been used include magnetization transfer imaging and T2 relaxation separation.[1] In clinical practice, conventional anatomic imaging is the mainstay because it can be easily performed. Quantification of myelin can be achieved in multicomponent relaxation (MCR) analysis.[5] MCR is a volume-weighted summation of distinct

A

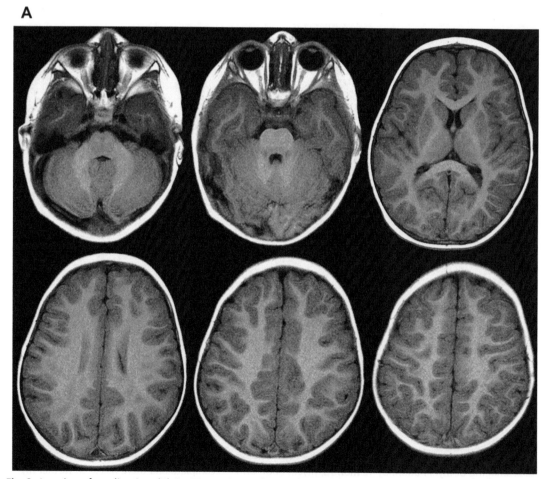

Fig. 8. Imaging of myelination. (A) On T1, at 18 months, myelin is complete and similar in appearance to that of 12 months. There is further thickening and "bulking up" of the central and deep white matter.

microanatomic water compartments. This analysis has revealed 2 water subdomains, namely, a slow relaxing species with free intracellular and extracellular water and a faster relaxing species of molecules from the water trapped between the lipid bilayer sheath.[5,6]

Currently, standard MR imaging techniques do not specifically have the ability to quantitate myelin. Instead, these techniques study a combination of the following: changes in axonal size and density, changes in membrane structure including lipid and protein content, and water and macromolecule content.[5] DTI is not a reliable indicator of the total amount of myelin, but it can give some information on changes in myelin.[1]

As reviewed by Barkovich[6] there are 2 distinct populations of water molecules that play a direct role in the signal characteristics of myelin on MR imaging. These populations are water located within the myelin sheath and that located outside the myelin sheath. On conventional imaging, mature myelin is hyperintense to the gray matter cortex on T1 and hypointense to the gray matter cortex on T2. However, on T1, this increase in signal is most likely because of increasing glycolipids, predominantly galactocerebroside[13] and cholesterol,[6,14] within the myelin membranes.[6,15] The T2 hypointensity is thought most likely due to the reduced water content as more myelin is laid down[7,16] with greater maturation of the myelin

B

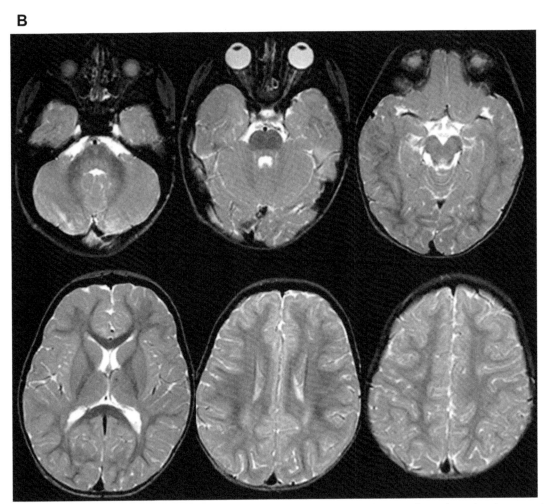

Fig. 8. (B) By 18 months, on T2, there is almost complete myelination except for the inferior frontal and temporal lobes as well as the terminal zones of myelination in the peritrigonal regions.

sheath, and tightening of the myelin spiral around the axon.[6,15]

The Normal Progression of Myelination

The general rule of progression of normal myelination as outlined by Barkovich[8] is that myelination begins in the fifth fetal month and continues throughout life. Myelination commences with the cranial nerves, which makes sense because we need these to rely on for survival. Generally, myelination progresses from bottom to top (caudocranial), back to front (posterior to anterior), and central to peripheral (deep to superficial) (**Fig. 2**).[17,18] It therefore makes sense that the brainstem and cerebellum myelinate before the cerebrum and that the basal ganglia and thalami commence myelination before the white matter. In addition, the posterior limb of the internal capsule myelinates before the anterior limb, splenium before the genu, and the central corona radiata before the subcortical regions.[19]

Counsell and colleagues[20] described myelination in the very preterm infant and confirmed myelination in the cerebellar vermis, vestibular nuclei, cerebellar peduncles, dentate nucleus, medial longitudinal fasciculus, medial geniculate bodies, subthalamic nuclei, inferior olivary nuclei, ventrolateral nuclei of the thalamus, medial and lateral lemnisci and inferior colliculi, as well as gracile

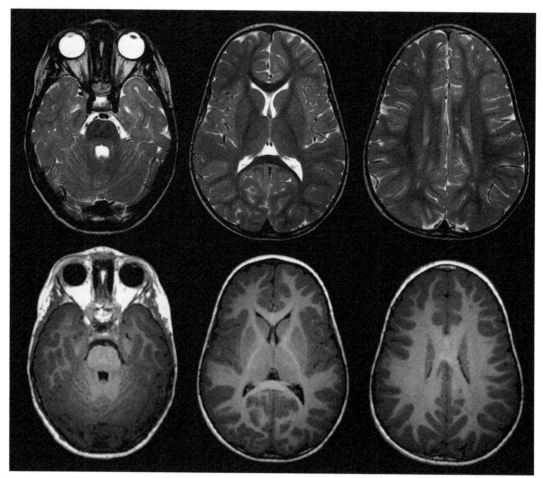

Fig. 9. Imaging of myelination. By 2 years, myelination is complete on T1 and T2 with some residual T2 hyperintensity parallel to the lateral ventricles as well as to the inferior frontal and temporal lobes.

and cuneate nuclei and fasciculi. The investigators did not find any new myelin sites between 28 and 36 weeks, after which there were again new myelin sites at the posterior limb of internal capsule, corona radiata, and the corticospinal tracts of the precentral and postcentral gyrus.

Histologic studies demonstrate myelination at birth in the brainstem, cerebellar white matter, and posterior limb of the internal capsule with extension to the thalamus and basal ganglia.[21]

Bird and colleagues[19] (1989) reviewed 60 patients on MR imaging and found that there was wide variation in the rate, onset, and appearance of changes associated with myelination. The investigators studied marker sites for certain ages in determining normal myelin. For example, at birth (term), there was mature myelination in the posterior limb of the internal capsule, the cerebellar

peduncles, and the corona radiata around the central sulcus. The slowest areas to myelinate were the central white matter of the supratentorial lobes.[19] The investigators again consistently confirmed progression of myelination in the posterior limb before the anterior limb, splenium before genu, and central corona radiata before poles in all subjects. This posterior to anterior sequence has been seen in autopsy subjects.[22]

Paus and colleagues[23] (2001) described 3 developmental patterns seen with respect to gray–white matter differentiation in the first 12–24 months of life. These patterns are the infantile pattern for less than 6 months with a reversal of the normal adult pattern, the isointense pattern (8–12 months) in which there is poor differentiation between gray and white matter, and the early adult pattern (greater than 12 months) in which gray matter

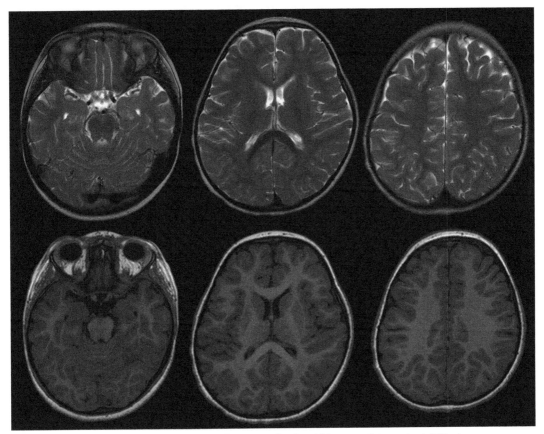

Fig. 10. Imaging of myelination. By 3 years of age, myelin should be complete and adultlike in appearance on both T1-weighted and T2-weighted sequences.

signal is greater than that of white matter on T2 and less than that of white matter on T1. This change is thought to be related to changes in relaxation times with rapid shortening in the first 12 months because of a rapid decrease in the water content of gray and white matter.[23]

Welker and Patton (2011)[15] recently published a table of age-specific progression of myelination on MR imaging with reference to T1, T2, Fluid-attenuated inversion recovery (FLAIR), and DTI sequences (Figs. 3–11). The reader is referred to this article for further detail.

The corpus callosum also undergoes a fairly uniform pattern of thickening and myelination. The splenium myelinates first by approximately 3 months followed by the body at 4 to 5 months and the genu by 5 to 6 months. There are changes in both the shape and signal intensity throughout development. These changes occur mainly in the first year of life.[24] As a neonate, the corpus callosum is thin in its entirety with thickening first seen in the genu (by 2–3 months) followed by the splenium, which demonstrates rapid thickening at about 5–6 months reaching the size of the genu by the end of the seventh month.[24] The corpus callosum enlarges gradually over 12 months (Figs. 12 and 13).[24] With respect to myelination on T1, the splenium of the corpus callosum demonstrates increased signal intensity by 4 months, and the genu by 6 months.[17] Thus

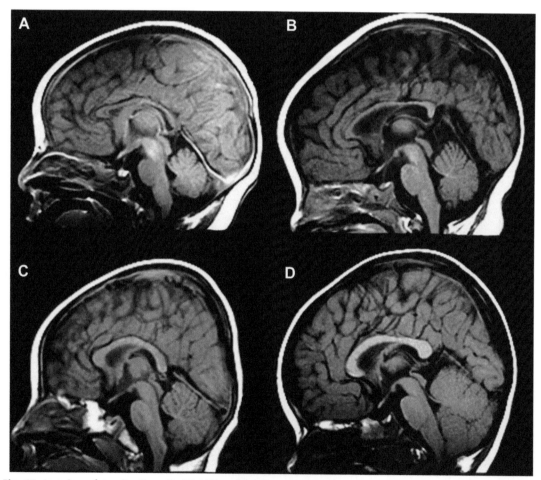

Fig. 11. Imaging of myelination. Sagittal T1-weighted sequences demonstrating normal development of the corpus callosum. (A) term, (B) 4 months, (C) 6 months, and (D) 16 months.

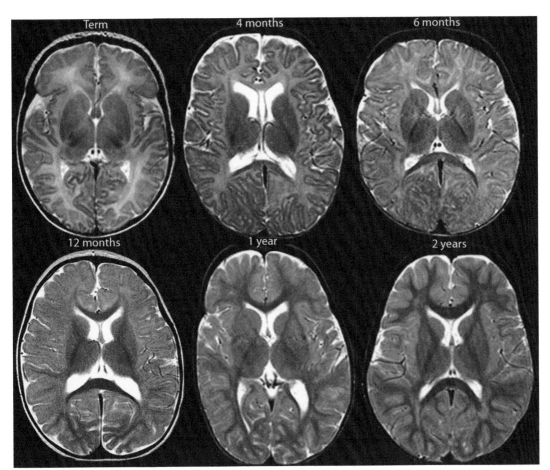

Fig. 12. Summary slide of progression of normal myelination. Progression of normal myelination on MR imaging from birth (term) to 2 years of age on a T2-weighted sequence.

the splenium myelinates before the genu.[19] By 8 to 9 months, the corpus callosum appears identical to that of an adult.[24,25]

Terminal Zones of Myelination

The last associative area to mature on MR imaging is the peritrigonal zone, which is the region posterosuperior to the trigones of the lateral ventricles.[26] This region maintains a persistent T2 hyperintensity, but not brighter than the gray matter on T2-weighted sequences (**Fig. 14**). Parazzini and colleagues,[26] also described terminal zones of myelin maturation on T2 in the frontotemporal subcortical regions. The investigators determined that these areas can exhibit subcortical T2 hyperintensity until 36 to 40 months (see **Fig. 14**).

With respect to idiopathic developmental delay, Maricich and colleagues[27] studied 93 children and found no definite evidence for correlation between idiopathic developmental delay and delay in myelination on T2-weighted imaging.

SUMMARY

MR imaging is to date the best modality for noninvasive assessment of myelin and myelination in the pediatric brain. To allow diagnosis of disorders with permanent hypomyelination or delayed myelin deposition, the normal progression of myelination should be known. For this reason, a pictorial review and discussion of normal MR imaging progression of myelination has been performed. In addition, normal progression of the development of the corpus callosum as well as recognition of the normal terminal zones of myelination is vital in understanding imaging of the pediatric brain.

ACKNOWLEDGMENTS

The author acknowledges the MR technologists without whom none of this work could be performed and Dr E. Bartlett for his schematic of a neuron and myelin.

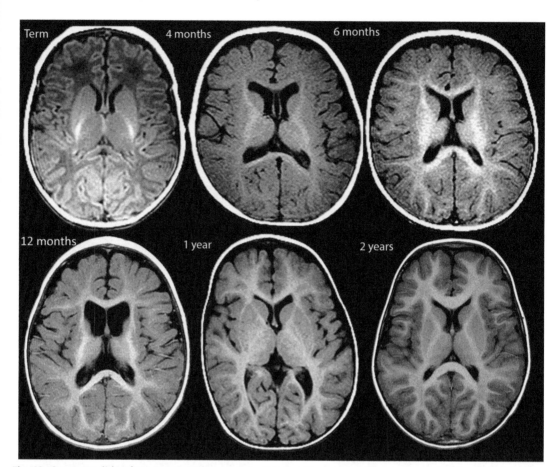

Fig. 13. Summary slide of progression of normal myelination. Progression of normal myelination on MR imaging from birth (term) to 2 years of age on a T1-weighted sequence.

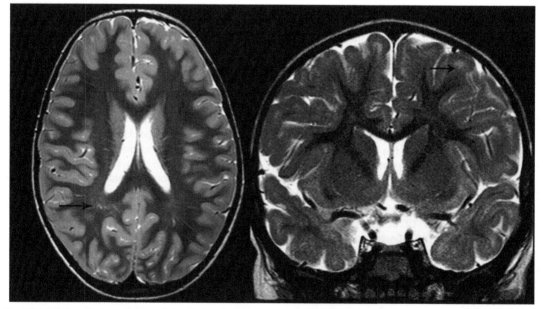

Fig. 14. Axial and coronal T2-weighted sequences demonstrate normal terminal zones of myelination (*black arrows*). These zones are classically located in the posterior periventricular region as well as the frontotemporal subcortical regions.

REFERENCES

1. Laule C, Vavasour IM, Kolind SH, et al. Magnetic resonance imaging of myelin. Neurotherapeutics 2007;4(3):460–84.
2. Edgar JM, McLaughlin M, Yool D, et al. Oligodendroglial modulation of fast axonal transport in a mouse model of hereditary spastic paraplegia. J Cell Biol 2004;166:121–31.
3. Edgar JM, Garbern J. The myelinated axon is dependent on the myelinating cell for support and maintenance: molecules involved. J Neurosci Res 2004;76:593–8.
4. Dyer CA. The structure and function of myelin: from inert membrane to perfusion pump. Neurochem Res 2002;27(11):1279–92.
5. Deoni SC, Mercure E, Blasi A, et al. Mapping infant brain myelination with magnetic resonance imaging. J Neurosci 2011;31(2):784–91.
6. Barkovich AJ. Concepts of myelin and myelination in neuroradiology. AJNR Am J Neuroradiol 2000;21: 1099–109.
7. Dietrich RB, Bradley WG, Zaragoza EJ IV, et al. MR evaluation of early myelination patterns in normal and developmentally delayed infants. AJR Am J Roentgenol 1988;150:889–96.
8. Barkovich AJ. Magnetic resonance techniques in the assessment of myelin and myelination. J Inherit Metab Dis 2005;28:311–43.
9. Van der Knaap M, Valk J. Myelin and white matter. In: Van der Knapp M, Valk J, editors. Magnetic resonance of myelination and myelin disorders. 3rd edition. Berlin, Heidelberg (Germany), New York: Springer; 2005. p. 1–19.
10. Brady ST, Witt AS, Kirkpatrick LL, et al. Formation of compact myelin is required for maturation of the axonal cytoskeleton. J Neurosci 1999;19(17): 7278–88.
11. Morell P, Quarles RH. Myelin formation, structure, and biochemistry. In: Siegel GJ, editor. Basic neurochemistry: molecular, cellular, and medical aspects. 6th edition. New York: Raven Press; 1999. p. 69–94.
12. Ledeen RW. Enzymes and receptors of myelin. In: Martenson RE, editor. Myelin: biology and chemistry. Boca Raton (FL): CRC Press; 1992. p. 531–70.
13. Kucharczyk W, MacDonald PM, Stanisz GJ, et al. Relaxivity and magnetization transfer of white matter lipids at MR imaging: importance of cerebroside and pH. Radiology 1994;192:521–9.
14. Koenig SH, Brown RD III, Spiller M, et al. Relaxometry of brain: why white matter appears bright in MRI. Magn Reson Med 1990;14(3):521–9.
15. Welker KM, Patton A. Assessment of normal myelination with magnetic resonance imaging. Semin Neurol 2012;32:15–28.
16. Holland BA, Haas DK, Norman D, et al. MRI of normal brain maturation. AJNR Am J Neuroradiol 1986;7:201–8.
17. Barkovich AJ, Kjos BO, Jackson DE Jr, et al. Normal maturation of the neonatal and infant brain: MR imaging at 1.5T. Radiology 1988;166:173–80.
18. Ballasteros MC, Hansen PE, Soila K. MR imaging of the developing human brain. Part 2. Postnatal developmental. Radiographics 1993;13:611–22.
19. Bird CR, Hedberg M, Drayer BP, et al. MR assessment of myelination in infants and children: usefulness of marker sites. AJNR Am J Neuroradiol 1989;10:731–40.
20. Counsell SJ, Maalouf EF, Fletcher AM, et al. MR imaging assessment of myelination in the very preterm brain. AJNR Am J Neuroradiol 2002;23: 872–81.
21. Van der Knaap M, Valk J. MR imaging of the various stages of normal myelination during the first year of life. Neuroradiology 1990;31:459–70.
22. Kinney HC, Brody BA, Kloman AS, et al. Sequence of central nervous system myelination in human infancy. II. Patterns of myelination in autopsied infants. J Neuropathol Exp Neurol 1988;47(3):217–34.
23. Paus T, Collins DL, Evans AC, et al. Maturation of white matter in the human brain: a review of magnetic resonance studies. Brain Res Bull 2001; 54(3):255–66.
24. Barkovich AJ, Kjos BO. Normal postnatal development of the corpus callosum as demonstrated by MR imaging. AJNR Am J Neuroradiol 1988;9:487–91.
25. Parazzini C, Bianchini E, Triulzi F. Myelination. In: Tortori-Donati P, Rossi A, Biancheri R, editors. Pediatric neuroradiology brain. Berlin: Springer-Verlag; 2005. p. P21–40.
26. Parazzini C, Baldoli C, Scotti G, et al. Terminal zones of myelination: MR evaluation of children aged 20–40 months. AJNR Am J Neuroradiol 2002;23: 1669–73.
27. Maricich SM, Azizi P, Jones JY, et al. Myelination as assessed by conventional MR imaging as normal in young children with idiopathic developmental delay. AJNR Am J Neuroradiol 2007;28:1602–5.

White Matter Anatomy
What the Radiologist Needs to Know

Victor Wycoco, MBBS, FRANZCR[a],
Manohar Shroff, MD, DABR, FRCPC[a],*,
Sniya Sudhakar, MBBS, DNB, MD[b], Wayne Lee, MSc[a]

KEYWORDS

- Diffusion tensor imaging (DTI) • White matter tracts • Projection fibers • Association Fibers
- Commissural fibers

KEY POINTS

- Diffusion tensor imaging (DTI) has emerged as an excellent tool for in vivo demonstration of white matter microstructure and has revolutionized our understanding of the same.
- Information on normal connectivity and relations of different white matter networks and their role in different disease conditions is still evolving. Evidence is mounting on causal relations of abnormal white matter microstructure and connectivity in a wide range of pediatric neurocognitive and white matter diseases.
- Hence there is a pressing need for every neuroradiologist to acquire a strong basic knowledge of white matter anatomy and to make an effort to apply this knowledge in routine reporting.

INTRODUCTION

DTI has allowed in vivo demonstration of axonal architecture and connectivity. This technique has set the stage for numerous studies on normal and abnormal connectivity and their role in developmental and acquired disorders. Referencing established white matter anatomy, DTI atlases, and neuroanatomical descriptions, this article summarizes the major white matter anatomy and related structures relevant to the clinical neuroradiologist in daily practice.

MR IMAGING OF WHITE MATTER TRACTS

White matter is seen well on the T1, T2, and fluid-attenuated inversion recovery (FLAIR) sequences used in routine MR imaging. Certain white matter tracts are reasonably well demonstrated particularly on T2 and FLAIR images[1] because of their location and in the pediatric age group, because of the differences in water content and myelination (Fig. 1). However, the use of specific DTI sequences provides far more detailed and clinically useful information.

DIFFUSION TENSOR IMAGING: THE BASICS

Using appropriate magnetic field gradients, diffusion-weighted sequences can be used to detect the motion of the water molecules to and from cells. This free movement of the water molecules is random and thermally driven in neurons. In the axons, the axonal membranes and myelin sheaths act as barriers to the random motion of the water molecules, and this motion thus becomes directionally dependent or anisotropic, with the direction of maximum diffusivity aligning with the direction of white matter tract orientation.[2] With DTI, this degree of anisotropy and fiber direction can be mapped voxel by voxel, allowing for the in vivo assessment of white matter tract architecture.

Financial disclosures: None.
[a] Division of Neuroradiology, Department of Diagnostic Imaging, The Hospital for Sick Children, University of Toronto, 555 University Avenue, Toronto, Ontario M5G 1X8, Canada; [b] Department of Radiology, Christian Medical College, Vellore 632002, Tamil Nadu, India
* Corresponding author.
E-mail address: Manohar.shroff@sickkids.ca

neuroimaging.theclinics.com

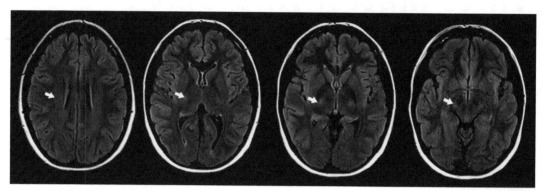

Fig. 1. Axial FLAIR images in a normal 14-year-old boy show that the corticospinal tract is mildly hyperintense, as marked with white arrows.

A diffusion tensor is a mathematical model containing diffusion measurements from at least 6 noncollinear directions, from which diffusivity in any direction as well as the direction of maximum diffusivity can be estimated.[3] Using more than 6 encoding directions will improve the accuracy of the tensor measurements,[4] and DTI is more often obtained with 30 to 60 directions. The tensor matrix is ellipsoid, with its principal axis oriented in the direction of maximum diffusivity. Via a linear algebraic procedure called matrix diagonalization, 3 *eigenvalues* are obtained, which represent apparent diffusivity in the 3 principal axes of the ellipsoid, namely the *major, medium,* and *minor* axes, also known as the *eigenvectors*.[3]

The x-, y-, and z-coordinate system to which the scanner is oriented is rotated to a new coordinate system, dictated by diffusivity information. Fractional anisotropy (FA) is derived from the standard deviation of the 3 eigenvalues and ranges from 0 (isotropy) to 1 (maximum anisotropy). The orientation of maximum diffusivity may be mapped using red, green, and blue color channels and color brightness, modulated by FA, and this can result in the formation of a color map demonstrating the degree of anisotropy and local fiber direction.

The conventional color coding is green for fibers oriented anteroposterior (mainly the association fibers), red for right–left oriented fibers (mainly commissural fibers), and blue for superior–inferior fibers (in particular as projection fibers). In 2D images (**Fig. 2**), mixed color is seen when fibers overlap, resulting in yellow (green and red), magenta (red and blue), and cyan (green and blue), and with changes in orientation (see **Fig. 2**).[5]

CLASSIFICATION OF WHITE MATTER TRACTS

The white matter tracts are broadly classified into 3 groups according to their connectivity (**Table 1**):

1. *Projection fibers*: These fibers connect the cortical areas with the deep gray nuclei, brainstem, cerebellum, and spinal cord or vice versa. Corticospinal fibers, corticobulbar fibers, corticopontine fibers, thalamic radiations, and geniculocalcarine fibers (optic radiations) are tracts identifiable on DTI.
2. *Association fibers*: These fibers connect different cortical areas within the same hemisphere. The fibers can be long range or short range, the latter including subcortical U fibers. The major long tracts include cingulum, superior and inferior occipitofrontal fasciculus; uncinate fasciculus; superior longitudinal fasciculus (SLF), including arcuate fasciculus; and inferior longitudinal fasciculus (occipitotemporal).
3. *Commissural fibers*: These fibers connect similar cortical areas in the 2 hemispheres, including the corpus callosum and the anterior commissure.

Other tracts and fibers, which can be seen in DTI maps, include the optic pathway, fornix, and many fibers within the cerebellum and brainstem. These tracts and fibers are described separately.

PROJECTION FIBERS

Projection fibers are afferent and efferent tracts that interconnect areas of the cortex with the brainstem, deep nuclei and cerebellum, and spinal cord. Of these, the main ones identifiable on DTI include the corticospinal, corticobulbar, corticopontine, and geniculocalcarine tracts (optic radiations).

Corticospinal Tracts

Corticospinal tracts are descending projection tracts connecting the motor area to the spinal cord (see **Fig. 2**; **Fig. 3**). Corticospinal tracts have long been believed to arise from the motor

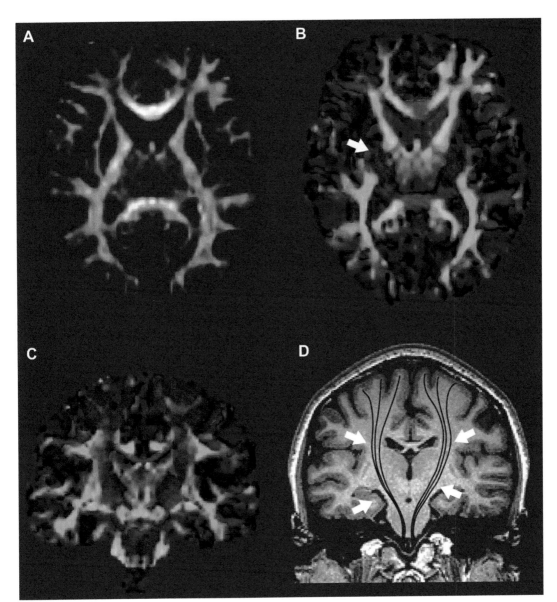

Fig. 2. Fractional anisotropy (*A*) and corresponding color maps (*B* and *C*) and Coronal T1 with schematic overlay of the corticospinal tract (*D*). Note that the horizontal fibers of the genu and splenium of the corpus callosum at this level are represented in red, whereas the vertically orientated corticospinal tracts in the posterior limb are represented in blue (*arrow, B*). Anteroposterior fibers such as the SLF are represented in green (*B*). Likewise because the corticospinal tracts enter the cerebral peduncles and take a medial course, their color value mixes red and blue into magenta (*arrows, D*).

cortex of the precentral gyrus. In a study of 42 healthy children using DTI, Kumar and colleagues[6] showed that the fibers originate in both precentral and postcentral gyrus in 71% of older children, followed by precentral gyrus, and least commonly from the postcentral gyrus. This pattern was not influenced by hand preference.

From the cortices, the fibers converge into the *corona radiata*. Here the more anterior fibers represent those servicing the face and the posterior fibers represent those that connect to the lower limb with fibers in between representing the hand.[7] Fibers then occupy the posterior aspect of the *posterior limb of internal capsule* (PLIC), beginning more anteriorly at the middle of the PLIC and then shifting more posteriorly as the tracts descend. Fibers representing the hand are anterior to those of the feet.[2]

At the level of the cerebral peduncles, the corticospinal tracts occupy the middle third of the *crus*

Table 1
White matter tracts, their connections and main functions

White Matter Tracts	Connection	Function
Cingulum	Cingulate gyrus to the entorhinal cortex	Affect, visceromotor control; response selection in skeletomotor control; visuospatial processing and memory access
Fornix	Hippocampus and the septal area to hypothalamus	Part of the Papez circuit; critical in formation of memory; damage or disease resulting in anterograde amnesia
Superior longitudinal fasciculus	Frontotemporal and frontoparietal regions	Integration of auditory and speech nuclei
Inferior longitudinal fasciculus	Ipsilateral temporal and occipital lobes	Visual emotion and visual memory
Superior fronto-occipital fasciculus	Frontal lobe to ipsilateral parietal lobe—name being a misnomer	Spatial awareness, symmetric processing
Inferior fronto-occipital fasciculus	Ipsilateral frontal and occipital, posterior parietal and temporal lobes	Integration of auditory and visual association cortices with prefrontal cortex
Uncinate fasciculus	Frontal and temporal lobes	Auditory verbal and declarative memory
Thalamic radiations	Lateral thalamic nuclei to cerebral cortex through internal capsule	Relay sensory and motor data to precentral and postcentral cortex
Corticofugal fibers (descending projection fibers)	Motor cortex and cerebral peduncle through internal capsule	Descending motor fibers from primary motor cortex, ventral and dorsal premotor areas, and supplementary motor areas
Corpus callosum	Corresponding cortical areas of both hemispheres	Interhemispheric sensorimotor and auditory connectivity
Anterior commissure	Olfactory bulbs and nuclei and amygdala	Integral part of the neospinothalamic tract for nociception and pain sensation

Adapted from Hutchins T, Herrod HC, Quigley E, et al. Dissection of the white matter tracts: interactive diffusion tensor imaging teaching atlas. University of Utah, Department of Neuroradiology. Available at: http://www.asnr2.org/neurographics/7/1/26/White%20Matter%20Tract%20Anatomy/DTI%20tutorial%202.html. Accessed July 15, 2012.

cerebri. Here the face fibers run medial to the fibers representing the feet, with the fibers representing the hand once again in between.[8] The fibers travel within the *basis pontis* before passing through the anterior medulla, forming *the medullary pyramids.* At the level of the caudal medulla, most of the fibers (75%–90%) in the pyramids cross to the contralateral side, forming the *pyramidal decussation of Mistichelli.* These fibers then descend as *the lateral corticospinal tract* within the posterior part of the *lateral funiculus* of the *medulla spinalis.* Of the fibers that do not cross, the majority travel in the anterior column on either side of the median fissure as the *anterior corticospinal tracts,* historically known as the *bundle of Türck.* These tracts decussate where they terminate, at their respective spinal level within the contralateral anterior horn gray matter.[7]

There are variations in this anatomy with some fibers not crossing to form ipsilateral lateral corticospinal tracts and others decussating to form contralateral anterior corticospinal tracts. Approximately 2% of the corticospinal tract remains truly ipsilateral, running in the ventrolateral funiculus as the bundle of Barnes to supply axial muscles of the trunk and proximal limbs.[9]

Likewise, there may be some asymmetry in the corticospinal tracts. The left corticospinal tract has higher FA values and lower transverse diffusivity because of high myelin content.[4] There is an increase in FA within the corticospinal tracts with increasing age.[6] Partially uncrossed pyramidal tracts are very rare (**Fig. 4**) and have been described by Alurkar and colleagues[10] and have been described with horizontal gaze palsy and scoliosis by Mori and colleagues[11] in 2005.

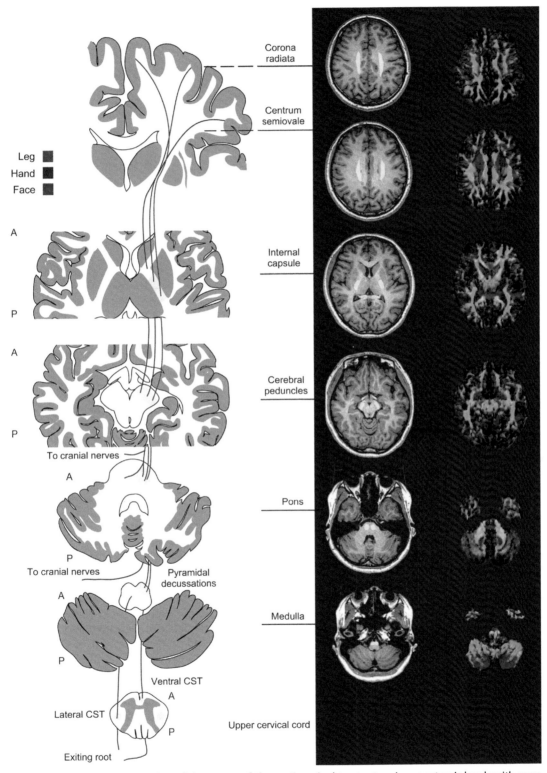

Fig. 3. A schematic representation of the course of the corticospinal tracts at various anatomic levels with corresponding T1-weighted MR image T1 and color FA (cFA) maps. Orientation of schematic illustrations match that of MR image (anterior [A] is the upper margin of each slice and posterior [P] is the lower margin.)

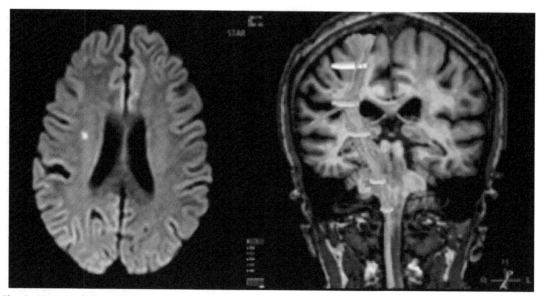

Fig. 4. Uncrossed pyramidal tracts: a previously normal young adult with acute weakness on the right side and focal-diffusion-restricted lesion in the right corticospinal tract. Weakness on the same side was well explained with diffusion tractography (coronal postprocessed tractography superimposed on T1-weighted image), which showed that most of the right-sided fibers were continuing down the same side below the level of the medulla. This patient did not have scoliosis or lateral gaze palsy, a syndrome that has been well described with uncrossed pyramidal tracts. (*Courtesy of* Ashish Atre, MD, STAR Imaging Center, Pune, India).

Corticobulbar Tracts

Corticobulbar tracts connect the motor cortex to cranial nerve nuclei in the brainstem. These fibers pass through the corona radiata and genu of internal capsule to run mediodorsal to the corticospinal tracts at the level of the cerebral peduncles.

Corticopontine Tracts

Corticopontine fibers arise from precentral and postcentral gyri with substantial contributions from premotor, supplementary motor, and posterior parietal cortices as well as from prefrontal and temporal cortices. The fibers course through the anterior limb of the internal capsule and medial cerebral peduncle before projecting into the pontine nuclei. Second-order neurons from the pontine nuclei decussate to the contralateral side and give rise to pontocerebellar pathways.

The corticospinal, corticopontine, and corticobulbar tracts run together and cannot be identified separately from each other using DTI but may be parcellated using advanced color maps.[12]

Internal Capsule

The internal capsule is the main conduit for projection fibers and is divided into 3 main sections. The anterior limb of internal capsule lies between the lentiform nucleus and the head of the caudate nucleus and carries the anterior thalamic radiations and frontopontine tracts. The PLIC separates the posterior aspect of the lentiform nucleus and the thalamus and contains corticospinal, corticobulbar, and frontopontine fibers; the superior thalamic radiation; and a smaller number of fibers connecting to the tectal, rubral, and reticular systems.

The PLIC can be further subdivided into thalamolenticular, sublenticular, and retrolenticular segments. Within the retrolenticular portion of the PLIC runs the posterior thalamic radiation (which includes the optic radiation) and the corticotectal, corticonigral, and corticotegmental fibers. The sublenticular portion of the PLIC contains the inferior thalamic radiation, auditory radiation, and temporal and parieto-occipital corticopontine fibers.[2]

The intervening genu of the internal capsule between the anterior and posterior limb contains corticobulbar and corticoreticular fibers as well as some frontopontine and superior thalamic radiation fibers.

Thalamic Radiations

The thalamus is known to have reciprocal connections (corticothalamic and thalamocortical fibers) to wide areas of the cortex. These fibers pass through the anterior and posterior limbs and retrolenticular segment of the internal capsule as the anterior, superior, and posterior thalamic radiations (Fig. 5) and fan out to form the corona radiata.[13]

Reciprocal connections include the *anterior nucleus* and *cingulate* cortex, *ventral lateral nucleus* and *motor* cortex, *ventral anterior nucleus* and *supplementary motor* area, *ventral posterior nucleus* and *sensory* cortex, *lateral geniculate body* (LGB) and *visual* cortex, *medial geniculate body* and *primary auditory* cortex, and *dorsomedial nucleus* and *prefrontal* cortex (Fig. 6).

Geniculocalcarine Tract (Optic Radiation)

The geniculocalcarine tract connects the LGB to the primary visual cortex and consists of 3 white matter bundles (Fig. 7). The *anterior bundle* corresponds to the lower retina fibers and projects from the LGB to run laterally then anteriorly across the roof of the anterior tip of the ipsilateral temporal horn. This bundle then makes a sharp turn to pass posteriorly forming the Meyer loop (Fig. 8) along the inferior lateral wall of the temporal horn through the temporal stem to converge on the lower lip of the calcarine fissure.[4] As it courses along the wall of the temporal horn, the Meyer loop lies deep to the inferior occipitofrontal fasciculus (Fig. 9).[4]

The Meyer loop is an important consideration in epilepsy surgery because damage during surgery can result in homonymous upper quadrantanopia. The anterior border of the Meyer loop and its relation to the tip of temporal horn and temporal pole has been a matter of controversy.[12]

Some studies have shown that the anterior extent of the Meyer loop may run more rostral than the tip of the temporal horn and may lie 20 mm from the tip of the temporal lobe.[4] Conversely, more recent studies with DTI have shown that the Meyer loop does not reach as far anteriorly as the tip of the temporal horn. The general consensus at present is that there is likely individual anatomic variation, making it difficult to give a generic recommendation on safe lengths of anterior temporal lobe resection without causing a visual field defect.[12] Because probabilistic tractographic studies are showing great promise in the delineation of the Meyer loop, this additional information could be used in neurosurgical planning to help avoid the risk of visual field defects.[12]

The *central bundle* serves the macular region and passes directly laterally, to cross the roof of the temporal horn before coursing along the lateral wall and roof of the trigone and occipital horn to the occipital pole. The *posterior bundle* corresponds to the superior retina and courses directly posteriorly, over the roof of the trigone and occipital horn, and ends at the upper lip of the calcarine fissure. The lateral walls of the temporal and occipital horns are formed by all the 3 bundles of optic radiation, separated from the ependyma by a thin layer of the corpus callosum, known as the tapetum. In conjunction with the inferior occipitofrontal fasciculus, inferior longitudinal fasciculus, and inferior aspect of the SLF, the optic radiation

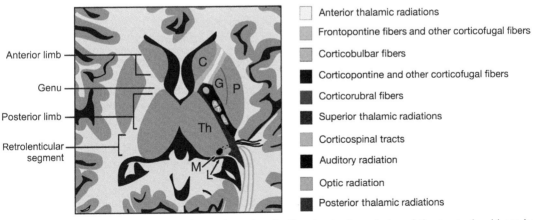

Fig. 5. Simplified illustration of internal capsule and main fiber tracts. Boundaries of the tracts should not be considered as definite because there is no precise distinction between some tracts. The corticospinal tracts are oriented such that the fibers representing arms (A) are anterior to the trunk (T), which in turn are anterior to the fibers representing the limbs (L). The auditory and optic radiations are shown arising, respectively, from the medial (M) and lateral (L) geniculate bodies (*arrows*). The gray matter structures: the caudate (C), globus pallidus (G), putamen (P), and thalamus (Th) are shown bounding the anterior and posterior limbs of the internal capsule.

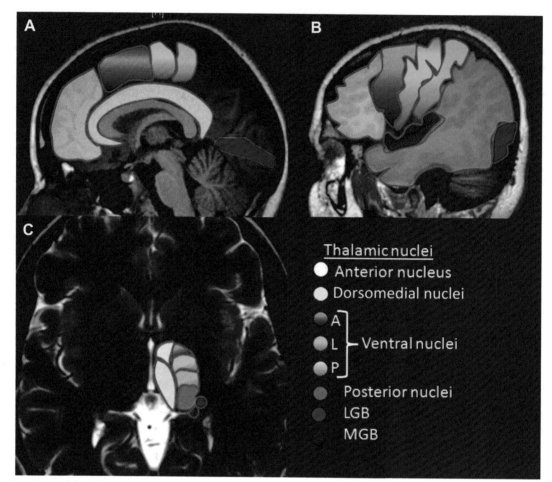

Fig. 6. Simplified illustration of reciprocal connections of thalamic nuclei to the cortical areas. Sagittal T1 midline (*A*), Sagittal T1 through the temporal lobe (*B*), axial T2 through the thalami (*C*). A, L, and P represent anterior, lateral, and posterior ventral nuclei, respectively; LGB, lateral geniculate body; MGB, medial geniculate body.

mingles posteriorly to form much of the sagittal stratum in the occipital lobe.

ASSOCIATION FIBERS

Association fibers unite different cortical areas within the same hemisphere and can be short or long. *Short association fibers* connect areas within the same lobe and include subcortical U fibers, which connect adjacent gyri (**Fig. 10**). The work by Oishi and colleagues[14] on a population-based atlas of the superficial white matter using DTI divides the cortical areas into 9 blade-type structures, further parcellated into 21 subregions. *Long association fibers* identifiable on DTI include the SLF, inferior longitudinal fasciculus, middle longitudinal fasciculus (MLF), uncinate fasciculus, superior fronto-occipital fasciculus, and inferior fronto-occipital fasciculus.

Superior Longitudinal Fasciculus

The SLF is the largest association bundle composed of bidirectional fibers connecting the frontal lobe to the parietal, temporal, and occipital lobes and includes the arcuate fasciculus (**Fig. 11**). Makris and colleagues[15] in their in vivo DTI study demonstrated that the SLF, as it is in primates, can be divided into 4 distinct components: SLF I, SLF II, SLF III, and the arcuate fascicle (AF).

SLF I

SLF I is located in the superior parietal lobe, precentral and postcentral gyri, superior precuneus, and posterior part of the superior frontal gyrus.[15] The medial and superior parietal involvement of SLF I suggests its contribution in regulating higher aspects of motor behavior, including conditional associative tasks (ie, selection of different motor tasks based on conditional rules).

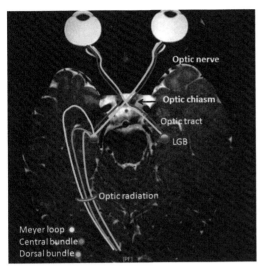

Fig. 7. MR image of visual pathway showing optic nerves, chiasm (*arrow*), optic tracts, lateral geniculate body (LGB), and optic radiations. Anterior, central, and posterior bundles of optic radiation as they course to the occipital cortex are also shown.

SLF II

SLF II connects the prefrontal cortex with the caudal inferior parietal cortex and is located in the angular gyrus, supramarginal gyrus, precentral and postcentral gyrus, middle frontal gyrus, and occipito-temporo-parietal region. SLF II provides bidirectional information and feedback between the prefrontal and posterior parietal regions with information regarding perception of visual space, with lesions resulting in disorders of spatial working memory.

SLF III

SLF III may function to transfer somatosensory information, including language articulation and monitoring orofacial and hand motions. SLF III has possible connections between the pars opercularis and supramarginal gyrus, with bidirectional connections between the ventral prefrontal cortex and inferior parietal lobule.

AF

The AF connects the frontal lobe, supramarginal gyrus, posterior part of the superior temporal gyrus, and temporo-occipital region and can be subdivided into the following segments:

- *Frontotemporal (FT) segment*: connects the inferior frontal cortex (Broca area, in the dominant hemisphere) with the superior temporal cortex (Wernicke area in the dominant hemisphere).
- *Frontoparietal segment*: connecting the inferior frontal cortex and the parietal cortex.
- *Temporoparietal segment*: connecting the temporal cortex in the region of the superior and middle temporal gyri with the parietal cortex.[16] Eluvathingal and colleagues[16]

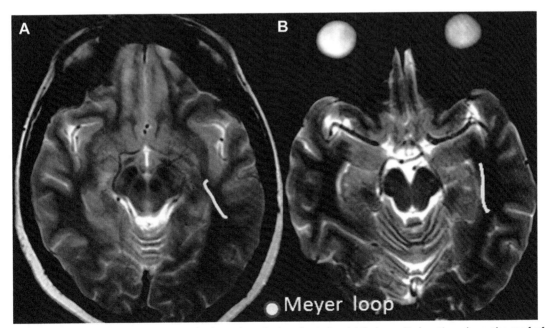

Fig. 8. Axial images of Meyer loop at the lateral geniculate body level (*A*) shows its location along the roof of temporal horn. At the level of hippocampus (*B*), it is seen along the lateral wall of temporal horn. Note that the anterior extent does not reach up to the tip of temporal horn.

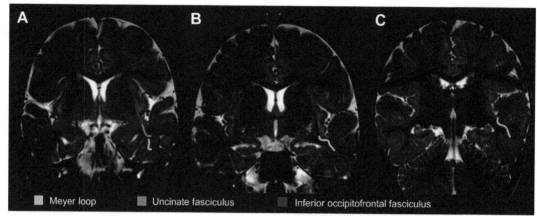

Meyer loop   Uncinate fasciculus   Inferior occipitofrontal fasciculus

Fig. 9. (A) Image at the level of the amygdala (A) showing anteriormost segment of the Meyer loop and its relation to the inferior occipitofrontal fasciculus (IOF) and uncinate fasciculus. (B) Image at the level of the hippocampus, showing the Meyer loop superolateral to temporal horn and passing through the temporal stem. At this level, the Meyer loop is deep to the IOF. (C) Image at the level of the lateral geniculate body shows the Meyer loop, located above and lateral to the temporal horn.

showed that the FT segment of the AF was not visible in 29% of normal cases and that the left FT segment demonstrates higher FA values than the right, consistent with functional and anatomic lateralization of language to the dominant hemisphere.

Interruption or insult to the SLF decreases the ability to repeat spoken language and can also cause unilateral neglect.

Inferior Longitudinal Fasciculus

The inferior longitudinal fasciculus connects the cortices of the anterior temporal and posterior occipital lobe and joins the inferior aspect of the

SLF, optic radiations, and inferior longitudinal fasciculus to form the sagittal stratum traversing the occipital lobe (**Figs. 12** and **13**). It has been shown that the inferior longitudinal fasciculus and the inferior fronto-occipital fasciculus share most of the projections from the posterior temporal and occipital lobes.[5] Interruption of this fasciculus may result in unilateral visual neglect, visual amnesia, and hallucinations and also visual hypoemotionality.[17,18]

Middle Longitudinal Fasciculus

Makris and colleagues[19] have delineated the MLF in humans and found it to be similar to the

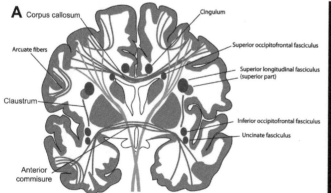
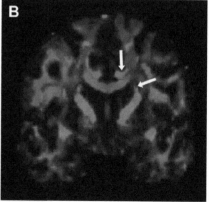

Fig. 10. Coronal illustration showing various association and commissural fibers and their relations. (A: Schematic, B: coronal color FA map at the level of the frontal horns) The corpus callosum is seen between the cingulum superomedially and the superior occipitofrontal fasciculus inferolaterally (arrows). The SLF courses along the superior margin of the claustrum in an arc and is separated from the SLF by internal capsule and corona radiata. The inferior occipitofrontal fasciculus lies along the inferolateral edge of the claustrum along the inferior insula. Uncinate fasciculus is seen inferomedial to the inferior occipitofrontal fasciculus.

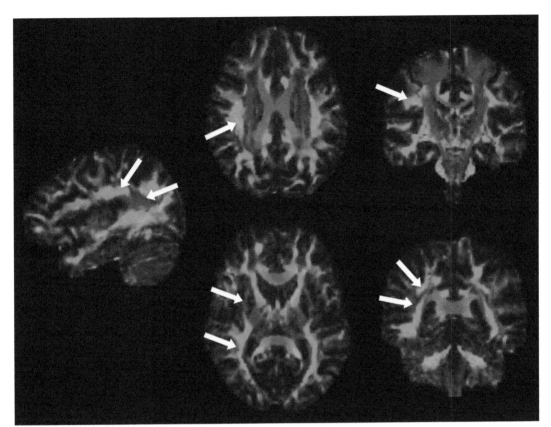

Fig. 11. The course (*arrows*) of the superior longitudinal fasciculus on color FA (cFA) DTI images.

described tracts in rhesus monkeys. The MLF extends from the caudal part of the inferior parietal lobule, specifically the angular gyrus, to the white matter of the superior temporal gyrus, remaining within the white matter of the superior temporal gyrus (Fig. 14).

The MLF is distinct from other adjacent fiber tracts such as the SLF II and the AF, which lie more laterally. Because of its location it is suggested that the MLF could have a central role in language (dominant hemisphere) and attention (nondominant hemisphere) functions.

Superior Occipitofrontal Fasciculus

The name superior occipitofrontal fasciculus is a misnomer because its fibers actually connect the frontal and parietal lobes (Fig. 15),[20] and hence it should probably be named the superior fronto-parietal fasciculus. This fasciculus lies deep to the corpus callosum, extending posteriorly along the dorsal border of caudate nucleus, and runs parallel to the SLF. Anteriorly it lies in the superior edge of the anterior limb of the internal capsule before projecting into the frontal lobe.[19] The functions of this fasciculus include spatial awareness and symmetric processing. A possible link between white matter hyperintensity burden and late life depression has been suggested.[21]

Inferior Occipitofrontal Fasciculus

This fasciculus connects the occipital and frontal lobes and also contains fibers connecting the frontal lobe with the posterior part of the parietal and temporal lobes. Fibers from the lateral frontal

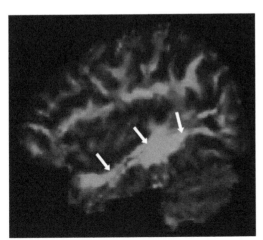

Fig. 12. Sagittal course (*white arrow*) of the inferior longitudinal fasciculus on color FA (cFA) DTI.

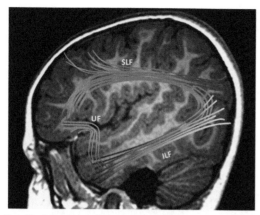

Fig. 13. MR image demonstrating relative trajectories of the SLF, uncinate fasciculus (UF), and inferior longitudinal fasciculus (ILF) to one another.

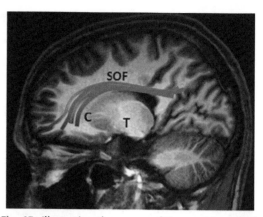

Fig. 15. Illustrating the course of the superior occipitofrontal fasciculus (SOF) arcing over the caudate nucleus and connecting frontal and parietal lobes. C, caudate nucleus; T, thalamus.

lobe converge into a single bundle to run along the inferolateral edge of the lentiform nucleus, at the inferior aspect of the claustrum, and may lie in the external as well as the extreme capsules. This fasciculus runs superior to the uncinate fasciculus in the temporal stem (**Fig. 16**).[4] Posteriorly, the inferior occipitofrontal fasciculus joins the inferior longitudinal fasciculus, the descending portion of the SLF, and portions of the geniculocalcarine tract to form most of the *sagittal stratum*, a large and complex bundle that connects the occipital lobe to the rest of the brain.[3]

This fasciculus may connect more superiorly located regions of the frontal lobe with more posterior areas of the temporal lobe, than those connected by the uncinate fasciculus. The fibers seem to connect auditory areas with visual

association cortex in the temporal lobe with prefrontal cortex.[21] Owing to the longer connections of the inferior occipitofrontal fasciculus, it may play a larger role of disease spread between the frontal and temporal lobes than the uncinate fasciculus. This tract may have a role in triggering temporal lobe syndromes in extratemporal lesions as well as be associated with amnesia, schizophrenia, and Alzheimer disease.

Uncinate Fasciculus

The uncinate fasciculus (of Russell) is a hook-shaped bundle of fibers and is also known as the temporofrontal (frontotemporal) fasciculus. This fasciculus connects the orbital and inferior frontal gyri and gyri rectus to the anterior temporal lobe, consisting of both afferent and efferent fibers. The fasciculus can be divided into 3 parts: temporal, insular, and frontal segments. Specifically it connects cortical nuclei of the uncus and amygdala to the subcallosal region and superior, medial, and inferior temporal gyri to the gyrus rectus and medial and lateral orbital gyri. In the temporal stem, the tract lies inferomedial to the inferior occipitofrontal fasciculus. Anteriorly the fibers curve upward behind and over the M1 segment of the middle cerebral artery (**Fig. 17**). The inner fibers pass through the external and extreme capsule, with part of the claustrum embedded in its fibers, before fanning horizontally in the frontal orbital white matter.[4]

The uncinate fasciculus has the longest period of development in terms of FA, and is the only major white fiber track that continues to develop beyond the age of 30 years.[22] In contrast to adults, FA values have not shown any asymmetry in diffusivities between right and left tracts in children.[16]

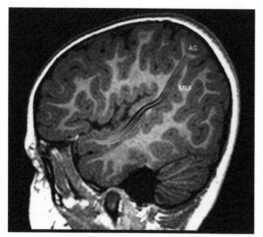

Fig. 14. MR image showing middle longitudinal fasciculus (MLF) extending from inferior parietal lobule to temporal pole. AG, angular gyrus.

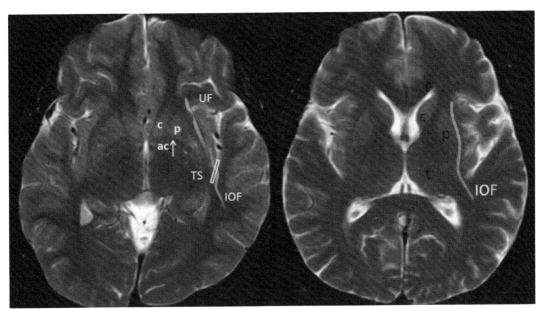

Fig. 16. Axial images showing the relation of uncinate fasciculus (UF) and inferior occipitofrontal fasciculus (IOF). The uncinate fasciculus courses through the anterior-most aspect of temporal stem (TS, shown as *small rectangle*) and the superior extent lies below the level of the frontal horns. IOF courses through the more posterior aspect of temporal stem, traverses its entire extent, and superiorly extends to the level of frontal horn. Uncinate fasciculus is inferior to the IOF and intermingles with it in the insula and frontal pole. C, caudate nucleus head; p, putamen; t, thalamus; ac, anterior commissure (shown with *arrow*); UF, uncinate fasciculus; IOF, inferior occipitofrontal fasciculus.

Traditionally considered to be part of the limbic system, the exact function of the uncinate fasciculus remains unknown. The integrity of the left uncinate fasciculus has been related with proficiency in auditory–verbal memory and declarative memory.[23] Review of many experimental studies supports the role of the uncinate fasciculus as one of the several connections whose disruption results in severe memory impairment, particularly in posttraumatic retrograde amnesia.[4]

The normal left-greater-than-right asymmetry in the anisotropy in this fasciculus has been shown to be absent in patients with schizophrenia, supporting the theory that patients with schizophrenia have abnormalities of myelin and reduced neuronal integrity of the uncinate fasciculus.[4]

COMMISSURAL FIBERS

Commissural fibers are the white matter tracts connecting corresponding homologous regions between the 2 hemispheres. The main structures discussed are the corpus callosum and anterior commissure.

Corpus Callosum

The corpus callosum is the largest white matter fiber bundle in the brain with more than 300 million axons connecting the corresponding areas of the 2 hemispheres. Although many of these fibers connect homologous/mirror image areas of cortex, there is a significant proportion of asymmetry.

The fibers of the anterior body are transversely oriented. Fibers projecting from the genu and splenium tend to arch more anteriorly and posteriorly, forming the forceps minor and forceps major, respectively. Projections from the splenium, which

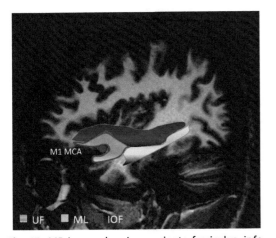

Fig. 17. MR image showing uncinate fasciculus, inferior occipitofrontal fasciculus (IOF), and the Meyer loop fibers projected to the cortical surface. Note the looping of the uncinate fibers around the M1 middle cerebral artery (MCA).

pass inferiorly along the lateral margin of the posterior horn of the lateral ventricle to the temporal lobes, are called the tapetum and are easily identifiable in midsagittal plane by their right–left orientation (**Fig. 18**). Near the cortex, corpus callosal fibers interdigitate with the association and projection fibers and are difficult to delineate.

The main function of the corpus callosum is interhemispheric sensorimotor and auditory connectivity. Embryologically, the corpus callosum appears at 15 weeks and extends in both anterior and posterior directions during the following weeks, before undergoing more anterior development at 19 weeks.[24] Agenesis may be associated with language delay, language task disconnection, and problems in integrating visual and tactile stimuli. The corpus callosum is specifically involved in multiple sclerosis, lymphoma, and interhemispheric spread of tumor (eg, glioblastoma multiforme).

Anterior Commissure

The anterior commissure is a small compact bundle of fibers between the anterior and posterior columns of the fornix.[25] This commissure contains decussating olfactory fibers connecting the olfactory bulb, anterior olfactory nucleus, and anterior perforated substance, and it also serves to connect the 2 temporal lobes; amygdala; inferior temporal, parahippocampal, and fusiform gyri; and inferior occipital cortex.

OTHER WHITE MATTER STRUCTURES
Temporal Stem

The temporal stem is the white matter bridge between temporal and frontal lobes and extends from the amygdala to the level of the LGB posteriorly (**Fig. 19**). The 3 main tracts passing through the temporal stem are the uncinate fasciculus, inferior occipitofrontal fasciculus, and the Meyer loop of the optic radiations. The temporal stem is an important structure because it is a possible route for tumor, infection, and seizure spread and also plays an important role in numerous disorders, including amnesia, Klüver-Bucy syndrome, traumatic brain injury, and Alzheimer disease (**Fig. 20**).[4] The close proximity of the temporal stem to the insula, basal ganglia, and external and extreme capsule makes it an important landmark during surgery of the temporal lobe.

Limbic System Fibers

Cingulum, fornix, and stria terminalis form the 3 major white matter tracts of the limbic system.

Cingulum

The fibers of the cingulum begin in the parolfactory area below the rostrum of the corpus callosum and arch over the corpus callosum, beneath the length of the cingulate gyrus, to reach the parahippocampal gyrus and uncus (**Fig. 21**). The cingulum carries afferent connections from the cingulate gyrus to

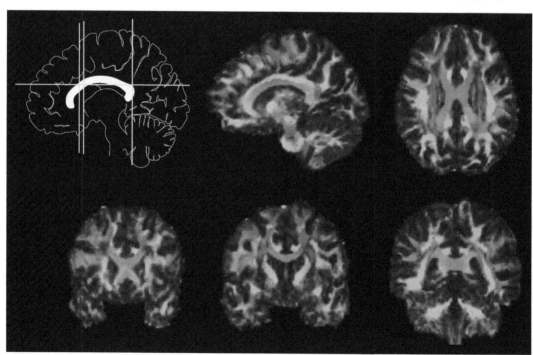

Fig. 18. The corpus callosum and directionality of fibers on color FA (cFA) DTI maps.

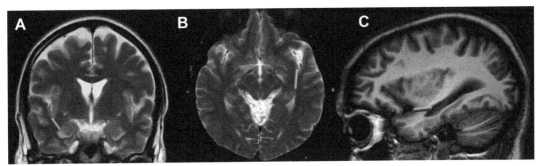

Fig. 19. MR illustration of location of temporal stem on coronal (*A*), axial (*B*), and sagittal (*C*) images.

the entorhinal cortex and connects portions of the frontal, parietal, and temporal lobes. The cingulum becomes appreciable only after 17 weeks' gestation.[24] Functionally the cingulate cortex is subdivided into at least 4 zones with a range of functions including affect, visceromotor and skeletomotor control, visuospatial processing, and memory access.[26]

Fornix

The fornix includes both afferent and efferent pathways between the hippocampus, the septal area (preanterior commissure segment of the fornix), and the hypothalamus and mammillary body (postcommissure). Similar to the cingulum, the fornix has a C-shaped trajectory consisting of the column, body, and crus. The fornix branches into 2 columns near the anterior commissure and projects into the dorsal regions of the hippocampi.

Stria terminalis

The stria terminalis is the innermost C-shaped trajectory of the 3 limbic fibers and provides afferent and efferent pathways between the amygdala and

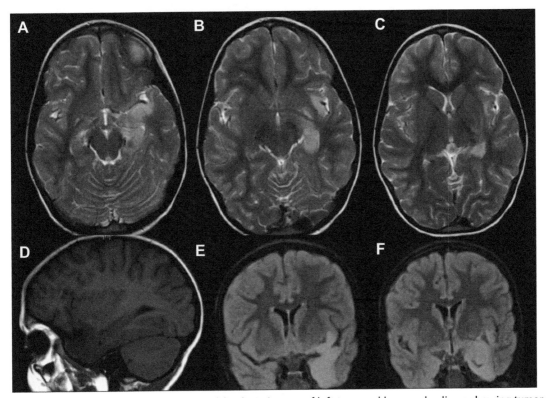

Fig. 20. Axial (*A–C*), sagittal (*D*), and coronal (*E, F*) MR images of left temporal low-grade glioma showing tumor extension through the temporal stem into the region of the external and extreme capsules and inferior frontal region.

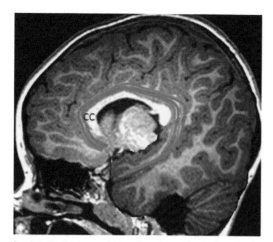

Fig. 21. Trajectory of the cingulum. Note that in this image, a midline image (through the [CC] corpus callosum) and a sagittal image (through the temporal lobe) are superimposed to show the complete trajectory of the cingulum.

the septal area and the hypothalamus. The major role of stria terminalis is in limbic interaction, amygdalar output, and hypothalamic-pituitary-adrenal axis input. Interruption disrupts gonadotropin secretion, and it is a target site for opiate withdrawal therapy. The stria terminalis and fornix are relatively small tracts in adult brains but can be seen as major tracts at 13 weeks' gestation.[24]

BRAINSTEM FIBERS

The 5 major white matter tracts that can be identified within the brainstem on DTI include the superior, middle, and inferior cerebellar peduncles; the corticospinal tract; and the medial lemniscus.[27] The cerebellum is connected to the brainstem by 3 main peduncles. Afferent fibers pass through the inferior cerebellar peduncle and middle cerebellar peduncle (MCP), whereas efferent fibers traverse the inferior and superior cerebellar peduncles.[9] Efferent fibers of the superior cerebellar peduncle originate from the dentate nucleus to connect with the thalamus, red nucleus,

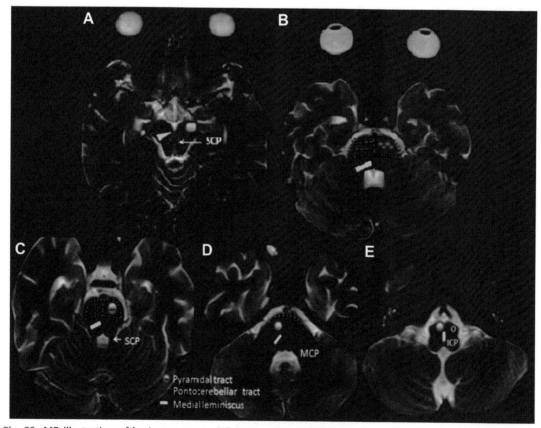

Fig. 22. MR illustration of brainstem tracts. (*A*) Decussation of SCP (*arrow*) at inferior colliculus level. (*B*) Pyramidal tracts being split by the transverse pontine fibers. Level of SCP (*C*), MCP (*D*), and ICP (*E*) showing topography and relations of various tracts. ICP, inferior cerebellar peduncle; O, olive; SCP, superior cerebellar peduncle.

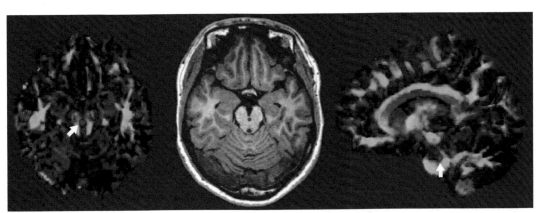

Fig. 23. "Focal red spot" (*arrow*) of the superior cerebellar peduncles' decussation at the level of the midbrain.

vestibular nuclei, and reticular formation. On axial DTI images, the superior cerebellar peduncle is identified at the dentate nucleus level, with a linear green/blue-colored course (**Figs. 22** and **23**). More superiorly, there is a "focal red spot," which is believed to represent the decussation of the superior cerebellar peduncle fibers. Merlini and colleagues[27] found that this decussation may also represent the ventral tegmental decussation.

The superior cerebellar peduncle functions as part of the motor coordination and balance network. Lesions can cause ipsilateral limb and trunk dystaxia. This peduncle is found to be atrophic in progressive supranuclear palsy, and there is an absence of normal decussation of fibers in Joubert syndrome.[21]

The fibers of the MCP are part of the pontocerebellar tracts and form "sheet-like" projections wrapping around the pons with dorsal anterioposterior (green) and ventral left–right (red)

directionality. The transverse pontine fibers (red) are also part of the MCP and are seen anteriorly and dorsally to the vertically oriented (blue) corticospinal tracts (**Fig. 24**).[27] These afferent fibers connect the contralateral pontine nuclei to the cerebellum and transmit impulses from the cerebral cortex to the intermediate and lateral zones of the cerebellum.[9] These fibers are involved in initiation, planning, and timing of volitional motor activity and have input from vestibular receptors, thus playing a role in posture, balance, and coordination. Lesions involving the MCP result in ipsilateral limb and gait ataxia.[21]

The *inferior cerebellar peduncle* carries both afferent and efferent fibers and connects the cerebellum and the medulla. Connections include the dorsal spinocerebellar tract and cuneocerebellar, olivocerebellar, vestibulocerebellar, reticulocerebellar, trigeminocerebellar, fastigiobulbar and cerebelloreticular tracts.[9] This peduncle can be

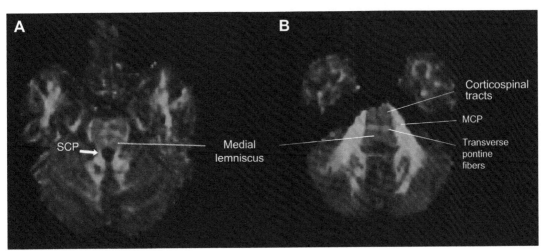

Fig. 24. Color FA (cFA) DTI maps at the level of the (*A*) superior cerebellar peduncle (SCP) (*arrow*) and (*B*) middle cerebellar peduncles (MCPs) demonstrating the position of the corticospinal tracts, transverse pontine fibers of the MCP, and the medial lemniscus.

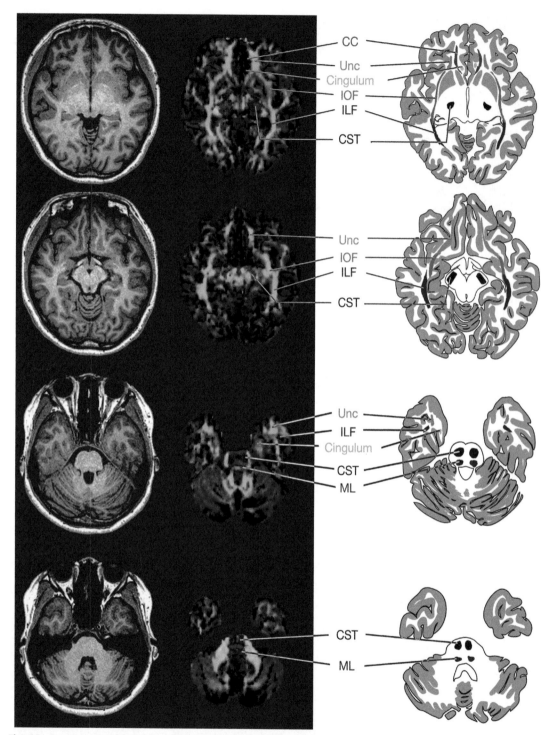

Fig. 25. A summary table of anatomic T1 MR images (first column) with corresponding color-coded FA maps (second column) and line diagrams (third column) depicting the major tracts is provided for quick reference. CC, corpus callosum; CST, corticospinal tract; ILF, inferior longitudinal fasciculus; IOF, inferior occipitofrontal fasciculus; ML, medial lemniscus; SOF, superior occipitofrontal fasciculus; Unc, uncinate fasciculus.

identified along the dorsal aspect of the medulla and pons and is represented by the color blue (inferior-superior direction) in its inferior half and by green in its superior half.[27]

The *medial lemniscus* serves as an important pathway for ascending sensory fibers to the ventroposterolateral thalamus and decussates at the level of the ventral medulla, becoming markedly dispersed at the midbrain level and thus limiting its identification on DTI. The medial lemniscus is best seen dorsal to the dorsal transverse pontine fibers at the level of the MCP[27] and functions to convey sensations of touch, vibration, proprioception, and 2-point discrimination.[21]

SUMMARY

DTI has emerged as an excellent tool for in vivo demonstration of white matter microstructure and has revolutionized our understanding of the same.

Information on normal connectivity and relations of different white matter networks and their role in different disease conditions is still evolving. Evidence is mounting on causal relations of abnormal white matter microstructure and connectivity in a wide range of pediatric neurocognitive and white matter diseases.

Hence there is a pressing need for every neuroradiologist to acquire a strong basic knowledge of white matter anatomy and to make an effort to apply this knowledge in routine reporting, along with being updated in this evolving field. A summary table of color-coded FA maps with corresponding anatomic T1 MR images and line diagrams depicting the major tracts is provided for quick reference of the reader (**Fig. 25**).

REFERENCES

1. Gawne-Cain ML, Silver NC, Moseley IF, et al. Fast FLAIR of the brain: the range of appearances in normal subjects and its application to quantification of white-matter disease. Neuroradiology 1987;39(4): 243–9.
2. Cowan FM, de Vries LS. The internal capsule in neonatal imaging. Semin Fetal Neonatal Med 2005; 10:461–74.
3. Jellison BJ, Field AS, Medow J, et al. Diffusion tensor imaging of cerebral white matter: a pictorial review of physics, fiber tract anatomy, and tumor imaging patterns. AJNR Am J Neuroradiol 2004;25:356–69.
4. Kier EL, Staib LH, Davis LM, et al. MR imaging of the temporal stem: anatomic dissection tractography of the uncinate fasciculus, inferior occipitofrontal fasciculus, and Meyer's loop of the optic radiation. AJNR Am J Neuroradiol 2004;25:677–91.
5. Wakana S, Jiang H, Nagae-Poetscher LM, et al. Fiber tract–based atlas of human white matter anatomy. Radiology 2004;230:77–87.
6. Kumar A, Juhasz C, Asano E, et al. Diffusion Tensor Imaging of study of the cortical origin, course of the corticospinal tract in healthy children. AJNR Am J Neuroradiol 2009;30(10):1963–70.
7. Al Masri O. An essay on the human corticospinal tract: history, development, anatomy, and connections. Neuroanatomy 2011;10:1–4.
8. Kwon HG, Hong JH, Jang SH. Anatomic location and somatotopic arrangement of the corticospinal tract at the cerebral peduncle in the human brain. AJNR Am J Neuroradiol 2011;32:2116–9.
9. Brazis PW, Masdeu JC, Biller J. Localization in clinical neurology. 5th Edition. Philadelphia: Lippincott Williams and Wilkins; 2007. ISBN-13: 978-0-7817-9552-2.
10. Alurkar A, Karanam SP, Atre A, et al. Ipsilateral stroke with uncrossed pyramidal tracts and underlying right internal carotid artery stenosis treated with percutaneous transluminal angioplasty and stenting. NRJ Digital 2012;2:267–72.
11. Mori H, Fijishiro T, Hayashi N, et al. Uncrossed pyramidal tracts shown by tractography in horizontal gaze palsy and scoliosis. AJR Am J Roentgenol 2005;84(Suppl 3):S4–6.
12. Mandelstam SA. Challenges of the anatomy and diffusion tensor tractography of the Meyer loop. AJNR Am J Neuroradiol 2012;33(7):1204–10.
13. Oishi K, Faria A, van Zijl PC, et al. MRI atlas of human white matter. Boston: Academic Press, Elsevier; 2011. ISBN: 97801238208–15.
14. Oishi K, Zilles K, Amunts K, et al. Human brain white matter atlas: identification and assignment of common anatomical structures in superficial white matter. Neuroimage 2008;43(3):447–57.
15. Makris N, Kennedy DN, McInerney S, et al. Segmentation of subcomponents within the superior longitudinal fascicle in humans: a quantitative, in vivo, DT-MRI study. Cereb Cortex 2005;15(6):854–69.
16. Eluvathingal TJ, Hasan KM, Kramer L, et al. Quantitative diffusion tensor tractography of association and projection fibers in normally developing children and adolescents. Cereb Cortex 2007;17(12):2760–8.
17. Ffytche DM, Blom JD, Catani M. Disorders of visual perception. J Neurol Neurosurg Psychiatry 2010; 81(11):1280.
18. Catani M, Jones DK, Donato R, et al. Occipito-temporal connections in the human brain. Brain 2003;126(9):2093–107.
19. Makris N, Papadimitriou GM, Kaiser JR, et al. Delineation of the middle longitudinal fascicle in humans: a quantitative, in vivo, DT-MRI study. Cereb Cortex 2009;19(4):777–85.
20. Mori S, Wakana S, Nagae-Poetscher LM, et al. MRI atlas of human white matter. Amsterdam: Elsevier; 2005.

21. Hutchins T, Herrod HC, Quigley E, et al. Dissecting the white matter tracts: interactive diffusion tensor imaging teaching atlas. University of Utah, Department of Neuroradiology. Available at: http://www.asnr2.org/neurographics/7/1/26/White%20Matter%20Tract%20Anatomy/DTI%20tutorial%202.html. Accessed July 15, 2012.

22. Lebel C, Walker L, Leemans A, et al. Microstructural maturation of the human brain from childhood to adulthood. Neuroimage 2008;40(3):1044–55.

23. Mabbott DJ, Rovet J, Noseworthy MD, et al. The relations between white matter and declarative memory in older children and adolescents. Brain Res 2009;1294:80–90.

24. Huang H. Structure of the fetal brain: what we are learning from diffusion tensor imaging. Neuroscientist 2010;16(6):634–49.

25. Kollias S. Parcelation of the white matter using DTI: Insights into the functional connectivity of the brain. Neuroradiology 2009;22(Suppl 1). Available at: http://www.whba1990.org/uploads/4/0/1/1/4011882/dti.pdf. Accessed July 15, 2012.

26. Vogt B. Cingulate neurobiology and disease. New York: Oxford University Press; 2009. ISBN 13: 9780198566960.

27. Merlini L, Vargas MI, De Haller R, et al. MRI with fibre tracking in Cogan congenital oculomotor apraxia. Pediatr Radiol 2010;40:1625–33.

Standardized Magnetic Resonance Imaging Acquisition and Reporting in Pediatric Multiple Sclerosis

Leonard H. Verhey, PhD[a,b], Sridar Narayanan, PhD[c],
Brenda Banwell, MD, FRCPC[d,*]

KEYWORDS

- Multiple sclerosis • Inflammatory CNS demyelination • Pediatric
- Standardized acquisition and reporting

KEY POINTS

- The value of MR imaging in the diagnosis and clinical management of children with multiple sclerosis (MS) rests in part on the use of a consistent and standard imaging protocol.
- Adopting a standard lexicon and reporting scheme for pediatric central nervous system (CNS) demyelination will be valuable for implementing structured reporting into radiological practice.
- We propose a standard MR imaging acquisition and reporting protocol based on the pediatric MS literature and experience and insights gained from following children with acute CNS demyelination and MS in the Canadian Pediatric Demyelinating Disease Network.
- Our goal is to provide a framework within which to refine the protocol to enhance its national and international applicability.

INTRODUCTION

Magnetic resonance (MR) imaging is perhaps one of the most important paraclinical tools for the diagnosis of multiple sclerosis (MS) and for monitoring disease progression and treatment response. However, the value of MR imaging in informing clinical management of MS patients largely depends on the use of a consistent and standard imaging protocol. The goals of MR imaging in MS include: confirmation of an MS diagnosis before a second clinical attack[1] in individuals with an acute demyelinating syndrome according to dissemination in time and space criteria[2,3]; exclusion of alternative diagnoses[4]; and prediction of outcome. In addition, clinicians caring for patients with MS rely on comparison of serial scans to qualitatively evaluate the rate of new lesion accrual for diagnosis, to inform on treatment decisions, and to monitor disease evolution apparent by formation of confluent lesions and atrophy. A standard MR imaging acquisition protocol and reporting method will improve the accuracy and reliability of MR imaging evaluation among radiologists and clinicians within and across centers, and will aid the clinician in managing patients with MS.

[a] Pediatric Demyelinating Disease Program, Program in Neuroscience and Mental Health, The Hospital for Sick Children, Room 11-105 Elm Wing, 555 University Avenue, Toronto, ON M5G 1X8, Canada; [b] Institute of Medical Science, University of Toronto, Medical Science Building, 1 King's College Circle, Room 2374, Toronto, ON M5S 1A8, Canada; [c] Department of Neurology and Neurosurgery, McConnell Brain Imaging Centre, Montreal Neurological Institute, McGill University, 3801 University Street, Montreal, Quebec H3A 2B4, Canada; [d] Division of Neurology, Department of Pediatrics, Research Institute, The Hospital for Sick Children, University of Toronto, 555 University Avenue, Toronto, Ontario M5G 1X8, Canada
* Corresponding author.
E-mail address: banwellb@email.chop.edu

Neuroimag Clin N Am 23 (2013) 217–226
http://dx.doi.org/10.1016/j.nic.2012.12.003
1052-5149/13/$ – see front matter © 2013 Elsevier Inc. All rights reserved.

neuroimaging.theclinics.com

An expert panel of adult MS radiologists and neurologists within the Consortium of MS Centers published a consensus-based MR imaging protocol for use in the investigation and monitoring of patients with MS.[5] However, the panel indicated that the applicability of the protocol to pediatric-onset MS requires further study. Although many of the MR imaging features of MS in children may overlap with those of adults, specific considerations unique to the imaging of children and the distinct MR imaging features of MS in prepubertal children[6] may necessitate a revised MR imaging protocol for pediatric MS.

The goal of this article is to provide clinicians and neuroradiologists caring for children with demyelinating disorders with a suggested standard MR imaging acquisition and reporting protocol, and to define a standard lexicon for lesion features typical of MS in children. Only conventional MR imaging sequences used in routine clinical practice and standard to most scanners are discussed; advanced MR imaging techniques are being increasingly applied in MS research, but are not yet applicable or feasible in the clinical setting. As considerable overlap exists between the features of pediatric-onset and adult-onset MS, these recommendations may be of relevance to adult clinicians and radiologists. The recommendations are based on recent MR imaging studies conducted in pediatric MS and on the expertise of pediatric MS neurologists and neuroradiologists at The Hospital for Sick Children (Toronto, Canada), the lead center for the Canadian Pediatric Demyelinating Disease Network, a prospective cohort study in which standardized clinical and MR imaging data and biological samples are collected at onset and serially in children with incident demyelination.

UNIQUE CONSIDERATIONS IN MR IMAGING OF CHILDREN

There are several considerations to be mindful of when imaging the child being investigated for MS.

1. In very young children, primary myelination is not yet complete. Use of T2-weighted sequences and, to a greater extent, fluid-attenuated inversion recovery (FLAIR) imaging, is not optimal for the assessment of the presence of inflammatory demyelinating lesions. The normal T2-weighted appearance of ongoing primary myelination in very young children may mimic the lesion appearance in children with a first attack of MS[6] or children with acute disseminated encephalomyelitis (ADEM),[7] in whom lesions are large, hazy, and ill defined.

2. Dental hardware, such as braces and retainers, can cause significant susceptibility artifact. Sequences especially prone to artifact are diffusion-weighted (DW) imaging and spoiled gradient-recalled echo imaging.

3. Tolerability of MR imaging scan length is a challenge in pediatrics, and often results in motion artifact–laden images. However, with the assistance of MR imaging–compatible movie goggles and headphones, children can tolerate lying still for longer durations of time. In very young children, sedation may be necessary to obtain sufficient imaging. Advances in MR imaging technology, such as parallel imaging, have significantly decreased scan time. However, situations may arise whereby a child has difficulty lying still for the total duration of the scan protocol; in these cases an abbreviated set of images without motion artifact is preferable to a complete protocol laden with motion artifact.

STANDARD MR IMAGING PROTOCOL FOR PEDIATRIC DEMYELINATION

Table 1 describes the suggested standard protocol for pediatric demyelinating disorders, and indicates a recommended minimum set of scans for situations whereby a child cannot tolerate the complete protocol. Consistent prescription of slice angulation is important for evaluation of new lesion formation across serial scans; oblique axial images, where the acquisition plane is parallel to the subcallosal line joining the inferior margin of the genu and inferior margin of the splenium, are recommended. Contiguous slices of 3-mm thickness are recommended to permit accurate lesion detection, given that minimum MS lesion diameter criteria are approximately 3 mm.[6,8] Attention should be given to ensure complete head coverage. To avoid distortions or edge blurring sometimes present in the first or last slice of a slab when the whole brain is not covered, acquisition of 1 to 2 slices of air outside the skull is recommended. This action is especially important when new lesions are present in regions of the brain omitted when whole brain coverage is not achieved, such as the juxtacortical region or brainstem (Fig. 1), both of which are important components of the 2010 revisions to the McDonald criteria for dissemination in space.[3]

The rationale for the sequences included in Table 1 is summarized as follows:

1. *Three-dimensional (3D) T1-weighted imaging.* A spoiled gradient-recalled echo sequence is recommended for its efficiency; that is, one

Table 1
Proposed MR imaging protocol for pediatric demyelinating disease

Order	Sequence	Recommendation	Comment
Brain Imaging			
1	3-plane localizer	Recommended	Prescribe oblique axial images[a]
2	3D T1-weighted spoiled gradient-recalled echo imaging	Recommended	By increasing TR to 30 ms, contrast is comparable with the contrast on SE imaging; important in assessment of T1-hypointense lesion formation
3	Sagittal FLAIR	Recommended[b]	
4	Axial T2-weighted FSE or TSE	Recommended[b]	
5	Axial DWI	Recommended	In children presenting with acute symptoms, DWI is important to rule out arterial ischemic stroke
6	Contrast Administration		
7	Axial FLAIR	Recommended	Acquired during 5-min delay between contrast injection and postcontrast imaging
8	Axial T1-weighted postcontrast spoiled gradient-recalled echo imaging	Recommended	By increasing the TR to 30 ms, the conspicuity of gadolinium enhancement is more comparable with that of SE imaging
Optional Orbital Imaging (Acquired Following Contrast Administration)			
1	3-plane localizer	If clinically indicated	Prescribe oblique axial images[a]
2	Coronal and axial T2-weighted fat-saturated imaging	If clinically indicated	Should include imaging of the optic nerves through to and including the optic chiasm
3	Coronal and axial T1-weighted postcontrast fat-saturated imaging	If clinically indicated	If acquired with brain protocol, acquire after sequence #8 under Brain Imaging
Optional Spinal Cord Imaging (Acquired Following Contrast Administration)			
1	3-plane localizer	If clinically indicated	
2	Sagittal T2-weighted FSE or TSE[c]	If clinically indicated	Acquire in superior, middle, and inferior sections
3	Axial T2-weighted FSE or TSE	If clinically indicated	Acquire only through regions of interest
4	Sagittal T1-weighted postcontrast SE	If clinically indicated	If acquired with the brain protocol, acquire after sequence #8 under Brain Imaging

Abbreviations: 3D, 3-dimensional; DWI, diffusion-weighted imaging; FLAIR, fluid-attenuated inversion recovery; FSE, fast spin-echo; SE, spin-echo; TR, repetition time; TSE, turbo spin-echo.
  [a] Axial images parallel to the genu-splenium subcallosal line.
  [b] May be omitted when child or adolescent cannot tolerate the scan.
  [c] A short-tau inversion recovery (STIR) sequence may be acquired either in place of or in addition to T2-weighted FSE images to enhance ability to detect inconspicuous intramedullary lesions.[24]

can achieve a higher signal-to-noise ratio (SNR) with a shorter acquisition time compared with spin-echo (SE) imaging. 3D imaging also enables reformatting of the data into axial, coronal, or sagittal planes, and is often used in centers performing volumetric analyses.

Acquiring T1-weighted imaging permits evaluation of black-hole accrual over time, the presence of which is highly predictive of MS in children with acute demyelination.[8] Black holes initially were defined on SE imaging.[9] However, increasing the repetition time (TR) of

A

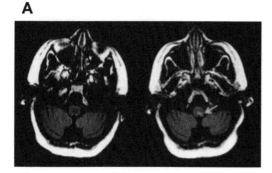

B

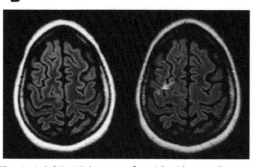

Fig. 1. Axial FLAIR images of a girl with MS who presented with a first attack of MS at age 11 years. (*A*) A new T2 lesion (*arrow*) is visible in the medulla when compared with the previous scan acquired 6 months earlier. (*B*) In the same patient, a new juxtacortical lesion (*arrow*) is visible when compared with the previous scan 2 years prior.

a T1-weighted 3D spoiled gradient-recalled echo sequence from the typical 20 milliseconds used for high-contrast, high-resolution applications to 30 milliseconds mutes the contrast to a level similar to that of an SE sequence. Lastly, T1-weighted imaging performed before contrast injection permits confirmation of lesion enhancement when present.

2. *Axial T2-weighted imaging.* Fast or turbo spin-echo imaging with an echo time (TE) between 80 and 120 milliseconds is recommended; a longer TE increases lesion conspicuity, at the cost of lower SNR. T2-weighted imaging provides better contrast than fluid-attenuated inversion recovery (FLAIR) for infratentorial lesion detection (**Fig. 2**). Infratentorial lesions and, specifically, brainstem lesions are important features of MS in children.[10,13] The presence of a "false lesion" in the pons caused by a deep interpeduncular cistern leading to a partial volume effect has been reported,[14] and warrants consideration when interpreting pontine lesions. An intermediate-weighted or proton density is not thought to contribute to lesion detection beyond that of combined T2-weighted and

FLAIR imaging, but may be used in some centers because it provides another contrast for automated lesion-detection techniques.

3. *Axial and sagittal FLAIR.* Juxtacortical and periventricular lesion detection may be obscured by the partial volume effect on T2-weighted imaging caused by cerebrospinal fluid. FLAIR imaging effectively suppresses the signal from cerebrospinal fluid, and therefore is a preferred sequence for MS lesion detection. Sagittal FLAIR imaging permits visualization of intracallosal lesions and lesions perpendicular to the long axis of the corpus callosum, a feature demonstrated to be predictive of MS in children.[15–17] A recommendation to reduce total examination time would be to acquire the axial FLAIR scan during the 5-minute delay time following gadolinium injection and before collection of contrast-enhanced imaging.[18] Caution should be taken when leptomeningeal hyperintensity is detected on FLAIR imaging, as this can be a normal finding in children imaged under sedation or general anesthetic.

4. *Axial DW imaging.* Given the broader differential in pediatric demyelination in comparison with adults, the ability to promptly rule out mimics of demyelinating disease is crucial. A short (<1 minute) DW imaging sequence provides sufficient information to assess the presence of a vascular occlusive disorder such as arterial ischemic stroke.

5. *Axial contrast-enhanced T1-weighted imaging.* "Muted-contrast" spoiled gradient-recalled echo imaging (ie, long TR), matched to the precontrast 3D T1-weighted spoiled gradient-recalled echo sequence described above, is recommended because it permits direct comparison with the precontrast 3D T1-weighted spoiled gradient-recalled echo images, and provides conspicuity of enhancing lesions that is roughly comparable with that of standard SE imaging. The contrast-enhanced T1-weighted scan should be the last sequence of the protocol, as gadolinium injection is sometimes not well tolerated in children and leads to motion artifacts. Although higher gadolinium doses, use of magnetization transfer contrast, and a longer postinjection delay before collecting the data may increase enhancement conspicuity,[19,20] these tactics are not essential for routine clinical imaging.[21] The presence of contrast-enhancing lesions indicates new lesion formation, which is important in establishing an MS diagnosis according to dissemination in time.[2,3] Along with markers of disease activity such as annualized relapse rate and formation of new T2 lesions, contrast enhancement is also used as

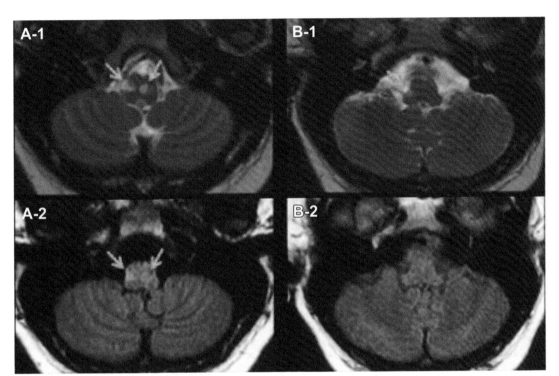

Fig. 2. Axial T2-weighted (*top row*) and axial fluid-attenuated inversion recovery (FLAIR) (*bottom row*) images of a child with multiple sclerosis. Two brainstem lesions (*arrows*) are visible on T2-weighted imaging in A-1, whereas both lesions (*arrows*) are more inconspicuous on FLAIR (A-2). At another level of the brainstem, the T2 lesion in B-1 (*arrow*) is not visible on FLAIR (B-2).

a surrogate marker of therapeutic efficacy in trials of MS treatment. Contrast-enhanced imaging is pivotal in excluding other diagnoses such as malignancy, infectious processes, or small-vessel primary angiitis of the central nervous system (CNS),[22] which may show leptomeningeal enhancement. A standard pediatric dose (0.1 mmol/kg) of gadolinium is recommended, with a 5-minute delay to acquisition of contrast-enhanced images. Autoinjection is not essential. For reasons of patient safety, a maximum of 5 mmol of contrast is recommended during a given MR imaging acquisition. Adherence to site-specific protocols around contrast administration in children with impaired renal function is necessary.[23]

Spinal Cord and Optic Nerve Imaging

Imaging of the spinal cord or optic nerves is recommended only to investigate symptoms referable to the optic nerves or spinal cord, or to aid in the diagnosis of MS when findings are equivocal on brain MR imaging. The additional scan time required may be tolerable for adolescent patients, but is often prohibitive in younger children. Considering that the spinal cord terminates at T12-L1 in children, sagittal T2-weighted superior and middle images are sufficient, and axial T2-weighted region-of-interest images are recommended. Both T1-weighted and T2-weighted short-tau inversion recovery (STIR) imaging may be more sensitive to spinal cord demyelinating lesions than fast SE and FLAIR imaging.[24–28] The increased sensitivity is due to the synergistic effect of prolonged T1 and T2 relaxation times in abnormal tissue, which increases lesion conspicuity. Compared with SE, STIR image quality tends to be noisy, but the contrast-to-noise ratio is high.[29] The STIR sequence may be more susceptible to motion artifacts and cerebrospinal fluid flow artifacts.[29] With respect to imaging of the optic nerves, axial and coronal fat-suppressed orbital imaging (ie, spectral attenuated inversion recovery [SPAIR]) is recommended. When spinal cord or optic nerve imaging and the brain MR imaging protocol are acquired simultaneously, additional gadolinium is not required.

STANDARD MR IMAGING LEXICON FOR PEDIATRIC DEMYELINATION

Standardization of terms used to describe MR imaging features of demyelination in children is important to help permit comparison of findings across studies and engage in multicenter collaborative studies. As pediatric-onset MS represents a smaller entity than adult-onset MS, multicenter studies are increasingly important in achieving sufficient power. Use of a consistently applied operative lexicon will facilitate the merging of data from multiple centers to inform on key questions related to the natural history of MS on MR imaging in children, evaluation of MR imaging surrogates of efficacy in treatment trials, and the study of MR imaging indicators of prognosis.

The proposed lexicon is applicable to children with incident CNS demyelination as well as those with established MS. It consists of parameters identified based on a review of the literature for

---

Box 1

MR imaging lexicon for pediatric acute central nervous system demyelination and MS

Detailed parameter definitions, including an atlas, are included in web appendix p. 226.e1–226.e7. All parameters are binary (ie, present or absent).

1. Bilateral lesion distribution: T2 lesions on either side of, or spanning across, the midline in the supratentorial or infratentorial regions

2. Gyral projection: T2 lesion continuously projecting from subcortical white matter at the depth of a sulcus into a gyrus, extending to abut the cortical ribbon at the gyral apex

3. (A) T1 hypointensity: T1 lesion present at incident demyelinating event with all or a portion of the lesion being hypointense relative to cortical gray matter; should be hyperintense on T2-weighted images. (B) Persistent T1 hypointensity: T1 hypointensity present at incident demyelinating event and persisting for at least 3 months, as assessed on serial scans

4. Lesional contrast enhancement: nodular or ring-link hyperintense signal on T1-weighted postcontrast imaging corresponding to a T2 lesion; not hyperintense on T1-weighted precontrast scan

5. Leptomeningeal contrast enhancement: linear or nodular hyperintense signal (minimum 3 mm in length or diameter) of the pia and arachnoid mater on T1-weighted postcontrast imaging; T2 hyperintensity of the leptomeninges may be a normal finding when scan is acquired under sedation or general anesthesia

6. Periventricular lesion: white matter T2 lesion abutting any portion of the lateral ventricles; lesions involving the corpus callosal white matter are included, but deep gray matter lesions (see parameters 10 and 11) are excluded

7. Cerebral white matter lesion: supratentorial nonjuxtacortical (see parameter 8) and nonperiventricular (see parameter 6) white matter T2 lesion; intracallosal lesions (see parameter 9) are excluded

8. Juxtacortical lesion: supratentorial white matter T2 lesion contiguous with the cortical ribbon (ie, involving subcortical U-fibers[11,12])

9. Intracallosal lesion: T2 lesion contained entirely within the margins of the corpus callosum (anatomic boundaries defined in web appendix p. 226.e3–226.e4; adapted from Callen and colleagues[10]); 1 mm of normal-appearing white matter surrounding the lesion is required to be confirmed as intracallosal and not periventricular (see parameter 6)

10. Thalamic lesion: T2 lesion either entirely or partially contained within the thalamus; bithalamic lesions counted as discrete lesions

11. Basal ganglia lesion: T2 lesion either entirely or partially contained within the caudate nucleus (includes head and tail), putamen, or globus pallidus (includes internal and external segments)

12. Internal capsule lesion: T2 lesion centered in the anterior or posterior limb of the internal capsule (anatomic boundaries defined in web appendix p. 226.e5; adapted from Callen and colleagues[10])

13. Brainstem lesion: T2 lesion within the brainstem, which extends from the most inferior aspect of the medulla oblongata (at the level of the pyramidal decussation) to the most superior portion of the midbrain (at the level of the red nuclei); posterior anatomic limits defined in web appendix p. 226.e6

14. Cerebellar lesion: T2 lesion involving any of the cerebellar white matter, cortices, dentate nuclei, vermis, or flocculus; anterior anatomic limits of the cerebellum defined in web appendix p. 226.e7

Data from Verhey LH, Branson HM, Shroff MM, et al. MRI parameters for prediction of multiple sclerosis diagnosis in children with acute CNS demyelination: a prospective national cohort study. Lancet Neurol 2011;10:1065–73. See full web appendix online at: www.mri.theclinics.com.

MR imaging features of MS and other demyelinating disorders, and characteristics that would aid in excluding the diagnosis of MS. An expert panel of pediatric neurologists and neuroradiologists at The Hospital for Sick Children (Toronto, Canada) met to refine the parameter definitions. The lexicon and accompanying atlas has been published by the authors as part of a study on MR imaging predictors of MS in children with acute demyelinating syndromes (Box 1).[8] The 14 parameters included describe the distribution and features of inflammatory demyelinating lesions on T1-weighted precontrast and postcontrast, and T2-weighted or FLAIR imaging. Use of this lexicon

by other groups will be essential to further refine or extend the parameters.

STANDARDIZED MR IMAGING REPORTING IN PEDIATRIC MS

A recommended template of an MR imaging report for children presenting with acute demyelination or those with established MS is provided in Box 2. MR imaging reports should be consistent to permit comparison of serial scans, and should conform to current diagnostic criteria for pediatric MS.[30] Published MR imaging diagnostic criteria for MS in children and adults are summarized in Table 2.

Box 2
MR imaging reporting template for pediatric demyelinating disease

Report Contents

1. Description of findings on a single scan

   a. Number of T2 lesions[a]

   b. T2 lesions located in regions considered characteristic for pediatric MS

      i. Periventricular

      ii. Juxtacortical

      iii. Corpus callosum

      iv. Brainstem or cerebellum

      v. Spinal cord (if acquired)

   c. Number of contrast-enhancing lesions

   d. Presence of T1-hypointense lesions, defined as hypointense to cortical gray matter on T1-weighted imaging

2. Summarizing change over serial scans

   a. Timing between scans being compared

   b. Number of new T2 lesions[a]

   c. Persistence of T1-hypointense lesions

   d. Number of contrast-enhancing lesions

   e. Changes in global brain volume

3. Statement of whether MR imaging features meet published MR imaging scoring criteria (see Table 2)

   a. McDonald MS criteria for DIS and DIT[2,3]

   b. Pediatric MS criteria for DIS[10]

   c. Pediatric criteria for differentiating MS from ADEM[31]

   d. Parameters predictive of MS in children with acute demyelination[8]

Abbreviations: DIS, dissemination in space; DIT, dissemination in time.
[a] T2 lesion count is a component of DIS criteria for MS diagnosis. The number of T2 lesions required to meet DIS has decreased as revisions to the diagnostic criteria have been published (see Table 2). However, it remains an important parameter for evaluating new T2 lesion accrual for DIT. Therefore, T2 lesion count, as much as practically possible, should be included when reporting.

Table 2
MR imaging criteria for MS diagnosis

	Pediatric-Onset MS	Adult-Onset MS
Polman et al,[2] 2005		*DIS*[a] Three of the following: 1. ≥9 T2 lesions *or* ≥1 contrast-enhancing lesion 2. ≥1 T2 infratentorial lesion 3. ≥1 T2 juxtacortical lesion 4. ≥3 T2 periventricular lesions DIT One of the following: 1. ≥1 contrast-enhancing lesion at least 3 mo after clinical onset 2. A new T2 lesion at any time compared with a reference scan acquired at least 30 d after clinical onset
Polman et al,[3] 2011	*DIS* Presence of ≥1 clinically silent T2 lesion in at least 2 of the 4 following CNS regions: 1. Periventricular 2. Juxtacortical 3. Infratentorial 4. Spinal cord *DIT* One of the following: 1. A new T2 or contrast-enhancing lesion on any serial scan with respect to a previous scan 2. Simultaneous presence of asymptomatic contrast-enhancing and nonenhancing lesions at any time	
Mikaeloff et al,[15] 2004	*MR imaging prognostic factors for MS in children with acute demyelination* Two of the following: 1. T2 lesions perpendicular to the long axis of the corpus callosum 2. Sole presence of well-defined T2 lesions	
Callen et al,[10] 2009	*MR imaging criteria to distinguish pediatric MS from relapsing nondemyelinating disease* Two of the following: 1. ≥5 T2 lesions 2. ≥2 T2 periventricular lesions 3. ≥1 T2 brainstem lesion	
Callen et al,[31] 2009	*MR imaging criteria to distinguish a first attack of MS from monophasic ADEM* Two of the following: 1. Absence of a diffuse bilateral T2 lesion pattern 2. Presence of black holes 3. ≥2 T2 periventricular lesions	
Verhey et al,[8] 2011	*MR imaging parameters that predict MS in children with acute demyelination* Two of the following: 1. ≥1 T2 periventricular lesion 2. ≥1 T1-hypointense lesion	

Abbreviations: ADEM, acute disseminated encephalomyelitis; CNS, central nervous system; DIS, dissemination in space; DIT, dissemination in time.

[a] A contrast-enhancing spinal cord lesion is equivalent to an enhancing lesion in the brain; individual spinal cord lesions and brain lesions can together contribute to the requirement of 9 or more T2 lesions.

SUMMARY

A standardized algorithm for MR imaging acquisition and reporting in pediatric MS that is based on the current literature and published diagnostic criteria is proposed. The use of this algorithm by other centers is vital for making consensus revisions and further refinement that will permit its implementation as a standard protocol. Adopting a standard lexicon and reporting scheme will inform the creation of structured reporting that is increasingly being proposed for diagnostic radiologists. Standard acquisition methods will be key in the collection of surrogate MR imaging treatment response data in pediatric clinical trials of disease-modifying therapy for MS.

ACKNOWLEDGMENTS

The authors acknowledge Dr Manohar Shroff, Dr Helen Branson, and Dr Suzanne Laughlin (Division of Pediatric Neuroradiology, The Hospital for Sick Children, Toronto, Canada) for their input and revisions to this work.

REFERENCES

1. Poser CM, Paty DW, Scheinberg L, et al. New diagnostic criteria for multiple sclerosis: guidelines for research protocols. Ann Neurol 1983;13:227–31.
2. Polman CH, Reingold SC, Edan G, et al. Diagnostic criteria for multiple sclerosis: 2005 revisions to the "McDonald Criteria". Ann Neurol 2005;58:840–6.
3. Polman CH, Reingold SC, Banwell B, et al. Diagnostic criteria for multiple sclerosis: 2010 revisions to the McDonald criteria. Ann Neurol 2011;69: 292–302.
4. Miller DH, Weinshenker BG, Filippi M, et al. Differential diagnosis of suspected multiple sclerosis: a consensus approach. Mult Scler 2008;14: 1157–74.
5. Simon JH, Li D, Traboulsee A, et al. Standardized MR imaging protocol for multiple sclerosis: consortium of MS Centers consensus guidelines. AJNR Am J Neuroradiol 2006;27:455–61.
6. Chabas D, Castillo-Trivino T, Mowry EM, et al. Vanishing MS T2-bright lesions before puberty: a distinct MRI phenotype? Neurology 2008;71:1090–3.
7. Tenembaum S, Chitnis T, Ness J, et al. Acute disseminated encephalomyelitis. Neurology 2007; 68:S23–36.
8. Verhey LH, Branson HM, Shroff MM, et al. MRI parameters for prediction of multiple sclerosis diagnosis in children with acute CNS demyelination: a prospective national cohort study. Lancet Neurol 2011;10:1065–73.
9. van Walderveen MA, Kamphorst W, Scheltens P, et al. Histopathologic correlate of hypointense lesions on T1-weighted spin-echo MRI in multiple sclerosis. Neurology 1998;50:1282–8.
10. Callen DJ, Shroff MM, Branson HM, et al. MRI in the diagnosis of pediatric multiple sclerosis. Neurology 2009;72:961–7.
11. Barkhof F, Filippi M, Miller DH, et al. Comparison of MRI criteria at first presentation to predict conversion to clinically definite multiple sclerosis. Brain 1997;120:2059–69.
12. Tintoré M, Rovira A, Martinez MJ, et al. Isolated demyelinating syndromes: comparison of different MR imaging criteria to predict conversion to clinically definite multiple sclerosis. AJNR Am J Neuroradiol 2000;21:702–6.
13. Ghassemi R, Antel SB, Narayanan S, et al. Lesion distribution in children with clinically isolated syndromes. Ann Neurol 2008;63:401–5.
14. Sener RN. A false lesion in the center of the pons on magnetic resonance images. Comput Med Imaging Graph 1998;22:413–6.
15. Mikaeloff Y, Adamsbaum C, Husson B, et al. MRI prognostic factors for relapse after acute CNS inflammatory demyelination in childhood. Brain 2004;127:1942–7.
16. Palmer S, Bradley WG, Chen DY, et al. Subcallosal striations: early findings of multiple sclerosis on sagittal, thin-section, fast FLAIR MR images. Radiology 1999;210:149–53.
17. Lisanti CJ, Asbach P, Bradley WG Jr. The ependymal "Dot-Dash" sign: an MR imaging finding of early multiple sclerosis. AJNR Am J Neuroradiol 2005;26: 2033–6.
18. Mathews VP, Caldemeyer KS, Lowe MJ, et al. Brain: gadolinium-enhanced fast fluid-attenuated inversion-recovery MR imaging. Radiology 1999;211: 257–63.
19. Filippi M, Yousry T, Campi A, et al. Comparison of triple dose versus standard dose gadolinium-DTPA for detection of MRI enhancing lesions in patients with MS. Neurology 1996;46:379–84.
20. Silver NC, Good CD, Barker GJ, et al. Sensitivity of contrast enhanced MRI in multiple sclerosis. Effects of gadolinium dose, magnetization transfer contrast and delayed imaging. Brain 1997; 120(Pt 7):1149–61.
21. Traboulsee A, Li DK. Conventional MR imaging. Neuroimaging Clin N Am 2008;18:651–73.
22. Cellucci T, Benseler SM. Diagnosing central nervous system vasculitis in children. Curr Opin Pediatr 2010;22:731–8.
23. Deo A, Fogel M, Cowper SE. Nephrogenic systemic fibrosis: a population study examining the relationship of disease development to gadolinium exposure. Clin J Am Soc Nephrol 2007;2:264–7.
24. Philpott C, Brotchie P. Comparison of MRI sequences for evaluation of multiple sclerosis of the cervical spinal cord at 3 T. Eur J Radiol 2011;80:780–5.

25. Rocca MA, Mastronardo G, Horsfield MA, et al. Comparison of three MR sequences for the detection of cervical cord lesions in patients with multiple sclerosis. AJNR Am J Neuroradiol 1999; 20:1710–6.

26. Campi A, Pontesilli S, Gerevini S, et al. Comparison of MRI pulse sequences for investigation of lesions of the cervical spinal cord. Neuroradiology 2000; 42:669–75.

27. Hittmair K, Mallek R, Prayer D, et al. Spinal cord lesions in patients with multiple sclerosis: comparison of MR pulse sequences. AJNR Am J Neuroradiol 1996;17:1555–65.

28. Dietemann JL, Thibaut-Menard A, Warter JM, et al. MRI in multiple sclerosis of the spinal cord: evaluation of fast short-tan inversion-recovery and spin-echo sequences. Neuroradiology 2000;42:810–3.

29. Ross JS. Newer sequences for spinal MR imaging: smorgasbord or succotash of acronyms? AJNR Am J Neuroradiol 1999;20:361–73.

30. Krupp LB, Banwell B, Tenembaum S. Consensus definitions proposed for pediatric multiple sclerosis and related disorders. Neurology 2007;68:S7–12.

31. Callen DJ, Shroff MM, Branson HM, et al. Role of MRI in the differentiation of ADEM from MS in children. Neurology 2009;72:968–73.

Pediatric Multiple Sclerosis
Pathobiological, Clinical, and Magnetic Resonance Imaging Features

Leonard H. Verhey, PhD[a,b],
Manohar Shroff, MD, DABR, FRCPC[c],
Brenda Banwell, MD, FRCPC[d,*]

KEYWORDS

- Multiple sclerosis • Pediatric • Clinical and pathobiological features • Magnetic resonance imaging

KEY POINTS

- Multiple sclerosis (MS) is an immune-mediated disease that is largely viewed to be initiated when a genetically-susceptible host is exposed to environmental risk factors, resulting in a dysregulated immune response that is targeted at the central nervous system (CNS).
- Pediatric-onset MS is increasingly recognized, with 2-4% of patients diagnosed prior to age 18 years.
- Epstein-Barr virus seropositivity, vitamin D deficiency, and the presence of an HLA-DRB1*15 allele are well-described environmental and genetic risk factors for pediatric MS.
- Essentially all children with MS follow a relapsing-remitting clinical course.
- MR features of MS in children are similar to that of adults; lesion features predictive of a subsequent MS diagnosis in children with acute demyelination have recently been defined.

INTRODUCTION

Multiple sclerosis (MS) is the most common autoimmune demyelinating disease of the central nervous system (CNS), characterized by immune-mediated inflammation and progressive neurodegeneration, causing intermittent and accumulating neurologic deficits. Pediatric-onset MS is being increasingly recognized worldwide, and it is estimated that approximately 2.2% to 4.4% of patients are diagnosed with MS before age 18 years.[1–6] Although the worldwide incidence of pediatric-onset MS is unknown, an American study reported an incidence rate of 0.51 per 100,000 children per year.[7] When considering acute CNS demyelinating events more broadly, 2 studies have reported an incidence ranging between 0.9 and 1.56 per 100,000 children per year.[7,8]

Historically, the first documented patient with MS was a girl living in the fourteenth century who, at 16 years of age, experienced a first attack of MS characterized by gait impairment and later developed optic neuritis (ON), upper extremity paresis, facial weakness, and pain.[9] However, it was not until 1958 that a cohort of patients with pediatric-onset MS was first described.[10]

[a] Pediatric Demyelinating Disease Program, Program in Neuroscience and Mental Health, The Hospital for Sick Children, Room 11-105 Elm Wing, 555 University Avenue, Toronto, Ontario M5G 1X8, Canada; [b] Institute of Medical Science, University of Toronto, Medical Science Building, 1 King's College Circle, Room 2374, Toronto, Ontario M5S 1A8, Canada; [c] Department of Diagnostic Imaging, The Hospital for Sick Children, 555 University Avenue, Toronto, Ontario M5G 1X8, Canada; [d] Division of Neurology, Department of Pediatrics, The Hospital for Sick Children, University of Toronto, 555 University Avenue, Toronto, Ontario M5G 1X8, Canada
* Corresponding author.
E-mail address: banwellb@email.chop.edu

Neuroimag Clin N Am 23 (2013) 227–243
http://dx.doi.org/10.1016/j.nic.2012.12.004
1052-5149/13/$ – see front matter © 2013 Elsevier Inc. All rights reserved.

That the onset of pediatric MS occurs in close temporal proximity to the inciting events believed to play a role in disease initiation uniquely permits exploration of the earliest aspects of disease pathobiology. The use of magnetic resonance (MR) imaging as a paraclinical tool to detect disease-related changes in the CNS of pediatric patients with MS permits exploration of the earliest aspects of inflammation and neurodegeneration. The sensitivity of MR imaging provides valuable information for MS diagnosis, assessment of disease activity and progression, and monitoring of treatment response.

In this article, after a summary of the pathobiological, clinical, and treatment aspects of pediatric-onset MS, the conventional MR imaging (ie, T1-weighted, proton-density, and T2-weighted imaging) features of MS in children are discussed, as well as the application of MR imaging in the diagnosis of pediatric-onset MS and in prediction of MS in children with an incident CNS demyelination. Insights gained from studies comparing MR imaging features of pediatric-onset and adult-onset MS are presented.

INTRODUCTION TO PEDIATRIC MS
Pathogenesis: Immunobiology and Risk Factors

MS is largely viewed as an immune-mediated disease that is initiated when a genetically susceptible host is exposed to environmental risk factors, resulting in a dysregulated immune response targeted at the CNS. T cells and B cells mature in the thymus and bone marrow, respectively, and enter the circulation as naive cells. These naive cells may encounter various antigens and contribute to memory and effector repertoires. Activation of these peripheral immune cells, such as CD4[+] and CD8[+] T cells, myeloid cells, and B cells, is dysregulated in patients with MS. Such aberrant immune cell activation leads to their more efficient adherence to the blood-brain barrier endothelium and increased trafficking into the CNS via matrix metalloproteinases, where the immune cells become reactivated.[11] The episodic cycles of immune cell infiltration into and reactivation within the CNS contribute to the development of the multifocal inflammatory lesions within the white and gray matter of patients with MS. Pathologic and imaging studies have shown that the CNS injury extends beyond the perivascular cuffs of inflammation and includes extensive neuroaxonal damage within the normal-appearing brain tissue.[12,13] Taken together, the underlying pathophysiology of MS involves a complex interaction of inflammatory and neurodegenerative processes

that are interrelated, with chronic inflammation leading to foci of neuronal destruction and neuronal or axonal damage inciting an immune response.

Interactions between genetic and environmental factors contribute to MS risk. The most well-established genetic component of MS susceptibility resides in the major histocompatibility complex (HLA), and HLA-DRB1 has specifically been associated with MS in adults.[14] A higher frequency of HLA-DRB alleles has been reported in patients with pediatric-onset MS.[15] In a cohort of children with incident CNS demyelination, those diagnosed with MS were more likely to have HLA-DRB1*15 alleles compared with those who remained monophasic, and this association was driven mainly by the presence of European ancestry.[16] In a multivariable analysis of HLA-DRB1*15 genotype, Epstein-Barr virus (EBV) seropositivity and 25-hydroxyvitamin D status in children with acute demyelination, the presence of at least 1 HLA-DRB1*15 allele was associated with a 2-fold increased risk of MS.[17]

Vitamin D insufficiency, remote infection with EBV and exposure to cigarette smoke have been proposed as environmental risk factors for MS in both pediatric-onset and adult-onset patients. Studies in animal models of MS have shown that vitamin D has a role in regulating immune cell activity via the vitamin D receptor on T lymphocytes,[18–20] suggesting the role of vitamin D as a mediator of immune-mediated inflammation. In a cohort of children with MS, every 10-ng/mL increase in serum 25-hydroxyvitamin D_3 (the active form of vitamin D) was associated with a 34% decrease in relapse rate.[21] When considering several predisposing factors for MS in children with acute demyelinating syndromes (ADSs), a 10-nmol/L increase in serum 25-hydroxyvitamin D concentration was independently associated with a risk reduction of 0.9.[17] Trials of vitamin D in children with MS are being planned. One study has reported that children exposed to parental cigarette smoke are at an increased risk for MS.[22] When comparing serum titers of cytomegalovirus (CMV), herpes simplex virus type 1, varicella zoster virus, parvovirus B19, and EBV in children with MS to those of age-matched controls, seropositivity to EBV was associated with a 3-fold increased likelihood of MS.[23] Several other studies have shown a higher EBV titer in children with MS compared with controls, and this association seems stronger for the Epstein-Barr nuclear antigen (EBNA1) than for the Epstein-Barr viral capsid antigen.[24–28] In children with ADSs, risk of MS is increased by more than 2-fold in those with remote EBV infection.[17] Intrathecal EBV antibodies have been reported in children with MS.[29] One study[30] reported that, in addition to the increased risk of MS in children seropositive for EBV, remote CMV infection lowers the odds of MS, suggesting that risk for MS depends in part on the viral infections acquired during the early-life window of exposure.

The pathobiology of pediatric-onset MS has many resemblances to that of adult-onset disease. When compared with adults with MS, inflammatory responses in children with MS, measured in studies of T-cell proliferation[31] and B-cell-derived antibodies,[32] are as robust and in some cases stronger than those observed in adult patients.[33] With respect to genetic and environmental risk factors, presence of HLA-DRB1*15 alleles, remote infection with EBV, vitamin D insufficiency, and exposure to cigarette smoke have all also been implicated as risk factors for adult-onset disease.[34]

Chronic Cerebrospinal Venous Insufficiency

Beginning in 2007, the Italian vascular surgeon Paolo Zamboni proposed the theory of chronic cerebrospinal venous insufficiency (CCSVI) as the underlying cause of MS.[35] It was hypothesized that MS results from chronically impaired venous drainage of the CNS caused by stenoses in the neck. The investigators implied that this state of CCSVI led to venous reflux, causing extravasation of iron and its accumulation in the CNS parenchyma; they proposed that iron accumulation may represent the inciting event in MS pathobiology, triggering immune-mediated inflammatory injury.[36] CCSVI was defined as the presence of at least 2 of the following criteria: (1) reflux in the internal jugular veins (IJVs) or vertebral veins (VV) in the upright and supine positions, (2) reflux in the deep cerebral veins, (3) high-resolution B-mode evidence of IJV stenoses, (4) lack of Doppler-detectable flow in the IJVs or VVs, and (5) reverted postural control of main cerebral venous outflow pathways.[37]

Using transcranial color-coded Doppler sonography and extracranial color Doppler sonography, Zamboni and colleagues[37] found that MS was associated with venous outflow anomalies and that patients with MS met the criteria for CCSVI with 100% sensitivity, 100% specificity, 100% positive predictive value (PPV), and 100% negative predictive value (NPV).[38] Interpretation of these results is challenged by the possibility of spectrum bias (sampling conditions for evaluation of the diagnostic test are not clinically representative), lack of blinding of the sonographer to patient diagnosis, uncertain reproducibility of ultrasonography results given the dependency on patient positioning and angle of insonation, and the possible risk of pulsation artifact from adjacent vascular structures.[39]

Led by Professor Zamboni, an open-label study was conducted in which patients underwent a percutaneous transluminal angioplasty to treat the neck venous stenoses.[40] During the 18-month period of follow-up after the procedure, improvement in clinical outcomes was noted in relapsing-remitting patients, although such improvements were not clearly defined. However, the small sample size, lack of a control group, unblinded neurologic evaluations, significant IJV restenosis rate (47%), and the confound that treated patients remained on disease-modifying therapies limit interpretation of these findings and make tenuous the interpretation of efficacy.[39]

Using ultrasound and MR imaging techniques, several international studies have been performed to compare venous structure between patients with relapsing-remitting or progressive forms of MS, those with a first attack of CNS demyelination, patients with other nondemyelinating CNS disorders, and healthy controls. The findings challenge the theory that CCSVI plays a causative role in MS pathogenesis.[41–44] Iron accumulation and iron-mediated CNS injury are not unique to MS and have been reported in many neurologic disorders,[45,46] and cerebrospinal ferritin levels have been found to be normal in patients with MS and do not change over time,[47] suggesting that CCSVI is not an inciting factor in MS. For CCSVI to be causative in MS pathobiology, it should be observed in the earliest stages of disease. The presence of anomalous venous drainage patterns in children with MS is being evaluated.

Several centers worldwide are conducting endovascular procedures for treatment of CCSVI. Anecdotal reports indicate serious injury and in some cases death as a result of endovascular procedures to treat CCSVI in patients with MS.[48] It is critical that patient safety remain foremost and that the findings of CCSVI be rigorously replicated in independent cohorts before the implementation of trials to evaluate the efficacy of balloon angioplasty as a treatment of MS.

Demographic and Clinical Characteristics

Onset of MS before the age of 10 years occurs in only 17% of all pediatric-onset patients.[49] Gender ratios vary according to age at onset. The ratio of girls to boys in children younger than 6 years is 0.8:1 and increases to 1.6:1 between the ages of 6 and 10 years. The female preponderance, similar to that seen in adults with MS, emerges only in adolescence, at about 10 years of age[49,50] which may indicate a hormonal influence on MS risk or a gender-defined genetic influence on immunologic activity.

An ADS represents the first presentation of MS in 20% to 30% of children; for the remaining 70% to 80%, the demyelinating event occurs as a monophasic illness.[17,51,52] An ADS can be classified into one of several clinical presentations: ON, acute transverse myelitis (TM), monofocal or polyfocal neurologic deficits extrinsic to the optic nerves or spinal cord, or acute disseminated encephalomyelitis (ADEM). Whereas monofocal presentations are more common in adolescents and adults, children typically present with polyfocal symptoms.[50] A polyfocal presentation of MS, characterized by neurologic symptoms referable to multiple areas within the CNS, occurs in 50% to 70% of children,[2,52,53] whereas 30% to 50% present with monofocal symptoms.[49] Approximately 10% to 23% of children with MS present with ON,[2,51,54] and bilateral ON carries an increased MS risk compared with unilateral ON.[55] Acute isolated TM occurs as a first attack of MS in only 2% to 14% children[51,52,56]; more frequently, acute TM represents a monophasic illness, or when co-occurring with ON, may represent the heralding features of neuromyelitis optica. Monofocal presentations of motor dysfunction occur in 30% of children with MS, sensory symptoms in 15% to 30%, ataxia in 5% to 15%, and brainstem symptoms in 25% to 41%.[49,52]

ADEM, defined by the International Pediatric MS Study Group (IPMSSG) as multifocal neurologic deficits and encephalopathy (change in behavior or consciousness),[57] is the most frequent ADS, occurring in 25% to 40% of children,[17,52] and represents a monophasic illness in up to 80% of children, with symptoms lasting approximately 3 months.[58] Recurrent and multiphasic forms of ADEM have been described but are rare.[57] Because younger children are more likely to experience a first attack of MS characterized by multifocal neurologic deficits, the distinction from monophasic ADEM can be difficult, but is important for prognosis. ADEM has been reported as a first attack of MS in as many as 18% of children,[58] and in as few as 2% to 6%.[17,51] These discrepant findings may be a result of inconsistent application of criteria for altered mental status or encephalopathy across studies. To mitigate this inconsistency and permit comparison of multiple cohorts, the IPMSSG proposed MS diagnostic criteria for children whose first attack met criteria for ADEM, requiring 2 non-ADEM events (which must exclude encephalopathy) more than 3 months after first attack.[57]

An MS relapse is defined as neurologic symptoms that persist for at least 24 hours and are separated from a previous attack by a minimum of 28 days.[59] Most children with MS experience complete recovery after the first demyelinating episode,[60] remaining clinically stable between subsequent MS relapses. More than 95% of children with MS follow a relapsing-remitting disease course[49,50]; primary progressive MS is extremely rare in children. Annualized relapse rate, estimated between 0.38 and 0.87,[3,54] is higher in children compared with adults.[61] On average, the secondary progressive stage of MS occurs 10 years later in children compared with adults, but pediatric-onset patients are 10 years younger than adult-onset patients when they reach this phase of the disease.[50]

Treatment

Corticosteroids are typically used to manage acute symptoms or relapses in children with MS,[62] and intravenous immunoglobulin or plasma exchange may be administered to treat severe or life-threatening symptoms.[63,64] Most disease-modifying therapies act on the immune-mediated inflammatory component of the disease. First-line immunomodulatory therapies used to treat pediatric MS include glatiramer acetate (GA), intramuscular and subcutaneous interferon (IFN) β1a, and subcutaneous IFN-β1b. At present, most treatment decisions for use of these first-line therapies in children are based on studies performed in adults. Recently, a European consensus for the use of IFN-β and GA in children with MS was published.[65] Initiation of MS-targeted therapy should commence promptly after confirmation of MS diagnosis, because efficacy is higher early on in the disease, both IFN-β and GA are safe and tolerable in children and seem effective at reducing relapse rate in the early stages of the disease; relapses interfere with school attendance and negatively affect quality of life.[33] Serious adverse effects to first-line therapies are rare in children,[66] and flulike symptoms, increased liver enzyme levels, and reduced white blood cell counts are most common.[33] Data on adequate treatment response are lacking; however, a reduction in relapse rate during the first 2 years of disease from 1.0 to less than 0.6 would be comparable to the 30% to 40% relapse rate reductions observed in adults.[33]

Two second-line therapies, natalizumab and fingolimod, have recently been approved for use in adult patients. Natalizumab has shown relapse rate reductions of 68% in adult MS trials and more than 90% reductions in contrast-enhancing lesions compared with placebo[67]; however, it is associated with an increased risk for infection with JC virus, leading to progressive multifocal leukoencephalopathy (PML).[68] Stringent monitoring and PML management guidelines are now in place. Fingolimod is the first orally administered disease-modifying therapy and has been shown to reduce MR imaging activity and clinical relapses in adults with MS.[69,70] Fingolimod acts by binding to sphingosine-1-phosphase receptors on immune cells, impeding their ability to emigrate from the thymus. Whether this sequestration of immune cells in the thymus (a particularly active tissue in children that is responsible for educating the T-cell repertoire) results in premature immune senescence must be understood before it can be considered for treatment of pediatric MS.[33]

Physical and Cognitive Outcome

Long-term outcome in children with MS is largely determined by rate of physical and cognitive disability accrual. The Expanded Disability Status Scale (EDSS)[71] is a widely used measure of physical disability, ranging from 0 to 10, with increasing scores referring to increased disability. Children reach a disability score of 4 (deficits, but able to ambulate 500 m without aid or rest) a median of 20 years from onset, a score of 6 (able to walk with unilateral aid no more than 100 m without rest) after 28.9 years, and a score of 7 (able to walk no more than 10 m without rest) after 37 years.[5] Compared with adults with MS, pediatric-onset patients take 10 years longer to reach irreversible disability scores, but do so at an age of 10 years younger.[5]

Longitudinal studies have shown that more than half of children with MS show cognitive impairment at 10 years of follow-up.[72,73] Compared with healthy controls, cross-sectional studies have shown that more than 30% of patients have cognitive impairment in the form of deficits in attention, memory, processing speed, expressive language, and visuomotor integration.[74–77] Over 2 years of follow-up, 70% of children with MS enrolled in a multicenter longitudinal study showed worsening of cognitive impairment.[78] Given that cognitive impairment affects quality of life and negatively affects school performance, special attention to school-related accommodations and emotional well-being is imperative to the multidisciplinary care of children with MS.

MR IMAGING APPEARANCE OF RELAPSING-REMITTING MS
Typical MR Imaging Features of MS

Conventional MR imaging has high sensitivity for macroscopic tissue abnormalities in MS, but low pathologic specificity within the lesions, because edema, inflammation, demyelination, remyelination, gliosis, and neuroaxonal loss all appear as hyperintense on dual-echo proton-density/T2-weighted, and fluid-attenuated inversion recovery (FLAIR) imaging. Dual-echo, FLAIR, and precontrast and postcontrast T1-weighted sequences provide important information for diagnosing MS, understanding the natural history of lesion accrual, and assessing whether treatment reduces accrual of new lesions.

MS lesions typically appear as focal ovoid areas of hyperintensity on dual-echo and FLAIR images, ranging from a few millimeters to more than 1 cm in diameter. White matter lesions, such as those involving the juxtacortical and periventricular regions, the corpus callosum, as well as the brainstem and cerebellum, can be visualized on conventional T2-weighted or FLAIR images (**Fig. 1**). In an analysis of supratentorial T2 lesion distribution in children with established MS, lesions have the highest probability of being located in the occipital periventricular white matter, followed by the frontal periventricular white matter, whereas cortical and deep gray matter T2 lesions are less commonly detected (**Fig. 2**).[79] T2 hypointensity has been detected in deep gray matter structures of pediatric patients with MS, specifically in the head of the caudate nucleus,[80] and may suggest abnormal iron deposition related to diffuse underlying MS. Tumefactive lesions, defined as large lesions (>2 cm) with marked perilesional edema, may be difficult to distinguish from malignancy at onset, and therefore biopsy may be required for diagnosis.[81] The presence of tumefactive lesions has been reported in children with acute demyelination who have subsequently been diagnosed with MS (**Fig. 3**).[82,83]

Gadolinium-enhanced T1-weighted imaging permits differentiation of active or newly formed lesions from inactive ones, because contrast enhancement occurs as a result of increased blood-brain barrier permeability and corresponds to active immune cell transmigration into the CNS.[84] Enhancing lesions are typically focal or ringlike in contour (**Fig. 4**). In a prospective cohort study of children with ADS,[51] contrast-enhancing lesions were present in 22% of patients (10% of patients who had a monophasic illness and 70% of children subsequently diagnosed with MS). Lesions typically enhance for approximately 3 weeks,[85] but the duration may be shorter in the context of treatment with methylprednisolone. Both number and volume of new T2 and contrast-enhancing lesions are often used as an outcome measure of in vivo inflammatory activity in treatment trials, because they capture subclinical disease activity with a higher frequency than clinical relapses.

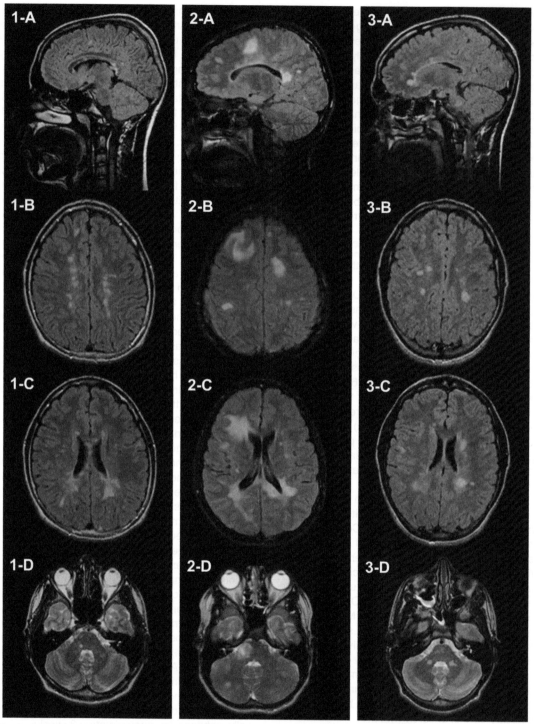

Fig. 1. Sagittal (*A*) and axial (*B* and *C*) FLAIR and axial T2-weighted (*D*) images of children with MS. All children were older than 10 years at the time of first demyelinating attack. Images acquired 4 months after onset (*column 1*) and at the time of onset (*column 2*) are presented from 2 boys, both of whom presented with polyfocal neurologic deficits, without encephalopathy. Column 3 contains images acquired from a boy 6 months after presentation with brainstem symptoms.

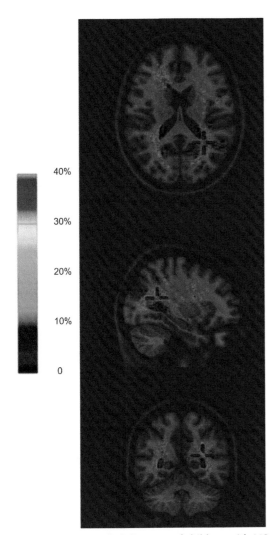

Fig. 2. T2 lesion probability map of children with MS. The highest probability for lesion accrual in the supratentorial region is in the occipital periventricular white matter followed by the frontal periventricular white matter. (*Courtesy of* D.L. Collins, PhD, and B. Aubert-Broche, PhD, McConnell Brain Imaging Center, Montreal Neurologic Institute, McGill University, Montreal, Canada.)

A subset of T2 hyperintense lesions appears hypointense on T1-weighted imaging, ranging in intensity from isointense to gray matter to isointense to cerebrospinal fluid.[86] These T1 lesions, or black holes, which may enhance with gadolinium initially but persist as nonenhancing lesions on serial T1-weighted images, represent focal areas of severe tissue damage and irreversible axonal loss (Fig. 5). Decreasing brain volume over time can be observed in children when comparing serial MR imaging scans (see Fig. 5).

MR Imaging Features of MS in Very Young Children

Whereas the MR imaging appearance of MS in children older than 11 years may be similar to that of adults, younger children (<11 years of age) present with atypical MR imaging features. MR imaging acquired at first attack in young children with MS may show large confluent T2 lesions, with poorly defined borders.[87] These large, ill-defined lesions may disappear on serial scans, unlike the more typical ovoid lesions in adolescents and adults, which persist on serial imaging. This difference in lesion appearance may relate to differences in an age-related capacity for lesional edema.

MR Imaging Features of the Spinal Cord in MS

Spinal cord lesion features in children with MS resemble that seen in adults. In a study of 36 children with MS (mean onset age 13.1 ± 3.5 years; disease duration 7.5 ± 3.3 years) who had spine imaging acquired as a result of intercurrent spinal cord symptoms or to aid in MS diagnosis, the median lesion count was 1 and lesions preferentially involved the cervical region. Lesions involved only a portion of the transverse diameter of the spinal cord (70% located in the posterior region), and 90% of lesions were focal, spanning less than 3 vertebral body segments in the rostral-caudal length.[88] When comparing spinal cord MR imaging features in children with MS with those with monophasic TM, both groups had a median lesion count of 1, but 88% of patients with TM had lesions extending 3 vertebral body segments or more compared with only 17% of children with MS. Focal lesions (<3 vertebral body segments) were rare (9%) in patients with monophasic TM compared with those with MS (75%).[89] The frequency of clinically silent spinal cord involvement in children with MS is not known, and will be important in determining the added value of spinal cord MR imaging in MS diagnosis in children. The length of time required to image both the brain and spinal cord, the difficulty for children to lie still for this time without anesthesia, and the poor imaging resolution as a result of a small spinal cord coupled with artifacts from cardiothoracic motion and cerebrospinal fluid pulsatility challenge the applicability of spine imaging as a routine component of the evaluation of children with MS.

MR IMAGING AND THE DIAGNOSIS OF MS

MR imaging diagnostic criteria for MS and parameters predictive of MS in patients with acute demyelination are summarized in Table 1.

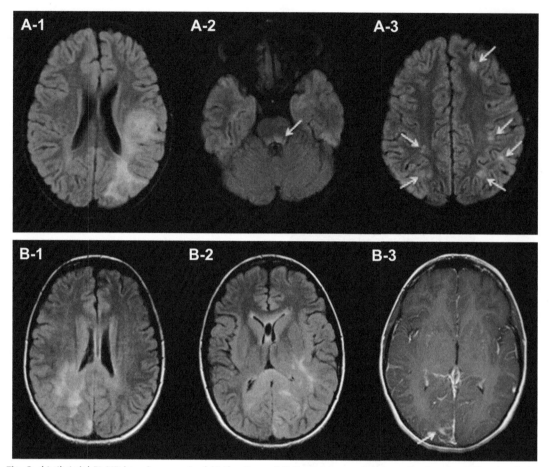

Fig. 3. (*A-1*) Axial FLAIR imaging acquired at the time of first attack reveals a tumefactive demyelinating lesion involving the posterior hemispheric white matter in a child with MS; postcontrast T1-weighted imaging was not acquired at the time of onset. (*A-2, A-3*) Axial FLAIR images acquired 15 months after baseline MR imaging (*A-1*) showing new brainstem, juxtacortical, and cerebral white matter lesions (*arrows*). (*B-1, B-2*) Axial FLAIR imaging shows a tumor involving the cortex, posterior hemispheric white matter, and splenium of the corpus callosum in a child initially evaluated for demyelination. (*B-3*) Postcontrast T1-weighted imaging reveals enhancement (*arrow*) of the tumor in the juxtacortical region of the occipital white matter.

International Pediatric Consensus Criteria

In 2007, the IPMSSG met to propose consensus definitions for MS in children (patients younger than 18 years of age at onset).[57] After the exclusion of alternative explanations for the neurologic symptoms,[90] the diagnosis of MS in children requires at least 2 episodes of neurologic dysfunction involving distinct regions of the CNS (dissemination in space [DIS]) and separated by at least 28 days (dissemination in time [DIT]), as is specified for adults.[59] The IPMSSG proposed that the 2005 McDonald criteria for adults[91–93] may be used to satisfy the requirements of DIS on MR imaging in children.[57] The MR imaging scan must show 3 of the following 4 features: (1) at least 1 gadolinium-enhancing lesion or at least 9 T2 hyperintense lesions if there is no gadolinium-enhancing lesion, (2) at least 3 periventricular lesions, (3) at least 1 juxtacortical lesion, and (4) at least 1 infratentorial lesion. The combination of an abnormal cerebrospinal fluid result (presence of oligoclonal bands or an increased IgG index) and at least 2 T2 lesions on MR imaging (1 of which is located in the brain) meet criteria for DIS.

The IPMSSG also agreed with the diagnostic criteria proposed for adult-onset MS, in which MR imaging can be used to satisfy the criteria for DIT following an initial attack (ie, ADS), even in the absence of a second clinical attack. According to the 2005 McDonald criteria, DIT on MR imaging may be shown in 1 of 2 ways: (1) gadolinium enhancement at least 3 months after onset of an ADS, or (2) detection of a new T2 lesion appearing at any timepoint compared with a reference scan performed at least 30 days after the onset of an ADS.[91]

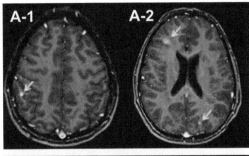

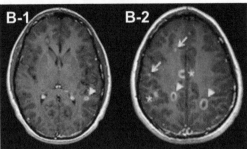

Fig. 4. Axial postgadolinium T1-weighted images from 2 children with MS (*A* and *B*). Focal enhancing lesions are depicted by arrows in (*A-1*), (*A-2*) and (*B-2*). Closed ringlike enhancing lesions are denoted by arrowheads in (*B-1*) and (*B-2*), and open ringlike enhancing lesions by asterisks in (*B-2*).

2010 McDonald Criteria for MS Diagnosis

In May, 2010, the International Panel on Diagnosis of MS met in Dublin, Ireland to revise the McDonald criteria.[94] Revisions to the DIS criteria were based on work of the European MAGNIMS (Magnetic Resonance Imaging in Multiple Sclerosis) multicenter collaborative network, which studies MR imaging in MS, and indicate that DIS can be shown by the presence of at least 1 clinically silent T2 lesion in at least 2 of the following 4 regions: periventricular, juxtacortical, infratentorial, and spinal cord.[95,96] The DIT criteria can be met by showing either: (1) at least 1 new T2 or gadolinium-enhancing lesion on a serial MR imaging scan, about a baseline scan, irrespective of the timing of the baseline scan, or (2) simultaneous presence of asymptomatic gadolinium-enhancing and nonenhancing lesions on any scan.[97,98] These revisions represent the first iteration of the McDonald criteria by which, in some circumstances, both DIS and DIT may be met on the scan acquired at time of incident demyelination. The 2010 McDonald criteria revisions included a focus on the pediatric population. Consensus of the Panel was that most pediatric patients with MS would meet DIS criteria at the time of ADS, because most patients have 2 lesions in at least 2 of the 4 specified locations. However,

application of the criteria to children with ADEM was not recommended. Validation studies of the revised criteria in the pediatric population, including in children presenting with ADEM, have yet to be performed.

MR IMAGING DIAGNOSTIC CRITERIA DEVELOPED FOR PEDIATRIC-ONSET MS
Adult Criteria Applied to Scans of Pediatric-Onset Patients

The adult McDonald criteria for DIS proposed in 2001 and revised in 2005[91,99] are 93% to 100% specific for MS diagnosis in children,[100,101] but only about 53% to 61% of children with MS meet criteria at the time of first attack.[102,103] The sensitivity of the McDonald DIS criteria for MS diagnosis is only 45% in children younger than 10 years at onset, but is 67% (similar to that observed in adults) in those older than 10 years,[101] supporting the notion of an atypical lesion pattern in younger children diagnosed with MS.[87] That approximately half of children with MS are not identified as such according to the McDonald criteria suggests the need for new or revised criteria specific to pediatric-onset MS.

Pediatric-Specific MR Imaging Criteria for MS Diagnosis

In a study of 38 children with MS and 45 with non-demyelinating relapsing CNS disease (migraine and CNS lupus), patients with MS were distinguished from patients with nondemyelinating disease by the presence of at least 2 of the following: at least 5 T2 lesions, at least 2 periventricular lesions, and at least 1 brainstem lesion on MR imaging acquired at second attack (sensitivity 85%, specificity 98%, PPV 97%, NPV 90%).[100] These criteria perform well at distinguishing established MS disease from nondemyelinating disease in children; however, the accuracy of these criteria decreases when used to differentiate children with MS from those with monophasic demyelination at the time of first attack.[51,102]

MR Imaging Predictors of MS Diagnosis in Children at Risk for MS

The usefulness of MR imaging in predicting a subsequent MS diagnosis in children with ADS has important implications for identifying children at highest risk for chronic relapsing disease, and therefore early intervention with disease-modifying therapy. The French Kid Sclerose en Plaques (KIDSEP) Study Group evaluated MR imaging scans of 116 children with ADS, and identified 2 features on initial MR imaging that

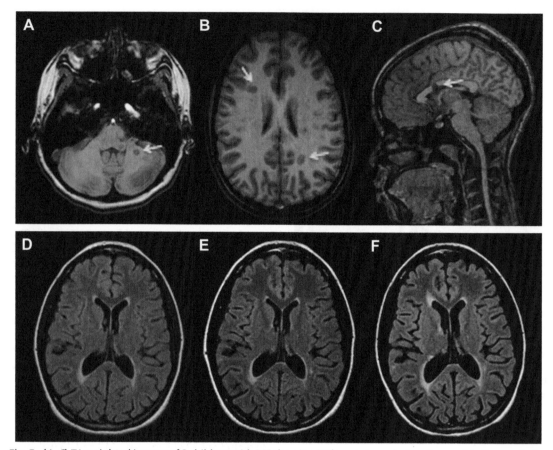

Fig. 5. (A–C) T1-weighted images of 3 children with MS showing T1 hypointense lesions (arrows) in the cerebellar (A) and cerebral (B) white matter and in the corpus callosum (C). (D–F) Serial FLAIR images from a child with MS acquired 4.9 years (D), 5.9 years (E), and 8.4 years (F) from onset; evidence of brain volume loss is depicted by enlargement of the lateral ventricles and widening of the sulci over time.

predicted subsequent MS diagnosis (Kids with Multiple Sclerosis [KIDMUS] criteria): at least 1 lesion perpendicular to the long axis of the corpus callosum (hazard ratio [HR] 2.89; 95% confidence interval [CI] 1.65–5.06) and the sole presence of well-defined lesions (HR 1.71; 95% CI 1.29–2.27).[104] Another study that evaluated prognostic factors for MS in children with acute demyelination showed that both the KIDMUS criteria[104] and the 2005 McDonald criteria for DIS[91] had a high PPV and specificity but low sensitivity for distinguishing children with a first attack of MS from those with monophasic ADS.[101] Although the KIDMUS criteria were 100% specific for an MS diagnosis, only 11% to 21% of children diagnosed with MS had these features at onset.[102,104] Therefore, applicability of the KIDMUS criteria for predicting MS in the clinical setting of acute demyelination is limited.

In a recent Canadian cohort study of determinants of MS in 302 children with acute demyelination, the presence of 1 or more T2 lesions on MR imaging was the most strongly associated with MS diagnosis (HR 37.9; 95% CI 5.25–273.85) when compared with other predictors, such as the presence of HLA-DRB1*15 alleles, previous infection with EBV, 25-hydroxyvitamin D insufficiency, and cerebrospinal fluid oligoclonal bands.[17]

Although the presence of even 1 brain lesion is strongly associated with MS outcome,[17] the ability of 1 or more T2 lesions at onset to discriminate between children destined for MS from those with monophasic illness is not sufficiently strong to serve as a diagnostic feature.[51] Therefore, to better understand the MR imaging features that predict MS in children with ADS, a study was conducted in which a standardized MR imaging scoring tool was developed and applied to MR imaging scans acquired in a cohort of 284 children with incident demyelination. In this cohort, 57 (20%) were diagnosed with MS, 75% of which showed MR imaging evidence of new lesions within 12 months of symptom onset.[51] The

Table 1
MR imaging criteria for MS diagnosis

References	Pediatric-Onset MS	Adult-Onset MS
Polman et al,[91] 2005		DIS[a] Three of the following: 1. ≥9 T2 lesions or ≥1 contrast-enhancing lesion 2. ≥1 T2 infratentorial lesion 3. ≥1 T2 juxtacortical lesion 4. ≥3 T2 periventricular lesions DIT One of the following: 1. ≥1 contrast-enhancing lesion at least 3 mo after clinical onset 2. A new T2 lesion at any time compared with a reference scan acquired at least 30 d after clinical onset
Polman et al,[94] 2011	DIS Presence of ≥1 clinically silent T2 lesion in at least 2 of the 4 following CNS regions: 1. Periventricular 2. Juxtacortical 3. Infratentorial 4. Spinal cord DIT One of the following: 1. A new T2 or contrast-enhancing lesion on any serial scan with respect to a previous scan 2. Simultaneous presence of asymptomatic contrast-enhancing and nonenhancing lesions at any time	
Mikaeloff et al,[104] 2004	MR imaging prognostic factors for MS in children with acute demyelination: Two of the following: 1. T2 lesions perpendicular to the long axis of the corpus callosum 2. Sole presence of well-defined T2 lesions	
Callen et al,[100] 2009	MR imaging criteria to distinguish pediatric MS from relapsing nondemyelinating disease Two of the following: 1. ≥5 T2 lesions 2. ≥2 T2 periventricular lesions 3. ≥1 T2 brainstem lesion	
Callen et al,[107] 2009	MR imaging criteria to distinguish a first attack of MS from monophasic ADEM Two of the following: 1. Absence of a diffuse bilateral T2 lesion pattern 2. Presence of black holes 3. ≥2 T2 periventricular lesions	
Verhey et al,[51] 2011	MR imaging parameters that predict MS in children with acute demyelination: Two of the following: 1. ≥1 T2 periventricular lesion 2. ≥1 T1-hypointense lesion	

Abbreviations: DIS, dissemination in space; DIT, dissemination in time.
[a] A contrast-enhancing spinal cord lesion is equivalent to an enhancing lesion in the brain; individual spinal cord lesions and brain lesions can together contribute to the requirement of ≥9 T2 lesions.

presence of at least 1 T1 hypointense lesion (HR 20.31; 95% CI 5.52–74.72) and at least 1 T2 periventricular lesion (HR 3.34; 95% CI 1.27–8.83) identified children who were more likely to go on to have clinical or MR imaging evidence of early MS relapse (sensitivity 94%, specificity 93%, PPV 76%, NPV 96%). Seven children were diagnosed with MS before age 10 years. The frequency of T1-hypointense lesions and T2 periventricular lesions was similar between children younger than 10 years (71%) and those 10 years and older (86%; P = .30). Including children with ADEM in this cohort did not affect the ability to identify children at highest risk for MS, suggesting that the clinical distinction of monophasic ADEM from an ADEM-like first attack of MS may not be relevant. The presence of T1-hypointense lesions to predict MS supports the concept that MS biology is already well established at the time of a first clinical attack.

DISTINGUISHING MONOPHASIC ADEM FROM A FIRST ATTACK OF RELAPSING-REMITTING MS

Up to 18% of children with MS present with an ADEM-like first attack.[58] Therefore, the ability to distinguish children with monophasic ADEM from those destined for MS has important prognostic value. According to the IPMSSG consensus criteria, in a child whose initial ADS is consistent with the clinical features of ADEM (polyfocal neurologic deficits and encephalopathy), a second non-ADEM event alone is not sufficient for an MS diagnosis. Rather, further evidence of DIT is required, either by new T2 lesions developing at least 3 months after the second event, or by evidence of a new (third) clinical non-ADEM event.[57] This recommendation is based on the concern that a second non-ADEM episode in children who initially present with ADEM might still reflect a transient demyelinating illness. Serial clinical and MR imaging studies are necessary to understand the rate of MS diagnosis in children presenting with ADEM. Biomarkers that distinguish ADEM from a first attack of MS are also needed to identify children destined for recurrent chronic demyelinating disease as opposed to monophasic illness.

MR imaging features of monophasic ADEM include focal or multifocal T2-weighted lesion(s) without evidence of neuroaxonal degeneration on T1-weighted imaging (black holes). Brain lesions are typically large (>1–2 cm in diameter), are confluent through the supratentorial and infratentorial white matter, have ill-defined borders, and involve the deep gray matter with a predilection

for the thalami (Fig. 6). In some cases, the spinal cord may also be involved.[105,106] The MR imaging criteria for pediatric MS diagnosis proposed by Callen and colleagues[100] do not perform well when used to distinguish children with monophasic ADEM from those with MS at the time of first attack.[102,107] To this end, Callen and colleagues conducted a parallel study in which they evaluated MR imaging scans obtained at first attack in 28 children with MS and 20 with monophasic ADEM and proposed that patients with MS were distinguished from those with ADEM by any 2 of the following criteria: (1) absence of diffuse bilateral pattern, (2) presence of black holes, and (3) presence of at least 2 periventricular lesions (sensitivity 81%, specificity 95%, PPV 95%, NPV 79%).[107] The performance of these criteria has been replicated in an independent Dutch cohort.[102]

COMPARISON OF MR IMAGING FEATURES OF ADULT-ONSET AND PEDIATRIC-ONSET MS

Intuitively, because of the short period of subclinical disease activity in children with MS by virtue of their young age, pediatric-onset patients would be expected to show fewer lesions on MR imaging at the time of first attack compared with adults. However, several studies have shown that children show similar or higher levels of disease activity

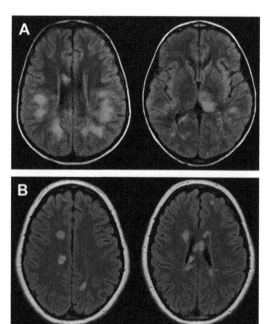

Fig. 6. Axial FLAIR images acquired at onset in a child with monophasic ADEM (A) and a child diagnosed with MS (B). T2-weighted lesions in ADEM may appear larger and have hazy margins, compared with the focal lesions typically seen in patients with MS.

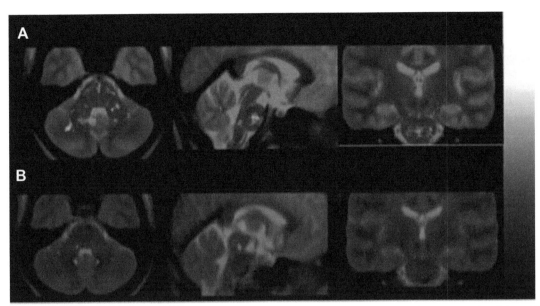

Fig. 7. Infratentorial T2 lesion distribution in patients with pediatric-onset MS (A) compared with adults with MS (B). (*Courtesy of* R. Ghassemi, McConnell Brain Imaging Center, Montreal Neurologic Institute, McGill University, Montreal, Canada.)

when compared with adults matched for disease duration.[61,108–110] Clinical relapses are significantly more common in the early stages of disease in patients with pediatric-onset MS (annualized relapse rate 1.13) compared with patients with adult-onset disease (annualized relapse rate 0.40), and this association persists when adjusting for proportion of disease spent on disease-modifying therapy.[61] In children with established MS, T2 and gadolinium-enhancing lesion volumes are similar to those of adult patients matched for disease duration, and the number of T2 lesions, gadolinium-enhancing lesions, and large T2 lesions on initial MR imaging is higher in children compared with adults.[108–110] Supratentorial T2 lesion distribution is similar, and infratentorial (specifically brainstem) lesion count is greater when comparing children with either ADS or MS with adults with MS matched for disease duration, implying that lesion accrual does not require a lengthy subclinical disease phase (**Fig. 7**).[109,110] The level of T1-hypointense lesion burden may be higher in children than adults early in the disease, given that the T1-lesion/T2-lesion volume ratio and the T1-lesion volume/brain parenchymal volume ratio are significantly higher in children.[108]

SUMMARY AND FUTURE DIRECTIONS

Conventional MR imaging has played a key role in identifying the imaging features of MS in children, and in predicting MS outcome in children at risk. Because only 30% of children with an acute

demyelinating episode herald further attacks leading to a diagnosis of MS, MR imaging is important in aiding the clinician to identify children who do not experience relapsing disease. With the mandate of pediatric investigation plans for all new drug trials, treatment trials for pediatric MS are soon to be launched. The ability to identify children at highest risk for MS diagnosis will be important in determining eligibility for such therapeutic trials. There remains a need to understand the natural history of lesion accrual on MR imaging, because these metrics will inform definitions of optimal therapeutic response in children with MS. Whether MR imaging can serve as a surrogate marker for prognosis is an important research question that has yet to be addressed and will require long-term clinical follow-up and standardized serial MR imaging evaluation.

REFERENCES

1. Ghezzi A, Deplano V, Faroni J, et al. Multiple sclerosis in childhood: clinical features of 149 cases. Mult Scler 1997;3:43–6.
2. Simone IL, Carrara D, Tortorella C, et al. Course and prognosis in early-onset MS: comparison with adult-onset forms. Neurology 2002;59:1922–8.
3. Boiko A, Vorobeychik G, Paty D, et al. Early onset multiple sclerosis: a longitudinal study. Neurology 2002;59:1006–10.
4. Deryck O, Ketelaer P, Dubois B. Clinical characteristics and long term prognosis in early onset multiple sclerosis. J Neurol 2006;253:720–3.

5. Renoux C, Vukusic S, Mikaeloff Y, et al. Natural history of multiple sclerosis with childhood onset. N Engl J Med 2007;356:2603–13.

6. Chitnis T, Glanz B, Jaffin S, et al. Demographics of pediatric-onset multiple sclerosis in an MS center population from the Northeastern United States. Mult Scler 2009;15:627–31.

7. Langer-Gould A, Zhang JL, Chung J, et al. Incidence of acquired CNS demyelinating syndromes in a multiethnic cohort of children. Neurology 2011;77:1143–8.

8. Banwell B, Kennedy J, Sadovnick D, et al. Incidence of acquired demyelination of the CNS in Canadian children. Neurology 2009;72:232–9.

9. Medaer R. Does the history of multiple sclerosis go back as far as the 14th century? Acta Neurol Scand 1979;60:189–92.

10. Gall J, Hayles A, Siekert R, et al. Multiple sclerosis in children: a clinical study of 40 cases with onset in childhood. Pediatrics 1958;21:703–9.

11. Bar-Or A. The immunology of multiple sclerosis. Semin Neurol 2008;28:29–45.

12. Trapp BD, Ransohoff R, Rudick R. Axonal pathology in multiple sclerosis: relationship to neurologic disability. Curr Opin Neurol 1999;12:295–302.

13. Trapp BD, Ransohoff R, Rudick R. Neurodegeneration in multiple sclerosis: relationship to neurological disability. Neuroscientist 1999;5:48–57.

14. Lincoln MR, Montpetit A, Cader MZ, et al. A predominant role for the HLA class II region in the association of the MHC region with multiple sclerosis. Nat Genet 2005;37:1108–12.

15. Boiko AN, Gusev EI, Sudomoina MA, et al. Association and linkage of juvenile MS with HLA-DR2(15) in Russians. Neurology 2002;58:658–60.

16. Disanto G, Magalhaes S, Handel AE, et al. HLA-DRB1 confers increased risk of pediatric-onset MS in children with acquired demyelination. Neurology 2011;76:781–6.

17. Banwell B, Bar-Or A, Arnold DL, et al. Clinical, environmental, and genetic determinants of multiple sclerosis in children with acute demyelination: a prospective national cohort study. Lancet Neurol 2011;10:436–45.

18. Mayne CG, Spanier JA, Relland LM, et al. 1,25-Dihydroxyvitamin D3 acts directly on the T lymphocyte vitamin D receptor to inhibit experimental autoimmune encephalomyelitis. Eur J Immunol 2011;41:822–32.

19. Pedersen LB, Nashold FE, Spach KM, et al. 1,25-dihydroxyvitamin D3 reverses experimental autoimmune encephalomyelitis by inhibiting chemokine synthesis and monocyte trafficking. J Neurosci Res 2007;85:2480–90.

20. Spach KM, Nashold FE, Dittel BN, et al. IL-10 signaling is essential for 1,25-dihydroxyvitamin D3-mediated inhibition of experimental autoimmune encephalomyelitis. J Immunol 2006;177:6030–7.

21. Mowry EM, Krupp LB, Milazzo M, et al. Vitamin D status is associated with relapse rate in pediatric-onset multiple sclerosis. Ann Neurol 2010;67:618–24.

22. Mikaeloff Y, Caridade G, Tardieu M, et al. Parental smoking at home and the risk of childhood-onset multiple sclerosis in children. Brain 2007;130:2589–95.

23. Banwell B, Krupp L, Kennedy J, et al. Clinical features and viral serologies in children with multiple sclerosis: a multinational observational study. Lancet Neurol 2007;6:773–81.

24. Petkau J. Statistical methods for evaluating multiple sclerosis therapies. Semin Neurol 1998;18:351–75.

25. Mowry EM, James JA, Krupp LB, et al. Vitamin D status and antibody levels to common viruses in pediatric-onset multiple sclerosis. Mult Scler 2011;17(6):666–71.

26. Lunemann JD, Huppke P, Roberts S, et al. Broadened and elevated humoral immune response to EBNA1 in pediatric multiple sclerosis. Neurology 2008;71:1033–5.

27. Pohl D, Krone B, Rostasy K, et al. High seroprevalence of Epstein-Barr virus in children with multiple sclerosis. Neurology 2006;67:2063–5.

28. Alotaibi S, Kennedy J, Tellier R, et al. Epstein-Barr virus in pediatric multiple sclerosis. JAMA 2004;291:1875–9.

29. Pohl D, Rostasy K, Jacobi C, et al. Intrathecal antibody production against Epstein-Barr and other neurotropic viruses in pediatric and adult onset multiple sclerosis. J Neurol 2010;257:212–6.

30. Waubant E, Mowry EM, Krupp L, et al. Common viruses associated with lower pediatric multiple sclerosis risk. Neurology 2011;76:1989–95.

31. Banwell B, Bar-Or A, Kennedy J, et al. T-cell proliferation against myelin, pancreatic, and dietary antigens in children: autoimmunity is detectable early in CNS demyelination and type I diabetes. Neurology 2006;66:A310.

32. McLaughlin KA, Chitnis T, Newcombe J, et al. Age-dependent B cell autoimmunity to a myelin surface antigen in pediatric multiple sclerosis. J Immunol 2009;183:4067–76.

33. Banwell B, Bar-Or A, Giovannoni G, et al. Therapies for multiple sclerosis: considerations in the pediatric patient. Nat Rev Neurol 2011;7:109–22.

34. Giovannoni G, Ebers G. Multiple sclerosis: the environment and causation. Curr Opin Neurol 2007;20:261–8.

35. Zamboni P, Menegatti E, Bartolomei I, et al. Intracranial venous haemodynamics in multiple sclerosis. Curr Neurovasc Res 2007;4:252–8.

36. Singh AV, Zamboni P. Anomalous venous blood flow and iron deposition in multiple sclerosis. J Cereb Blood Flow Metab 2009;29:1867–78.

37. Zamboni P, Galeotti R, Menegatti E, et al. Chronic cerebrospinal venous insufficiency in patients with multiple sclerosis. J Neurol Neurosurg Psychiatry 2009;80:392–9.

38. Zamboni P, Menegatti E, Galeotti R, et al. The value of cerebral Doppler venous haemodynamics in the assessment of multiple sclerosis. J Neurol Sci 2009;282:21–7.

39. Khan O, Filippi M, Freedman MS, et al. Chronic cerebrospinal venous insufficiency and multiple sclerosis. Ann Neurol 2010;67:286–90.

40. Zamboni P, Galeotti R, Menegatti E, et al. A prospective open-label study of endovascular treatment of chronic cerebrospinal venous insufficiency. J Vasc Surg 2009;50:1348–58.

41. Doepp F, Wurfel JT, Pfueller CF, et al. Venous drainage in multiple sclerosis: a combined MRI and ultrasound study. Neurology 2011;77:1745–51.

42. Doepp F, Paul F, Valdueza JM, et al. No cerebrocervical venous congestion in patients with multiple sclerosis. Ann Neurol 2010;68:173–83.

43. Sundstrom P, Wahlin A, Ambarki K, et al. Venous and cerebrospinal fluid flow in multiple sclerosis: a case-control study. Ann Neurol 2010;68:255–9.

44. Zivadinov R, Marr K, Cutter G, et al. Prevalence, sensitivity, and specificity of chronic cerebrospinal venous insufficiency in MS. Neurology 2011;77:138–44.

45. Benarroch EE. Brain iron homeostasis and neurodegenerative disease. Neurology 2009;72:1436–40.

46. Zecca L, Youdim MB, Riederer P, et al. Iron, brain ageing and neurodegenerative disorders. Nat Rev Neurosci 2004;5:863–73.

47. Worthington V, Killestein J, Eikelenboom MJ, et al. Normal CSF ferritin levels in MS suggest against etiologic role of chronic venous insufficiency. Neurology 2010;75:1617–22.

48. Experimental multiple sclerosis vascular shunting procedure halted at Stanford. Ann Neurol 2010;67:A13–5.

49. Banwell B, Ghezzi A, Bar-Or A, et al. Multiple sclerosis in children: clinical diagnosis, therapeutic strategies, and future directions. Lancet Neurol 2007;6:887–902.

50. Yeh EA, Chitnis T, Krupp L, et al. Pediatric multiple sclerosis. Nat Rev Neurol 2009;5:621–31.

51. Verhey LH, Branson HM, Shroff MM, et al. MRI parameters for prediction of multiple sclerosis diagnosis in children with acute CNS demyelination: a prospective national cohort study. Lancet Neurol 2011;10:1065–73.

52. Mikaeloff Y, Suissa S, Vallee L, et al. First episode of acute CNS inflammatory demyelination in childhood: prognostic factors for multiple sclerosis and disability. J Pediatr 2004;144:246–52.

53. Ozakbas S, Idiman E, Baklan B, et al. Childhood and juvenile onset multiple sclerosis: clinical and paraclinical features. Brain Dev 2003;25:233–6.

54. Ghezzi A, Pozzilli C, Liguori M, et al. Prospective study of multiple sclerosis with early onset. Mult Scler 2002;8:115–8.

55. Wilejto M, Shroff M, Buncic JR, et al. The clinical features, MRI findings, and outcome of optic neuritis in children. Neurology 2006;67:258–62.

56. Pidcock FS, Krishnan C, Crawford TO, et al. Acute transverse myelitis in childhood: center-based analysis of 47 cases. Neurology 2007;68:1474–80.

57. Krupp LB, Banwell B, Tenembaum S. Consensus definitions proposed for pediatric multiple sclerosis and related disorders. Neurology 2007;68:S7–12.

58. Mikaeloff Y, Caridade G, Husson B, et al. Acute disseminated encephalomyelitis cohort study: prognostic factors for relapse. Eur J Paediatr Neurol 2007;11:90–5.

59. Poser CM, Paty DW, Scheinberg L, et al. New diagnostic criteria for multiple sclerosis: guidelines for research protocols. Ann Neurol 1983;13:227–31.

60. Duquette P, Murray TJ, Pleines J, et al. Multiple sclerosis in childhood: clinical profile in 125 patients. J Pediatr 1987;111:359–63.

61. Gorman MP, Healy BC, Polgar-Turcsanyi M, et al. Increased relapse rate in pediatric-onset compared with adult-onset multiple sclerosis. Arch Neurol 2009;66:54–9.

62. Dale RC, Brilot F, Banwell B. Pediatric central nervous system inflammatory demyelination: acute disseminated encephalomyelitis, clinically isolated syndromes, neuromyelitis optica, and multiple sclerosis. Curr Opin Neurol 2009;22:233–40.

63. Hahn JS, Siegler DJ, Enzmann D. Intravenous gammaglobulin therapy in recurrent acute disseminated encephalomyelitis. Neurology 1996;46:1173–4.

64. Nishikawa M, Ichiyama T, Hayashi T, et al. Intravenous immunoglobulin therapy in acute disseminated encephalomyelitis. Pediatr Neurol 1999;21:583–6.

65. Ghezzi A, Banwell B, Boyko A, et al. The management of multiple sclerosis in children: a European view. Mult Scler 2010;16:1258–67.

66. Tenembaum SN, Segura MJ. Interferon beta-1a treatment in childhood and juvenile-onset multiple sclerosis. Neurology 2006;67:511–3.

67. Polman CH, O'Connor PW, Havrdova E, et al. A randomized, placebo-controlled trial of natalizumab for relapsing multiple sclerosis. N Engl J Med 2006;354:899–910.

68. Clifford DB, DeLuca A, Simpson DM, et al. Natalizumab-associated progressive multifocal leukoencephalopathy in patients with multiple sclerosis: lessons from 28 cases. Lancet Neurol 2010;9: 438–46.

69. Cohen JA, Barkhof F, Comi G, et al. Oral fingolimod or intramuscular interferon for relapsing multiple sclerosis. N Engl J Med 2010;362:402–15.

70. Kappos L, Radue EW, O'Connor P, et al. A placebo-controlled trial of oral fingolimod in relapsing multiple sclerosis. N Engl J Med 2010; 362:387–401.

71. Kurtzke JF. Rating neurologic impairment in multiple sclerosis: an expanded disability status scale (EDSS). Neurology 1983;33:1444–52.

72. Amato MP, Ponziani G, Pracucci G, et al. Cognitive impairment in early-onset multiple sclerosis. Pattern, predictors, and impact on everyday life in a 4-year follow-up. Arch Neurol 1995;52:168–72.

73. Amato MP, Ponziani G, Siracusa G, et al. Cognitive dysfunction in early-onset multiple sclerosis: a reappraisal after 10 years. Arch Neurol 2001;58: 1602–6.

74. Till C, Ghassemi R, Aubert-Broche B, et al. MRI correlates of cognitive impairment in childhood-onset multiple sclerosis. Neuropsychology 2011; 25:319–32.

75. MacAllister WS, Belman AL, Milazzo M, et al. Cognitive functioning in children and adolescents with multiple sclerosis. Neurology 2005;64:1422–5.

76. Banwell BL, Anderson PE. The cognitive burden of multiple sclerosis in children. Neurology 2005;64: 891–4.

77. Amato MP, Goretti B, Ghezzi A, et al. Cognitive and psychosocial features of childhood and juvenile MS. Neurology 2008;70:1891–7.

78. Amato MP, Goretti B, Ghezzi A, et al. Cognitive and psychosocial features in childhood and juvenile MS: two-year follow-up. Neurology 2010;75: 1134–40.

79. Aubert-Broche B, Fonov V, Ghassemi R, et al. Regional brain atrophy in children with multiple sclerosis. Neuroimage 2011;58:409–15.

80. Ceccarelli A, Rocca MA, Perego E, et al. Deep grey matter T2 hypo-intensity in patients with paediatric multiple sclerosis. Mult Scler 2011;17:702–7.

81. Lucchinetti CF, Gavrilova RH, Metz I, et al. Clinical and radiographic spectrum of pathologically confirmed tumefactive multiple sclerosis. Brain 2008;131:1759–75.

82. McAdam L, Blaser S, Banwell B. Pediatric tumefactive demyelination: case series and review of the literature. Pediatr Neurol 2002;26:18–25.

83. Balassy C, Bernert G, Wober-Bingol C, et al. Long-term MRI observations of childhood-onset relapsing-remitting multiple sclerosis. Neuropediatrics 2001;32:28–37.

84. Katz D, Taubenberger JK, Cannella B, et al. Correlation between magnetic resonance imaging findings and lesion development in chronic, active multiple sclerosis. Ann Neurol 1993;34:661–9.

85. Cotton F, Weiner HL, Jolesz FA, et al. MRI contrast uptake in new lesions in relapsing-remitting MS followed at weekly intervals. Neurology 2003;60: 640–6.

86. van Walderveen MA, Kamphorst W, Scheltens P, et al. Histopathologic correlate of hypointense lesions on T1-weighted spin-echo MRI in multiple sclerosis. Neurology 1998;50:1282–8.

87. Chabas D, Castillo-Trivino T, Mowry EM, et al. Vanishing MS T2-bright lesions before puberty: a distinct MRI phenotype? Neurology 2008;71: 1090–3.

88. Verhey LH, Branson HM, Makhija M, et al. Magnetic resonance imaging features of the spinal cord in pediatric multiple sclerosis: a preliminary study. Neuroradiology 2010;52:1153–62.

89. Thomas T, Branson HM, Verhey LH, et al. The demographic, clinical, and magnetic resonance imaging (MRI) features of transverse myelitis in children. J Child Neurol 2012;27:11–21.

90. Charil A, Yousry TA, Rovaris M, et al. MRI and the diagnosis of multiple sclerosis: expanding the concept of "no better explanation". Lancet Neurol 2006;5:841–52.

91. Polman CH, Reingold SC, Edan G, et al. Diagnostic criteria for multiple sclerosis: 2005 revisions to the "McDonald Criteria". Ann Neurol 2005;58: 840–6.

92. Tintore M, Rovira A, Martinez MJ, et al. Isolated demyelinating syndromes: comparison of different MR imaging criteria to predict conversion to clinically definite multiple sclerosis. AJNR Am J Neuroradiol 2000;21:702–6.

93. Barkhof F, Filippi M, Miller DH, et al. Comparison of MRI criteria at first presentation to predict conversion to clinically definite multiple sclerosis. Brain 1997;120(Pt 11):2059–69.

94. Polman CH, Reingold SC, Banwell B, et al. Diagnostic criteria for multiple sclerosis: 2010 revisions to the McDonald criteria. Ann Neurol 2011; 69:292–302.

95. Swanton JK, Rovira A, Tintore M, et al. MRI criteria for multiple sclerosis in patients presenting with clinically isolated syndromes: a multicentre retrospective study. Lancet Neurol 2007;6:677–86.

96. Swanton JK, Fernando K, Dalton CM, et al. Modification of MRI criteria for multiple sclerosis in patients with clinically isolated syndromes. J Neurol Neurosurg Psychiatry 2006;77:830–3.

97. Rovira A, Swanton J, Tintore M, et al. A single, early magnetic resonance imaging study in the diagnosis of multiple sclerosis. Arch Neurol 2009;66: 587–92.

98. Montalban X, Tintore M, Swanton J, et al. MRI criteria for MS in patients with clinically isolated syndromes. Neurology 2010;74:427–34.

99. McDonald WI, Compston A, Edan G, et al. Recommended diagnostic criteria for multiple sclerosis: guidelines from the International Panel on the diagnosis of multiple sclerosis. Ann Neurol 2001; 50:121–7.

100. Callen DJ, Shroff MM, Branson HM, et al. MRI in the diagnosis of pediatric multiple sclerosis. Neurology 2009;72:961–7.

101. Neuteboom RF, Boon M, Catsman Berrevoets CE, et al. Prognostic factors after a first attack of inflammatory CNS demyelination in children. Neurology 2008;71:967–73.

102. Ketelslegers IA, Neuteboom RF, Boon M, et al. A comparison of MRI criteria for diagnosing pediatric ADEM and MS. Neurology 2010;74: 1412–5.

103. Hahn CD, Shroff MM, Blaser S, et al. MRI criteria for multiple sclerosis: evaluation in a pediatric cohort. Neurology 2004;62:806–8.

104. Mikaeloff Y, Adamsbaum C, Husson B, et al. MRI prognostic factors for relapse after acute CNS inflammatory demyelination in childhood. Brain 2004;127:1942–7.

105. Tenembaum S, Chamoles N, Fejerman N. Acute disseminated encephalomyelitis: a long-term follow-up study of 84 pediatric patients. Neurology 2002;59:1224–31.

106. Tenembaum S, Chitnis T, Ness J, et al. Acute disseminated encephalomyelitis. Neurology 2007; 68:S23–36.

107. Callen DJ, Shroff MM, Branson HM, et al. Role of MRI in the differentiation of ADEM from MS in children. Neurology 2009;72:968–73.

108. Yeh EA, Weinstock-Guttman B, Ramanathan M, et al. Magnetic resonance imaging characteristics of children and adults with paediatric-onset multiple sclerosis. Brain 2009;132:3392–400.

109. Waubant E, Chabas D, Okuda DT, et al. Difference in disease burden and activity in pediatric patients on brain magnetic resonance imaging at time of multiple sclerosis onset vs adults. Arch Neurol 2009;66:967–71.

110. Ghassemi R, Antel SB, Narayanan S, et al. Lesion distribution in children with clinically isolated syndromes. Ann Neurol 2008;63:401–5.

The Magnetic Resonance Imaging Appearance of Monophasic Acute Disseminated Encephalomyelitis
An Update Post Application of the 2007 Consensus Criteria

Samantha E. Marin, MD,
David J.A. Callen, MD, PhD, FRCP(C)*

KEYWORDS

- Acute disseminated encephalomyelitis • Consensus guidelines • Molecular mimicry
- Inflammatory cascade

KEY POINTS

- Acute disseminated encephalomyelitis (ADEM) typically occurs after a viral infection or recent vaccination.
- ADEM can represent a diagnostic challenge for clinicians, as many disorders (inflammatory and noninflammatory) have a similar clinical and radiologic presentation.
- The differential diagnosis for multifocal hyperintense lesions on neuroimaging includes an exhaustive list of potential mimickers, namely infectious, inflammatory, rheumatologic, metabolic, nutritional, and degenerative entities.

INTRODUCTION

Acute disseminated encephalomyelitis (ADEM) is an immunologically mediated inflammatory disease of the central nervous system (CNS) resulting in multifocal demyelinating lesions affecting the gray and white matter of the brain and spinal cord. ADEM is characteristically a monophasic illness that is commonly associated with an antigenic challenge (febrile illness or vaccination), which is believed to function as a trigger to the inflammatory response underlying the disease. It is most commonly seen in the pediatric population, but can occur at any age.[1–6] Symptoms are highly dependent on the area of the CNS affected, but are polyfocal in nature. Common symptoms include hemiparesis, cranial nerve palsy, seizures, cerebellar ataxia, and hypotonia.[3,7–9] The diagnosis of ADEM depends on the history, physical examination, and supplemental neuroimaging.

Despite the long-standing recognition of ADEM as a specific entity, no consensus definition of ADEM had been reached until recently. Historically, different definitions of ADEM have been used in

Division of Pediatric Neurology, Department of Pediatrics, McMaster Children's Hospital, 1280 Main Street West, Hamilton, Ontario L8S 4K1, Canada
* Corresponding author.
E-mail address: dcallen@mcmaster.ca

Neuroimag Clin N Am 23 (2013) 245–266
http://dx.doi.org/10.1016/j.nic.2012.12.005
1052-5149/13/$ – see front matter © 2013 Elsevier Inc. All rights reserved.

published cases of pediatric and adult patients, which varied as to whether events required (1) monofocal or multifocal clinical features, (2) a change in mental status, and (3) a documentation of previous infection or immunization.[3,8–17] To avoid further misdiagnosis and to develop a uniform classification, the International Pediatric Multiple Sclerosis (MS) Study Group[18] proposed a consensus definition for ADEM for application in both research and clinical settings (Box 1). One of the most significant changes proposed by this definition was the mandatory inclusion of encephalopathy as a clinical symptom in patients presenting with ADEM. Before the development of the consensus definition, although encephalopathy was included in the clinical description it was not considered an essential criterion for the diagnosis. Thus, many of the previous studies investigating the clinical and radiologic features of pediatric ADEM were performed on patients who may no longer meet the consensus criteria, and may have led to the classification of other neurologic disorders as ADEM (Table 1). It may be that there is an inherent difference in the patients who present with multifocal symptoms and encephalopathy as opposed to those without encephalopathy; therefore, this distinction is imperative. Because of the lack of uniform description and clear clinical and neuroimaging diagnostic criteria in ADEM, caution must be exercised when applying previous clinical and radiologic descriptions of patients with this disorder.

This review is intended to give an overview of ADEM in the pediatric population, focusing on differences that have emerged since the consensus definition was established. Although the focus is on neuroimaging in these patients, a synopsis of the clinical features, immunopathogenesis, treatment, and prognosis of ADEM is provided.

EPIDEMIOLOGY AND CLINICAL PRESENTATION

Considering that the diagnostic criteria for ADEM were not elucidated before 2007, the annual incidence rate and prevalence within the population is not precisely known. In addition, no analyses of worldwide distribution of ADEM have been completed; therefore, the reported prevalence and incidence taken within a single area may not be generalizable to the population as a whole. Before 2007, the prevalence of ADEM within the pediatric population was estimated at 0.8 to 1.1 per 100,000 in those younger than 10 years.[6,7] A study by Leake and colleagues[11] evaluated the incidence of ADEM in San Diego County, USA. The investigators estimated this to be 0.4 per 100,000 per year in those younger than 20 years. More recent studies completed after the definition of ADEM had been established have suggested that these rates may actually be higher. Visudtibhan and colleagues[26] reported the prevalence of children with definite ADEM in Bangkok, Thailand to be 4.1 per 100,000. Another study from Fukuoka Prefecture, Japan reported the annual incidence to be 0.64 per 100,000.[27] The overall frequency of ADEM in Canadian children with acquired demyelinating disorders had been estimated at 22%.[28]

Although ADEM may present at any age, it is most frequently described in the pediatric population. The mean age of onset in the pediatric population is reported to be 7.4 ± 1.3 years of age and the median age of onset is 8 years, according to a recent meta-analysis.[7] However, 12 of the 13 studies included in the analysis were performed before the revised ADEM definition.[3,7–9,11–14,16,17,29–31] More recent studies using the new criteria for ADEM have shown a similar mean age of onset,

---

Box 1
International MS Study Group monophasic ADEM criteria

- No history of prior demyelinating event
- First clinical event with presumed inflammatory or demyelinating cause
- Acute or subacute onset
- Affects multifocal areas of central nervous system
- Must be polysymptomatic
- Must include encephalopathy (ie, behavioral change or altered level of consciousness)
- Neuroimaging shows focal/multifocal lesion(s) predominantly affecting white matter
- No neuroimaging evidence of previous destructive white matter changes
- Event should be followed by clinical/radiologic improvements (although may be residual deficits)
- No other etiology can explain the event
- New or fluctuating symptoms, signs, or magnetic resonance imaging findings occurring within 3 months are considered part of the acute event

Data from Krupp LB, Banwell B, Tenembaum S. Consensus definitions proposed for pediatric multiple sclerosis and related disorders. Neurology 2007;68:S7–12.

Table 1
Summary of the lesion characterization in previous pediatric ADEM cohorts within the last 10 years

Authors,[Ref.] Year	N	New Criteria[a] (%)	White Matter (%)				Gray Matter (%)			Brainstem (%)	Cerebellum (%)	Enhancing[b] (%)
			Deep	Juxt	Peri	CC	Cort	BG	Thal			
Hynson et al,[9] 2001	31	68	90	—	29	29	61	39	32	42	—	8/28
Tenembaum et al,[13] 2002	84	69	—	—	—	—	—	—	12	—	—	8/27
Murthy et al,[12] 2002	18	44	100 8.0[c] (1–30)	—	60 2.5[c] (0–16)	7 0.1[c] (0–1)	80 4.9[c] (0–28)	20 0.3[c] (0–2)	27 0.3[c] (0–2)	47 1.1[c] (0–8)	13 0.1[c] (0–1)	4/15
Anlar et al,[14] 2003	33	48	42	—	12	12	—	45	—	45	42	2/31
Richer et al,[19] 2005	10	40	90	—	30	80	—	60	—	50	—	3/9
Madan et al,[20] 2005	7	43	86	—	—	—	—	43	14	14	14	—
Singhi et al,[21] 2006	52	56	54	—	19	13	—	17	30	17	26	—
Mikaeloff et al,[22] 2007	108	100	—	61	42 (>2)	—	18	58	—	63	—	14/85
Atzori et al,[23] 2009	20	65	—	60	20	5	15	50	—	60	—	10/14
Alper et al,[24] 2009	24	42	68	21	18	9	—	43	—	41	50	—
Callen et al,[25] 2009	20	100	80	90	65	80	80	70	—	70	70	5/11
Visudtibhan et al,[26] 2010	16	100	75	19	75	—	19	50	—	50	25	—
Pavone et al,[7] 2010	17	100	—	—	—	—	—	—	23	—	—	3/17

Abbreviations: BG, basal ganglia; CC, callosal; Cort, cortical gray matter; Juxt, juxtacortical; Peri, periventricular; Thal, thalamic.
[a] Consensus criteria of International Pediatric Multiple Sclerosis Society.[18]
[b] Number of patients showing enhancing lesions (numerator) over the number of study patients who received contrast (denominator).
[c] Mean lesion count in category and minimum and maximum lesion counts (in parentheses).

ranging from 5.7 to 7.6 years.[22,25,27] An equal sex distribution was previously suggested,[6,8,11] but more current studies show a slight male preponderance (1.4–2.3:1) in patients presenting with ADEM at.[7,22,25,27] A seasonal distribution of ADEM has been described, with an increased number of cases during the winter and spring months.[8,11,12]

ADEM typically occurs after a viral infection or recent vaccination. The frequency with which a preceding febrile illness is noted has widely varied in previous literature, ranging from 46% to 100%.[3,8,9,11–16,22,32] This variation is likely attributable to the lack of uniform diagnostic criteria, with some investigators using the term ADEM only when a preceding febrile illness has been documented, as well as different latency periods from febrile illness to ADEM being deemed clinically significant. A recent meta-analysis showed that a preceding triggering event occurred in 69% of 492 patients diagnosed with ADEM.[7] The most common preceding trigger is a nonspecific upper respiratory tract infection.[13] The duration between antigenic challenge and the first signs and symptoms of ADEM has been cited as ranging from 1 to 28 days with a mean of 6 to 12 days.[7,13,26,33,34] Pavone and colleagues[7] showed different latency periods depending on the triggering factor, with the shortest latency being seen for upper respiratory tract infections or gastroenteritis (2–4 days). Although a link between viral illness and ADEM is likely, it should be noted that there is a high frequency of viral episodes in childhood, and medical history is often positive regardless of whether a causal correlation exists.

The neurologic features of ADEM are often seen following a short prodromal phase consisting of fever, malaise, headache, nausea, or vomiting. Patients subsequently develop neurologic symptoms subacutely, within a mean period of 4.5 to 7.5 days (range: 1–45 days).[7,13] Occasionally there is rapid progression of symptoms and signs to coma and/or decerebrate posturing.[3] The clinical presentation of ADEM is widely variable, with the type and severity clinical features being determined by the distribution of lesions within the CNS. Although studies have previously reported an encephalopathy in 21% to 74% of patients[3,8,9,11–17,33,35] (with only 55% having altered mental status in a recent meta-analysis[7]), application of the new diagnostic criteria mandates that encephalopathy (either behavioral change or altered mental status) be present in 100% of cases. It should thus be noted that previous studies looking at the presenting signs and symptoms encompass patients who, today, would not meet diagnostic criteria for ADEM. With that in mind, the neurologic features that

have previously been noted in ADEM include: unilateral or bilateral pyramidal signs (60%–95%); cranial nerve palsies (22%–89%); hemiparesis (76%–79%); ataxia (18%–65%); hypotonia (34%–47%); seizures (10%–47%); visual loss due to optic neuritis (7%–23%); and speech impairment (5%–21%).[3,7–9,11,13,14,16,17] Peripheral nervous system involvement has been reported in the adult cohort (with frequencies up to 43.6% of patients), but is considered rare in childhood ADEM patients.[35–38]

Only 2 studies have looked at presenting signs and symptoms of patients with ADEM according to the new consensus definitions. Mikaeloff and colleagues[22] reported that 79% presented with long tract dysfunction, 48% presented with brainstem dysfunction, 32% presented with seizures, and 6% presented with optic neuritis. Pavone and colleagues[7] found the following signs and symptoms: ataxia (47%), hypotonia (41%), seizures (29%), thalamic syndrome (23%), hemiparesis (23%), cranial nerve palsy (18%), headache (18%), fever (12%), and ptosis (6%).

Respiratory failure secondary to brainstem involvement or severely impaired consciousness has been reported in 11% to 16% of patients in previous studies.[13,39] In a study where all children met the consensus definition of ADEM, the numbers of patients with respiratory failure were strikingly similar (11%).[7] A recent study investigating the necessity of intensive care unit (ICU) admissions for patients with ADEM found that 25% of patients with ADEM required an ICU admission, with an incidence of 0.5 per million children per year.[40] Rates of ICU admission may be higher than previously expected, considering the mandatory inclusion of altered mental status. In the study by Pavone and colleagues,[7] ICU admissions were necessary in 41% of patients with ADEM at some point during their clinical course.

IMMUNOPATHOGENESIS

The precise mechanisms implicated in ADEM are not well known, and the relationship between the pathogenesis of ADEM and MS continues to remain a matter of controversy. There is a general consensus that ADEM is an immune-mediated disorder resulting from an autoimmune reaction to myelin.[5] An autoimmune pathogenesis is supported by the pathologic similarities between ADEM and the experimental allergic encephalomyelitis (EAE) model,[41,42] which is a demyelinating disease that may be induced in a variety of animal species after immunization with myelin proteins or peptides.

There are 2 basic mechanisms proposed to cause ADEM,[5] both of which rely on the exposure of the immune system to an antigenic challenge (ie, viral, bacterial, or exposure to degradation products via immunization):

1. Molecular mimicry theory.[43] This theory relies on the idea that myelin antigens (for example, myelin basic protein [MBP], proteolipid protein, and myelin oligodendrocyte protein) could share a structural similarity with antigenic determinants on the infecting pathogen. The infected host mounts an immune response producing antiviral antibodies that are thought to cross-react with myelin antigens that share a similar structure, inadvertently producing an autoimmune response. Myelin proteins have shown resemblance to several viral sequences, and cross-reactivity of immune cells has been demonstrated in several studies. T cells to human herpesvirus-6 (HHV-6),[44] coronavirus,[45] influenza virus,[46] and Epstein-Barr virus (EBV)[47] have been shown to cross-react with MBP antigens. Furthermore, enhanced MBP reactive T-cell responses have been demonstrated in patients with postinfectious ADEM,[48,49] and enhanced anti-MBP antibodies have been shown in patients with postvaccinial ADEM following vaccination with Semple rabies vaccine.[50,51]

2. Inflammatory cascade theory. Nervous system tissue is thought to be damaged secondary to viral infection, resulting in the leakage of myelin-based antigens into the systemic circulation through an impaired blood-brain barrier.[5] These antigens promote a T-cell response after processing in the lymphatic organs, which in turn causes secondary damage to the nervous system tissue through an inflammatory response.[5] This theory is supported by the Theiler murine encephalomyelitis virus (TMEV)-induced demyelinating disease model,[52] which is a biphasic disease of the CNS whereby direct infection of neurotropic TMEV picornavirus results in an initial CNS injury followed by a secondary autoimmune response.[53,54] However, this model has been criticized for its superficial resemblance to ADEM, as ADEM is not thought to be due to a direct viral infection of the CNS. It is more likely that the nervous system tissue damage proposed by this theory is indirect, through the release of multiple cytokines and chemokines in response to the initial infection. The role of chemokines, particularly interleukin-6, tumor necrosis factor α, and matrix metalloproteinase 9, have been hypothesized to play a role in ADEM,[55,56] and the spectrum of chemokines found to be elevated in ADEM may differ from that in MS.[57]

As expected by the currently proposed mechanisms discussed here, ADEM is frequently preceded by an infection or recent vaccination.[58] However, in most cases investigations fail to identify the precise infectious agent responsible.[3] Viruses that have been implicated in promoting the immune response responsible for ADEM include herpes simplex virus, human immunodeficiency virus, HHV-6, mumps, measles, rubella, varicella, influenza, enterovirus, hepatitis A, coxsackie, EBV, and cytomegalovirus.[59–70] It has been proposed that the risk of ADEM is highest with measles and rubella, with the risk after infection with these viruses being 1:1000 and 1:20,000, respectively.[71] Other infectious agents that have been linked to ADEM include group A β-hemolytic streptococcal infection,[72,73] pertussis,[74] *Mycoplasma pneumonia*,[75,76] *Borrelia burgdorferi*,[77] *Legionella*,[75,78] Rickettsiae,[79] and *Plasmodium falciparum* and *Plasmodium vivax* malaria.[80]

Approximately 5% to 12% of patients with ADEM have a history of vaccination within the month before presentation.[11,13] The only vaccination that has been epidemiologically and pathologically proven to be associated with ADEM is the Semple form of the rabies vaccine.[81,82] Other vaccinations that have been reported to have a temporal association with the onset of ADEM include hepatitis B, pertussis, smallpox, diphtheria, measles, mumps, rubella, human papilloma virus, pneumococcus, varicella, influenza, Japanese B encephalitis, polio, and meningococcal A and C.[11,13,83–94] The rates at which these vaccinations are reported to cause ADEM are: 1 to 2 per million for measles[94]; 1 in 3000 to 1 in 7000 for Semple rabies[81]; 1 in 25,000 for duck embryo rabies[95]; less than 1 in 75,0000 for nonneural human diploid cell rabies[93]; 0.2 per 100,000 for inactivated mouse brain–derived Japanese B encephalitis[87]; 3 in 665,000 for smallpox[83]; and 0.9 per 100,000 for diphtheria, pertussis, and tetanus.[94] On rare occasions ADEM has been also reported following organ transplantation.[96,97]

Recently, studies have investigated the role of genetics in predisposing patients to ADEM. Multiple human leukocyte antigen (HLA) alleles have been found to occur at a higher frequency in patients with ADEM, including HLA-DRB1*1501, HLA-DRB5*0101, HLA-DRBQ*1503, HLA-DQA1*0102, HLA-DQB1*0602, HLA-DRB1*01, HLA-DRB*03, and HLA-DPA1*0301.[17,98,99] The exact frequency of expression of these alleles and their future clinical utility in ADEM is currently unknown.

LABORATORY FINDINGS

Laboratory findings are useful for ADEM, mainly to rule out other causes for the patient's presenting symptoms. Despite ADEM patients commonly reporting a recent infection before their neurologic presentation, only 17% have evidence of a recent infection on serology.[13]

Cerebrospinal fluid (CSF) is normal in up to 61.5% of patients with ADEM.[3,7] If patients are found to have abnormal CSF parameters, they are usually minor and nonspecific. A lymphocyte pleocytosis (usually between 50 and 180 cells/mm^2) and elevated protein (commonly 0.5–1.0 g/dL) can be seen.[7,13,22] Rarely a mild increase in glucose has been noted.[7] Oligoclonal bands, which are commonly positive in patients with MS, are less frequently observed in patients with ADEM (seen in 0%–29%).[3,7,9,13,18,22,100,101] Elevations in immunoglobulins have been reported in up to 13% of patients.[13]

An electroencephalogram (EEG) may be completed as part of the workup of a patient with ADEM following a presentation with seizures or to rule out nonconvulsive status epilepticus as a cause of the accompanying encephalopathy. Although 78% of patients with ADEM have a diffusely slow background (consistent with encephalopathy), focal slowing (10%) or focal epileptiform discharges (2%) may be seen.[13] EEG is seldom useful in establishing diagnosis.

Evoked potentials (including visual evoked potentials, brainstem auditory evoked potentials, and somatosensory evoked potentials) may be normal, depending on the location of brain lesions. Abnormal visual evoked potentials have been reported in up to 12% of patients.[7]

NEUROIMAGING
Computed Tomography of the Brain

There are few studies that comment on computed tomography (CT) findings in patients with ADEM, namely because these patients are more commonly imaged with more sensitive imaging modalities, in addition to the concern of radiation exposure in the pediatric population. Most studies indicate that CT is unrevealing when completed early in the disease and that this imaging modality is insensitive for smaller demyelinating lesions.[3,5,34] The most commonly reported abnormalities are discrete hypodense areas within cerebral white matter and juxtacortical areas.[7,13] However, some investigators have reported high rates of CT-scan abnormalities in patients with ADEM. Tenembaum and colleagues[13] reported abnormal findings in 78% of patients after a mean interval of 6.5 days from symptom onset. In an article by Pavone and colleagues,[7] where all patients met the new consensus criteria for ADEM, abnormal CT scans were reported in 86% of their patients when performed after a mean interval of 2.5 days from initial neurologic presentation.

Magnetic Resonance Imaging of the Brain and Spine

Magnetic resonance (MR) imaging of the brain is the most important paraclinical tool available to aid in the diagnosis of ADEM and to distinguish the clinical presentation from other inflammatory and noninflammatory neurologic diseases. Since the advent of MR imaging, many studies have evaluated the radiologic appearance of ADEM in children and adults.[2,5,7,9,12–14,19–26,34,102–110] From the listed studies, the typical MR imaging findings described in ADEM are widespread, bilateral, asymmetric patchy areas of homogeneous or slightly inhomogeneous increased signal intensity on T2-weighted imaging within the white matter, deep gray nuclei, and spinal cord. Within the white matter, juxtacortical and deep white matter is involved more frequently than is periventricular white matter, which is an important contrast to patients with MS. In addition, lesions involving the corpus callosum, which are considered typical in MS, are rarely seen in ADEM. Infratentorial lesions are common, including the brainstem and cerebellar white matter. With respect to lesion size and morphology, variation is seen, ranging from small, round lesions to large, amorphous, and irregular lesions. Unenhanced T1-weighted images reveal that lesions are typically inconspicuous unless the lesions are large, in which case a faint hypodensity is seen within the affected areas. These lesions typically appear simultaneously with clinical presentation. However, delayed appearance of abnormalities up to 1 month after clinical onset has been described, so a normal MR image within the first days after symptom onset suggestive of ADEM does not exclude the diagnosis. Contrast enhancement in ADEM is variable and has been reported in 30% to 100% of patients with ADEM, in nonspecific patterns (nodular, diffuse, gyral, complete, or incomplete ring).

In the past 10 years, only 4 studies have described the MR imaging appearance of cohorts of children who uniformly meet the current consensus criteria for ADEM. A summary of the neuroimaging findings of selected studies completed within the last 10 years is presented in **Table 1.** **Fig. 1** displays the potential location sites for demyelination as described below.

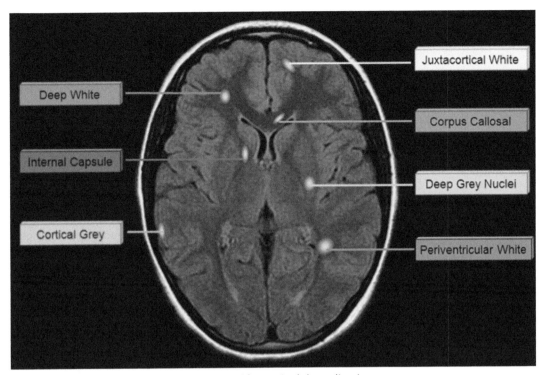

Fig. 1. Potential location of lesions in patients with acquired demyelination.

Mikaeloff and colleagues[22] qualitatively described the radiologic appearance of 108 children with monophasic ADEM. In their cohort, juxtacortical white matter, deep gray matter, and infratentorial structures were affected with approximately 60% frequency. Lesions were less commonly seen in periventricular white matter, cortical gray matter (18%), and spinal cord (12%). Deep white matter lesions and cerebellar lesions were not specifically described, thus their frequency of involvement cannot be commented on. Almost half of the children in their cohort had at least 9 lesions, but comprehensive lesion counts were not reported. Bilateral lesions were described in 81% of their patient cohort. "Large lesions" (>2 cm) were present in 72% of cases, but there was no comment made about other lesion sizes. Nearly half of their patients met at least 3 Barkoff criteria. Of the patients who received gadolinium, only 16% displayed enhancing lesions. However, there was no comment about the pattern of enhancement.

A smaller study was more recently published by Vistudtibhan and colleagues.[26] Although 16 patients met the initial criteria for ADEM, 3 of these patients subsequently fulfilled criteria for relapsing-remitting MS. Based on the reported imaging characteristics described for the remaining 13 patients with monophasic ADEM, the brain region most commonly involved was the subcortical/periventricular region (88%). A distinction was not made between subcortical lesions and periventricular lesions, which would have been useful considering that the literature seems to favor periventricular lesions as being more characteristic of MS in comparison with ADEM.[25,111] Similar to the results from Mikaeloff and colleagues,[22] brainstem and deep gray nuclei were also commonly affected, with a frequency of 69% and 50%, respectively. Lesions involving cortex and juxtacortex were seen less frequently (31%); however, there was no distinction made between these 2 areas. The cerebellum was involved in approximately one-third of the patients. Spinal cord involvement was much higher than that reported by Mikaeloff and colleagues,[22] with a frequency of approximately 60%. There was no comment made about lesion size, nor the frequency of gadolinium enhancement.

Data from the authors' group was published in 2009.[25] The characteristics of lesions in 20 children with monophasic ADEM were quantitatively assessed. When the data are viewed qualitatively (ie, displaying the number of patients having at least 1 lesion in any given location), lesions appear to be relatively common in all regions of the brain. However, when the mean lesion counts are evaluated for each region (**Table 2**), a difference in the

Table 2
Quantitative lesion parameters in children with ADEM from Callen and colleagues[25]

	Lesion Counts		
	Mean	Minimum[a]	Maximum
Deep white matter	6.8	0 (4)	29
Juxtacortical white matter	9.7	0 (2)	38
Periventricular white matter	1.4	0 (9)	10
Callosal white matter	1.1	0 (7)	4
Cortical gray matter	7.5	0 (4)	35
Deep gray matter	2.6	0 (6)	8
Brainstem	1.7	0 (6)	6
Cerebellar	0.8	0 (11)	4
Small	15.8	2	41
Medium	5.6	0 (3)	18
Large	3.5	0 (6)	18
Total	24.8	3	62

Small: <1 cm axial, <1.5 cm longitudinal; Medium: 1–2 cm axial, 1.5–2.5 cm longitudinal; Large: >2 cm axial, >2.5 cm longitudinal.

[a] Number in parentheses represents the number of children with ADEM (n = 20) who had zero lesions in this category.

Data from Callen DJ, Shroff MM, Branson HM, et al. Role of MRI in the differentiation of ADEM from MS in children. Neurology 2009;72:968–73.

lesion distribution is apparent. Similar to the findings by Mikaeloff and colleagues[22] and Vistudtibhan and colleagues,[26] lesions were more commonly seen in the deep white matter and juxtacortical white matter than in the periventricular white matter. In contrast to the previous studies by both groups, lesions were commonly found to impinge on the cortical ribbon. Another consistent result between all 3 studies was the frequent involvement of the deep gray nuclei. Although the mean lesion count was only 2.5, only 30% of the patients had no deep gray involvement. Infratentorial regions were commonly involved, as reported in the other studies, but the mean lesion counts in these regions were low. With respect to lesion size, small (<1 cm axial, <1.5 cm longitudinal) and medium (1–2 cm axial, 1.5–2.5 cm longitudinal) lesions were found in all patients, but 70% also had large (>2 cm axial, >2.5 cm longitudinal) lesions. This amount is nearly identical to the number of "large lesions" seen by Mikaeloff and

colleagues.[22] Finally, only 11 of the authors' patients received gadolinium, 5 of whom (45%) displayed enhancement.

In addition to describing lesion characteristics, many investigators have previously attempted to divide patients into groups showing similar radiologic features. Application of these classification criteria to the authors' cohort has proved to be unsuccessful. **Figs. 2–5** display the variety of lesion patterns displayed in selected cases of this patient population. When one considers the multitude of causes that have been reported to produce an ADEM phenotype, the lack of a consistent pattern is not surprising. However, despite the lack of subgroups, there do appear to be some consistent radiologic findings in ADEM (**Box 2**).

Most recently, a prospective study published by Pavone and colleagues[7] described the radiologic appearance of 17 patients with ADEM. It should be noted that patients who were included before 1998 received imaging on a 0.5-T machine, whereas those after 1998 received imaging on a 1.5-T machine. The patients were classified according to the pattern of abnormalities seen on MR imaging into the following groups previously described by Tenembaum and colleagues[13]: ADEM with large, confluent, or tumefactive lesions (23%); ADEM with small (<5 mm) lesions (53%); and ADEM with additional symmetric capsulobithalamic involvement (23%). The frequency of patients in each group is similar to that seen by Tenembaum and colleagues,[13] with the exception of an increased frequency of thalamic involvement (12% vs 23%), but is strikingly different to the frequency with which large lesions were seen by both Mikaeloff and colleagues[22] and the authors' group[25]; this may be secondary to the different size cutoff for "large lesions" used by Pavone and colleagues,[7] which was not specified. With respect to lesion number, it was noted that all patients had more than 3 identifiable lesions, but no further quantification was made. There was no comment on the specific location of these lesions, with the exception that spinal cord lesions were not identified in any of the patients in this series. Gadolinium enhancement was noted in 18% of the children, with all patients having an open-ring pattern of enhancement.

Imaging after a short period of treatment usually shows a decrease in the size and number of lesions and a change in signal intensity of lesions, paralleling clinical improvement (**Fig. 6**). Complete resolution has been noted in up to 70% of patients within months of presentation; however, residual deficits may persist in up to one-third of patients 2 years after ADEM onset.[25]

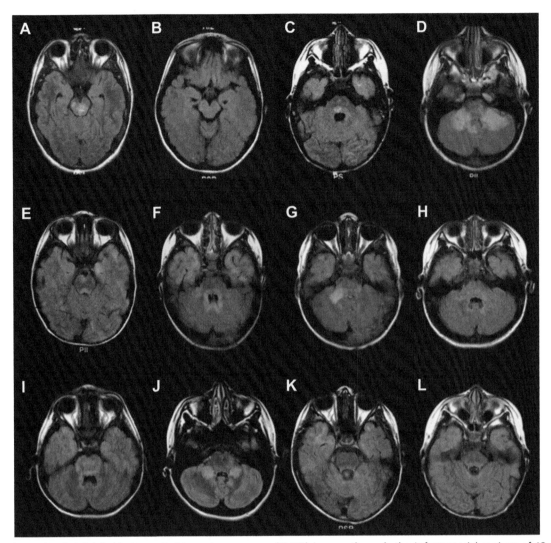

Fig. 2. (*A–L*) Axial fluid-attenuated inversion recovery (FLAIR) images through the infratentorial regions of 12 children with ADEM.

Advanced MR Imaging Modalities

Advanced MR imaging modalities, including magnetization transfer (MY) imaging, diffusion-weighted (DW) imaging, diffusion tensor (DT) imaging, MR spectroscopy, positron emission tomography (PET), and single-photon emission computed tomography (SPECT), have recently been introduced in the diagnostic workup in some settings where there is access to sophisticated neuroimaging. There is increasing literature available on the findings on these modalities in patients with ADEM; however, most studies were completed before the introduction of the new diagnostic criteria for the disorder.

MT imaging

It is widely becoming recognized in MS literature that conventional neuroimaging does not capture the extent of damage of the disorder. With newer imaging modalities, what appeared as "normal appearing" white matter on conventional imaging shows abnormalities on more advanced techniques, such as MT imaging.[112] In ADEM it was believed that MT imaging would play a role, particularly early in the disease course at a time when conventional imaging may be unrevealing. However, studies thus far have shown that, unlike in MS, MT imaging fails to reveal abnormalities in normal-appearing brain tissue in these patients.[113]

DW imaging

Studies investigating the role of DW imaging in patients with ADEM have shown that DW changes are variable and highly dependent on the stage of the disease.[103] If DW imaging is completed within the first 7 days of clinical onset, a pattern of

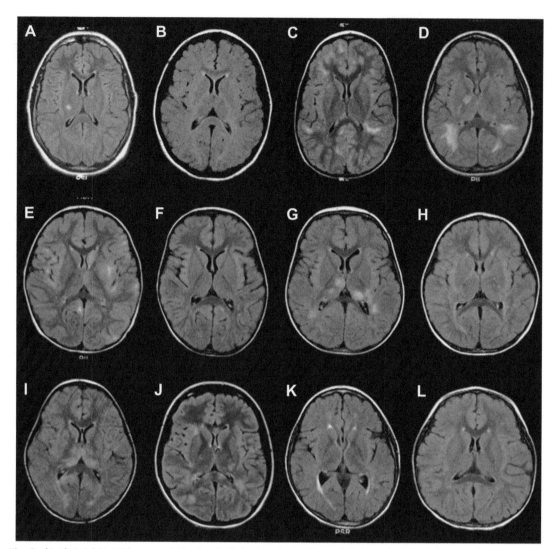

Fig. 3. (*A–L*) Axial FLAIR images at the level of the basal ganglia and thalamus of 12 children with ADEM.

restricted diffusion may sometimes be seen, which subsequently changes to a pattern of increased diffusion thereafter.[103,114] Balasubramanya and colleagues[103] hypothesized that during the acute stage (within the first 7 days of disease onset), there is swelling of myelin sheaths, reduced vascular supply, and dense inflammatory cell infiltration, which may account for the initial reduced diffusivity, whereas in the subacute stage (after 7 days), demyelination and edema cause expansion of the extracellular space resulting in increased diffusivity. In the authors' experience, diffusion changes are variable. Most commonly T2 shine-through is seen, rather than true restricted diffusion (**Fig. 7**).

DT imaging
Few studies have been completed that investigate the changes on DT imaging in patients with ADEM.

Recently, a study suggested that there was reduced fractional anisotropy in a patient with documented active inflammatory demyelination on neuropathology.[115] Further studies are needed to delineate the role of DT imaging in patients with ADEM.

MR spectroscopy
An increasing number of studies are being published on the role of MR spectroscopy in ADEM. Similar to findings on DW imaging, the changes on MR spectroscopy appear to be sensitive to the stage of the disease.[103,114,116,117] Within the acute phase, an elevation of lipids and reduction of myoinositol/creatinine ratio has been reported, with no change in the *N*-acetylaspartate (NAA) or choline values.[103,117] As the disease progresses, there is a reduction of NAA and an increase in

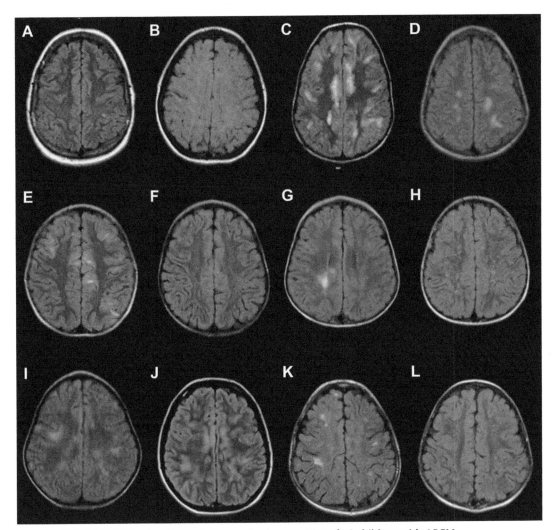

Fig. 4. (*A–L*) Axial FLAIR images through the cerebral convexities of 12 children with ADEM.

choline (with corresponding reductions in NAA/creatine and NAA/choline ratios) in regions corresponding to areas of high signal intensity on T2-weighted imaging.[103,116] These findings normalize as the clinical and conventional neuroimaging abnormalities resolve. This finding suggests a transient neuroaxonal dysfunction rather than irreversible neuroaxonal loss, and is in contrast to the situation in MS, whereby there is a prompt choline elevation caused by increased levels of the myelin breakdown products, glycerophosphocholine and phosphocholine.[116,118] These changes are also in stark contrast to those seen in intracranial tumors, which is particularly important in patients presenting with a tumefactive demyelinating lesion.

PET and SPECT

In patients with ADEM, studies investigating the role of PET have shown that despite conventional imaging showing only focal demyelinating lesions, there appears to be global and bilateral decreased cerebral metabolism.[119] SPECT imaging using ^{99m}Tc-HMPAO (D,L-hexamethylpropylene amine oxime) in patients with ADEM have consistently shown areas of hypoperfusion that are more extensive than lesions identified on conventional neuroimaging.[120–122] In one study, persistent cerebral circulatory impairment examined with SPECT using acetazolamide was thought to be a contributing factor to the persistent neurocognitive and language deficits observed in some patients within this cohort.[123] Considering that most conventional and unconventional imaging modalities do not seem to find the persistent abnormalities suggested by these studies, further investigation into the clinical role of PET and SPECT in patients with ADEM is warranted.

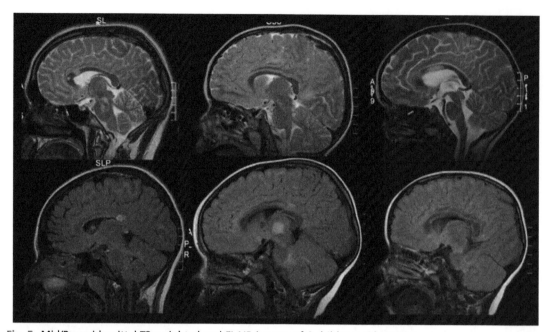

Fig. 5. Mid/Paramidsagittal T2-weighted and FLAIR images of 6 children with ADEM.

DIFFERENTIAL DIAGNOSIS

ADEM can represent a diagnostic challenge for clinicians, as many disorders (inflammatory and noninflammatory) have a similar clinical and radiologic presentation. The differential diagnosis for multifocal hyperintense lesions on neuroimaging includes an exhaustive list of potential mimickers, namely infectious, inflammatory, rheumatologic, metabolic, nutritional and degenerative entities. Despite the significant overlap in clinical and radiologic pictures of many conditions, neuroimaging can aid in narrowing the differential diagnosis.

Box 2
Proposed commonalities in ADEM MR imaging appearance

- Bilateral asymmetric/symmetric involvement (rarely unilateral)
- White matter > gray matter, but usually both affected
- Deep/juxtacortical white matter > periventricular white matter
- Both supratentorial and infratentorial lesions (less commonly either/or)
- Small > medium > large, but often all sizes are present in same patient
- Variable contrast enhancement

The first priority in a patient presenting with neurologic signs and symptoms and encephalopathy, particularly in the presence of a preceding febrile illness, is to rule out bacterial or viral infection of the CNS. Therefore, a lumbar puncture and MR imaging should be completed as soon as possible and empiric antimicrobial therapy should be considered. A lumbar puncture will likely provide the most important diagnostic clues of an infective process, but neuroimaging can also play a role. A diagnosis of meningoencephalitis can be suggested by leptomeningeal enhancement on postcontrast imaging (which is not a feature of ADEM) or stereotypical involvement of limbic structures in the case of limbic encephalitis.

After neuroimaging has been completed, the findings at the time of initial presentation may be useful. If a large tumor-like lesion is present in addition to tumefactive ADEM or MS, one should consider a benign or malignant tumor, one of the MS variants (including Schilder[124] and Marburg[125] variants), or brain abscess depending on the clinical picture. The differentiation of ADEM from tumor becomes particularly difficult in the case of ADEM-related brainstem lesions, as they are commonly associated with edema and can be easily misdiagnosed as a malignant process. In the case of tumefactive demyelination, it has been suggested that a combination of open-ring enhancement, peripheral restriction on DW imaging, venular enhancement, and presence of

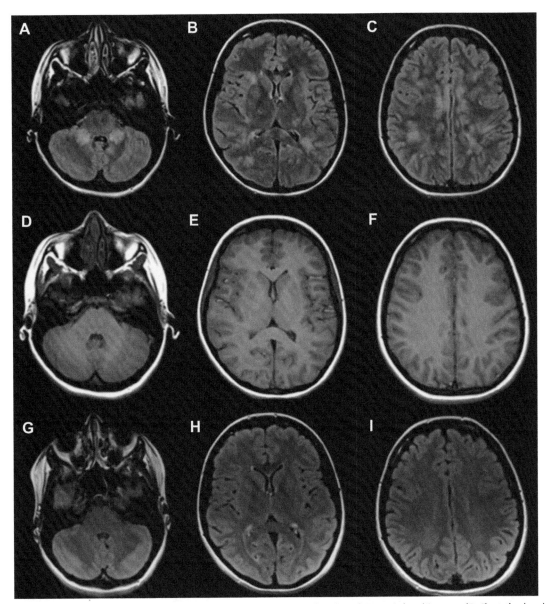

Fig. 6. Resolution of lesions on follow-up imaging. Axial FLAIR (*A–C*) and T1-weighted images (*D–F*) at the level of the cerebellar hemispheres (*A, D*), basal ganglia (*B, E*) and (*C, F*) cerebral convexities at time of presentation. Axial FLAIR images (*G–I*) depicting the same patient weeks after presentation, showing near complete resolution of lesions.

glutamine/glutamate (Glx) levels on MR spectroscopy may be helpful in differentiating ADEM from neoplastic lesions.[126]

If there is bithalamic involvement, in addition to ADEM with this radiologic representation (particularly in the case of ADEM after Japanese B encephalitis[127]) one should consider mitochondrial disorders (particularly Leigh syndrome), deep cerebral vein thrombosis, hypernatremia, Reye syndrome, Sandoff disease, and acute necrotizing encephalopathy of childhood (ANEC),

depending on the clinical picture. ANEC, which has mainly been described in Japan, Taiwan, and Korea, is an acute encephalopathy following 2 to 4 days of gastrointestinal or respiratory symptoms and fever.[128] Neuroimaging findings include multifocal, symmetric brain lesions involving the thalami, cerebral or cerebellar white matter, and brainstem.[128,129] Basal ganglia involvement, which is common in ADEM (particularly poststreptococcal ADEM[130]), may be consistent with many processes: for example, organic acidurias, mitochondrial

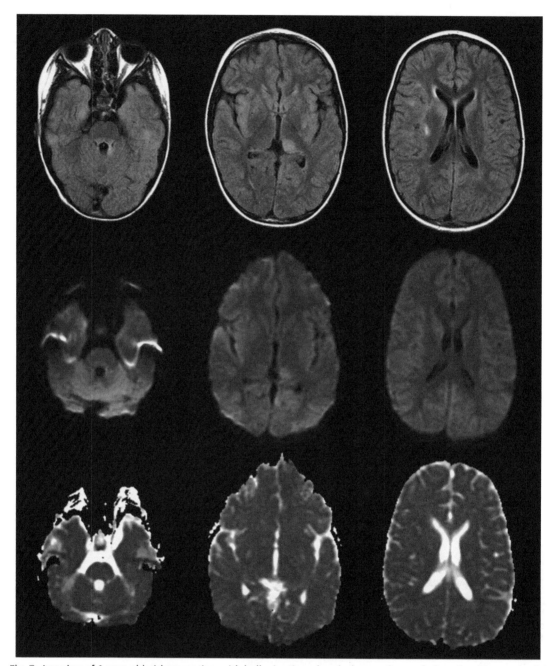

Fig. 7. Imaging of 4-year-old girl presenting with hallucinations, headaches, and encephalopathy. (*Top row*) axial FLAIR. (*Middle row*) Diffusion-weighted imaging (DWI). (*Bottom row*) Apparent diffusion coefficient map. Some of the lesions visualized on the FLAIR images are also hyperintense on DWI, but none show restricted diffusion.

disorders (particularly Leigh syndrome), and Wilson disease.

Another diagnostic consideration with a similar clinical presentation is posterior reversible encephalopathy syndrome (PRES). Although typically induced by hypertension, seizures, or immunosuppressants, a history of a preceding inciting factor may be lacking. PRES presents with reversible white matter edema that may or may not have a posterior predominance.

The enhancement pattern of the lesions may also suggest alternative diagnoses. Although ring enhancement has been reported in ADEM, one should consider brain abscess, tuberculomas, neurocystercosis, toxoplasmosis, or histoplasmosis, depending on the history.[131]

One of the most difficult differentiations is between ADEM and other demyelinating disorders, namely MS. The authors attempted to describe means by which patients with ADEM could be differentiated from patients with MS based on their radiologic findings.[25] Previous descriptive studies in which the MR imaging appearances of patients with ADEM were compared with MR imaging scans obtained during the first attack of MS determined that these two clinical scenarios could not reliably be distinguished. After retrospective analysis of MR imaging scans at first attack in 28 children with MS and 20 children with ADEM, the following criteria were reliable in distinguishing patients with MS from those with ADEM, with a sensitivity of 81% and specificity of 95%: any 2 of (1) absence of diffuse bilateral lesion pattern, (2) presence of black holes, and (3) presence of 2 or more periventricular lesions.[25]

TREATMENT

There is no standard treatment regimen for ADEM. Most of the data describing the treatment of patients with ADEM are derived from case reports and some small series. To date, no randomized controlled trials for treatment of ADEM have been completed in either the pediatric or adult population. Most treatment approaches use some form of nonspecific immunosuppressant therapy, including corticosteroids, intravenous immunoglobulin (IVIg), or plasmapheresis. There are no studies comparing the efficacy of the different immunomodulatory therapies.

Corticosteroids are the most widely used and most ubiquitously reported therapy for patients with ADEM. In a recently proposed algorithm for treatment in ADEM, steroids were considered the first line in therapy.[132] Throughout the literature, there is great variation in the dose and formulation of steroids used, the routes of administration followed (oral or intravenous), and tapering regimens described. Most groups use steroids at very high doses. The most commonly used treatment protocols include intravenous methylprednisolone, 10 to 30 mg/kg/d up to a maximum daily dose of 1 g or dexamethasone (1 mg/kg) for 3 to 5 days followed by an oral steroid taper over 4 to 6 weeks.[3,8,9,13,133] There is some suggestion in comparative studies that methylprednisolone-treated patients had significantly better Expanded Disability Status Scale scores after treatment than those administered dexamethasone.[13] It has also been reported that there is an increased risk of relapse with steroid tapers of less than 3 weeks.[8,14] Corticosteroids are very effective for symptom resolution in

ADEM, with 50% to 80% of patients having a full recovery.[8,9,13] Recovery is typically seen over a few days, with the more severely affected patients requiring weeks or months for recuperation. Despite their efficacy, steroids are not without risk. Side effects of corticosteroids include gastric hemorrhage and perforation, hyperglycemia, hypokalemia, hypertension, facial flushing, and mood lability, even with short-term use. Therefore, it is advisable to administer gastric protective measures during the short period that patients are being treated with corticosteroids.

There are multiple case reports of successful use of IVIg, either alone,[134,135] in combination with corticosteroids,[136] after failed intravenous pulse steroids,[137–139] or in recurrent demyelination.[69,140] The reported dosing for IVIg is more consistent than that for steroids, with a total dose of 1 to 2 g/kg as a single dose or over 3 to 5 days. IVIg is generally well tolerated.

Plasmapheresis theoretically works to remove autoantibodies that are presumably triggering demyelination seen in ADEM, or to shift the dynamics of the interactions of B and T cells within the immune system. Its use has been reported in several case studies, typically in severe cases of ADEM when steroid treatment has failed. Complete recovery has been reported in some patients with ADEM.[141–143] In patients with CNS demyelination (including patients with ADEM), 40% had moderate to marked improvement following a mean number of 7 exchanges.[144] It has been suggested that plasmapheresis is more effective when given early in the course.[145] Unfortunately, it is often used as a last resort, owing to the resources needed for treatment implementation. Side effects noted include hypotension, anemia, and headache.

Patients with ADEM have been symptomatically managed with decompressive hemicraniectomy as a life-saving measure when there is massive cerebral edema that is refractory to medical management; however, this is an uncommon scenario.[146,147]

PROGNOSIS

ADEM has a monophasic course in 70% to 90% of cases.[7–9,13,15,22,61,148–151] Typically prognosis is excellent in patients with ADEM.[8,13] In previous studies, a full recovery has been noted in approximately 70% to 90% of patients, characteristically within 6 months of onset.[3,8,9,11–17] Studies including patients who meet criteria according to Krupp and colleagues[18] have shown similar results.[7,22,26] Severe complications (including death) are rare in the pediatric population,[14,26,152] unless measles is the inciting factor.[62,153,154] The most common focal neurologic deficits following ADEM include focal motor deficits (ranging from mild clumsiness to hemiparesis), visual impairment, behavioral or cognitive problems, or epilepsy.[93] However, more recently there has been increased awareness regarding the frequency of behavioral and subtle neurocognitive deficits in patients with a previous diagnosis of ADEM. Subtle neurocognitive deficits have been identified in attention, executive function, and behavior when evaluated years after ADEM in up to 50% to 60% of patients.[7,155–157] These effects appear to be more prominent in patients who have a younger age of onset (<5 years).[155]

VARIANTS

More aggressive variants of ADEM have been described in the literature, including acute hemorrhagic leukoencephalitis, acute hemorrhagic encephalomyelitis, and acute necrotizing hemorrhagic leukoencephalitis of Weston Hurst. All of these variants describe hyperacutely presenting, rapidly progressive, fulminant inflammatory and hemorrhagic demyelinating disorders of the CNS that are usually triggered by an upper respiratory tract infection. In one large cohort, these hemorrhagic variants had been described in 2% of patients with ADEM.[13] On MR imaging, lesions tend to be large, with perilesional edema and mass effect.[158,159] Death had previously been described in a majority of these patients within 1 week of onset; however, there is increasing evidence of favorable outcomes if early and aggressive treatment with immunomodulatory agents is used.[13,160–162] These variants are covered in more detail elsewhere in this issue.

ADEM has a monophasic course in a majority of patients; however, recurrent and multiphasic cases have been documented.[8,9,13,15,22,61,148–151] As such, the International Pediatric MS Study Group[18] also proposed a consensus definition for recurrent ADEM (RADEM) and multiphasic ADEM (MADEM). The difference between recurrent and multiphasic ADEM hinges on whether there is involvement of a new brain region, as suggested by clinical history, examination, or neuroimaging (MADEM), or if there is recapitulation of the prior illness (RADEM). As with the first episode, polyfocal clinical symptoms and encephalopathy are mandatory.

Notwithstanding the new consensus definitions for RADEM and MADEM, there continues to be controversy regarding the existence of these entities, as the monophasic course of ADEM is considered by some to be a hallmark of this disorder. The rates of these entities reported in the literature have varied depending on the ADEM definition used, the period of inclusion or follow-up, and the study design. Considering that previous studies used dissimilar definitions of ADEM (which differ from the definition proposed), it may be that the inclusion of patients with monofocal presentation or those lacking encephalopathy will bias these studies toward describing a fundamentally different cohort. In addition, in the studies describing recurrent and multiphasic cases of ADEM, different diagnostic criteria for relapses were used. As the new definition for ADEM states that any new symptoms within 3 months from onset should be considered part of the initial attack, it is likely that some of the patients deemed to have relapsed may no longer meet criteria for either multiphasic or relapsing ADEM.[18]

Despite these issues, previously reported rates of a recurrent or multiphasic course have ranged from 5% to 30%.[3,8,9,11–17] Since implementation of the new consensus criteria, 3 studies have commented on recurrence rates in patients with ADEM. Visudtibhan and colleagues[26] followed their patients for a mean of 5.8 years and ultimately diagnosed 3 of 15 children with MS. None were diagnosed with MADEM or RADEM by the end of the follow-up period.[26] Mikaeloff and colleagues[22] found a recurrence rate in 18% of their patients after a mean follow-up period of 5.4 ± 3.3 years. All of these patients were noted to have a second attack at a different site in the CNS. An increased risk of a second attack has been associated with previous demyelination episodes in the family, first presentation with optic neuritis, fulfilling MS Barkoff criteria on initial neuroimaging, and absence of sequelae after the acute episode.[22] Considering that the first 3 risk factors are known predictive factors for further relapses in MS, it was surmised that this strengthened the link between relapsing disease after ADEM onset and MS.[22] The final study by Pavone and colleagues[7] found a relapse rate of 12% after a follow-up period ranging from 4.4 to 17.1 years. It is not clear whether these patients would have met criteria for either RADEM or MADEM considering that the presence of encephalopathy was not noted in either patient, nor was the location of their lesions on MR imaging. Considering the results of these 3 studies, it may be that Mikaeloff and colleagues[22] were correct in suggesting a strong link between recurrent ADEM and MS. Long-term prospective follow-up studies of patients diagnosed with ADEM by the new consensus criteria will provide important information regarding the natural history of ADEM and its potential relationship with MS.

REFERENCES

1. Nasr JT, Andriola MR, Coyle PK. ADEM: literature review and case report of acute psychosis presentation. Pediatr Neurol 2000;22:8–18.
2. Khong PL, Ho HK, Cheng PW, et al. Childhood acute disseminated encephalomyelitis: the role of brain and spinal cord MRI. Pediatr Radiol 2002; 32:59–66.
3. Gupte G, Stonehouse M, Wassmer E, et al. Acute disseminated encephalomyelitis: a review of 18 cases in childhood. J Paediatr Child Health 2003; 39:336–42.
4. Caldemeyer KS, Smith RR, Harris TM, et al. MRI in acute disseminated encephalomyelitis. Neuroradiology 1994;36:216–20.
5. Rossi A. Imaging of acute disseminated encephalomyelitis. Neuroimaging Clin N Am 2008;18: 149–61, ix.
6. Menge T, Hemmer B, Nessler S, et al. Acute disseminated encephalomyelitis: an update. Arch Neurol 2005;62:1673–80.
7. Pavone P, Pettoello-Mantovano M, Le Pira A, et al. Acute disseminated encephalomyelitis: a long-term prospective study and meta-analysis. Neuropediatrics 2010;41:246–55.
8. Dale RC, de Sousa C, Chong WK, et al. Acute disseminated encephalomyelitis, multiphasic disseminated encephalomyelitis and multiple sclerosis in children. Brain 2000;123(Pt 12):2407–22.
9. Hynson JL, Kornberg AJ, Coleman LT, et al. Clinical and neuroradiologic features of acute disseminated encephalomyelitis in children. Neurology 2001;56:1308–12.
10. Schwarz S, Mohr A, Knauth M, et al. Acute disseminated encephalomyelitis: a follow-up study of 40 adult patients. Neurology 2001;56:1313–8.
11. Leake JA, Albani S, Kao AS, et al. Acute disseminated encephalomyelitis in childhood: epidemiologic, clinical and laboratory features. Pediatr Infect Dis J 2004;23:756–64.
12. Murthy SN, Faden HS, Cohen ME, et al. Acute disseminated encephalomyelitis in children. Pediatrics 2002;110:e21.
13. Tenembaum S, Chamoles N, Fejerman N. Acute disseminated encephalomyelitis: a long-term follow-up study of 84 pediatric patients. Neurology 2002; 59:1224–31.
14. Anlar B, Basaran C, Kose G, et al. Acute disseminated encephalomyelitis in children: outcome and prognosis. Neuropediatrics 2003;34:194–9.
15. Mikaeloff Y, Suissa S, Vallee L, et al. First episode of acute CNS inflammatory demyelination in childhood: prognostic factors for multiple sclerosis and disability. J Pediatr 2004;144:246–52.
16. Hung KL, Liao HT, Tsai ML. The spectrum of postinfectious encephalomyelitis. Brain Dev 2001;23:42–5.
17. Idrissova Zh R, Boldyreva MN, Dekonenko EP, et al. Acute disseminated encephalomyelitis in children: clinical features and HLA-DR linkage. Eur J Neurol 2003;10:537–46.
18. Krupp LB, Banwell B, Tenembaum S. Consensus definitions proposed for pediatric multiple sclerosis and related disorders. Neurology 2007;68:S7–12.
19. Richer LP, Sinclair DB, Bhargava R. Neuroimaging features of acute disseminated encephalomyelitis in childhood. Pediatr Neurol 2005;32:30–6.
20. Madan S, Aneja S, Tripathi RP, et al. Acute disseminated encephalomyelitis—a case series. Indian Pediatr 2005;42:367–71.
21. Singhi PD, Ray M, Singhi S, et al. Acute disseminated encephalomyelitis in North Indian children: clinical profile and follow-up. J Child Neurol 2006; 21:851–7.
22. Mikaeloff Y, Caridade G, Husson B, et al. Acute disseminated encephalomyelitis cohort study: prognostic factors for relapse. Eur J Paediatr Neurol 2007;11:90–5.
23. Atzori M, Battistella PA, Perini P, et al. Clinical and diagnostic aspects of multiple sclerosis and acute monophasic encephalomyelitis in pediatric patients: a single centre prospective study. Mult Scler 2009; 15:363–70.
24. Alper G, Heyman R, Wang L. Multiple sclerosis and acute disseminated encephalomyelitis diagnosed in children after long-term follow-up: comparison of presenting features. Dev Med Child Neurol 2009;51:480–6.
25. Callen DJ, Shroff MM, Branson HM, et al. Role of MRI in the differentiation of ADEM from MS in children. Neurology 2009;72:968–73.
26. Visudtibhan A, Tuntiyathorn L, Vaewpanich J, et al. Acute disseminated encephalomyelitis: a 10-year cohort study in Thai children. Eur J Paediatr Neurol 2010;14:513–8.
27. Torisu H, Kira R, Ishizaki Y, et al. Clinical study of childhood acute disseminated encephalomyelitis, multiple sclerosis, and acute transverse myelitis in Fukuoka Prefecture, Japan. Brain Dev 2010;32: 454–62.
28. Banwell B, Kennedy J, Sadovnick D, et al. Incidence of acquired demyelination of the CNS in Canadian children. Neurology 2009;72:232–9.
29. Khurana DS, Melvin JJ, Kothare SV, et al. Acute disseminated encephalomyelitis in children: discordant neurologic and neuroimaging abnormalities and response to plasmapheresis. Pediatrics 2005; 116:431–6.
30. Suppiej A, Vittorini R, Fontanin M, et al. Acute disseminated encephalomyelitis in children: focus on relapsing patients. Pediatr Neurol 2008;39:12–7.
31. Weng WC, Peng SS, Lee WT, et al. Acute disseminated encephalomyelitis in children: one medical center experience. Acta Paediatr Taiwan 2006;47:67–71.

32. Lin CH, Jeng JS, Hsieh ST, et al. Acute disseminated encephalomyelitis: a follow-up study in Taiwan. J Neurol Neurosurg Psychiatry 2007;78:162–7.

33. Jayakrishnan MP, Krishnakumar P. Clinical profile of acute disseminated encephalomyelitis in children. J Pediatr Neurosci 2010;5:111–4.

34. Daoud E, Chabchoub I, Neji H, et al. How MRI can contribute to the diagnosis of acute demyelinating encephalomyelitis in children. Neurosciences (Riyadh) 2011;16:137–45.

35. Marchioni E, Ravaglia S, Piccolo G, et al. Postinfectious inflammatory disorders: subgroups based on prospective follow-up. Neurology 2005;65:1057–65.

36. Amit R, Shapira Y, Blank A, et al. Acute, severe, central and peripheral nervous system combined demyelination. Pediatr Neurol 1986;2:47–50.

37. Amit R, Glick B, Itzchak Y, et al. Acute severe combined demyelination. Childs Nerv Syst 1992;8:354–6.

38. Nadkarni N, Lisak RP. Guillain-Barré syndrome (GBS) with bilateral optic neuritis and central white matter disease. Neurology 1993;43:842–3.

39. Wingerchuk DM. Postinfectious encephalomyelitis. Curr Neurol Neurosci Rep 2003;3:256–64.

40. Absoud M, Parslow R, Wassmer E, et al. Severe acute disseminated encephalomyelitis: a paediatric intensive care population-based study. Mult Scler 2011;17:1258–61.

41. Rivers TM, Sprunt DH, Berry GP. Observations on attempts to produce acute disseminated encephalomyelitis in monkeys. J Exp Med 1933;58:39–53.

42. Rivers TM, Schwentker FF. Encephalomyelitis accompanied by myelin destruction experimentally produced in monkeys. J Exp Med 1935;61:689–702.

43. Wucherpfennig KW, Strominger JL. Molecular mimicry in T cell-mediated autoimmunity: viral peptides activate human T cell clones specific for myelin basic protein. Cell 1995;80:695–705.

44. Tejada-Simon MV, Zang YC, Hong J, et al. Cross-reactivity with myelin basic protein and human herpesvirus-6 in multiple sclerosis. Ann Neurol 2003;53:189–97.

45. Talbot PJ, Paquette JS, Ciurli C, et al. Myelin basic protein and human coronavirus 229E cross-reactive T cells in multiple sclerosis. Ann Neurol 1996;39:233–40.

46. Markovic-Plese S, Hemmer B, Zhao Y, et al. High level of cross-reactivity in influenza virus hemagglutinin-specific CD4+ T-cell response: implications for the initiation of autoimmune response in multiple sclerosis. J Neuroimmunol 2005;169:31–8.

47. Lang HL, Jacobsen H, Ikemizu S, et al. A functional and structural basis for TCR cross-reactivity in multiple sclerosis. Nat Immunol 2002;3:940–3.

48. Pohl-Koppe A, Burchett SK, Thiele EA, et al. Myelin basic protein reactive Th2 T cells are found in acute disseminated encephalomyelitis. J Neuroimmunol 1998;91:19–27.

49. Jorens PG, VanderBorght A, Ceulemans B, et al. Encephalomyelitis-associated antimyelin autoreactivity induced by streptococcal exotoxins. Neurology 2000;54:1433–41.

50. Ubol S, Hemachudha T, Whitaker JN, et al. Antibody to peptides of human myelin basic protein in post-rabies vaccine encephalomyelitis sera. J Neuroimmunol 1990;26:107–11.

51. O'Connor KC, Chitnis T, Griffin DE, et al. Myelin basic protein-reactive autoantibodies in the serum and cerebrospinal fluid of multiple sclerosis patients are characterized by low-affinity interactions. J Neuroimmunol 2003;136:140–8.

52. Lipton HL. Theiler's virus infection in mice: an unusual biphasic disease process leading to demyelination. Infect Immun 1975;11:1147–55.

53. Miller SD, Vanderlugt CL, Begolka WS, et al. Persistent infection with Theiler's virus leads to CNS autoimmunity via epitope spreading. Nat Med 1997;3:1133–6.

54. Clatch RJ, Lipton HL, Miller SD. Characterization of Theiler's murine encephalomyelitis virus (TMEV)-specific delayed-type hypersensitivity responses in TMEV-induced demyelinating disease: correlation with clinical signs. J Immunol 1986;136:920–7.

55. Ichiyama T, Shoji H, Kato M, et al. Cerebrospinal fluid levels of cytokines and soluble tumour necrosis factor receptor in acute disseminated encephalomyelitis. Eur J Pediatr 2002;161:133–7.

56. Ichiyama T, Kajimoto M, Suenaga N, et al. Serum levels of matrix metalloproteinase-9 and its tissue inhibitor (TIMP-1) in acute disseminated encephalomyelitis. J Neuroimmunol 2006;172:182–6.

57. Franciotta D, Zardini E, Ravaglia S, et al. Cytokines and chemokines in cerebrospinal fluid and serum of adult patients with acute disseminated encephalomyelitis. J Neurol Sci 2006;247:202–7.

58. Johnson RT. The pathogenesis of acute viral encephalitis and postinfectious encephalomyelitis. J Infect Dis 1987;155:359–64.

59. Stuve O, Zamvil SS. Pathogenesis, diagnosis, and treatment of acute disseminated encephalomyelitis. Curr Opin Neurol 1999;12:395–401.

60. Kanzaki A, Yabuki S. Acute disseminated encephalomyelitis (ADEM) associated with cytomegalovirus infection–a case report. Rinsho Shinkeigaku 1994;34:511–3 [in Japanese].

61. Shoji H, Kusuhara T, Honda Y, et al. Relapsing acute disseminated encephalomyelitis associated with chronic Epstein-Barr virus infection: MRI findings. Neuroradiology 1992;34:340–2.

62. Johnson RT, Griffin DE, Hirsch RL, et al. Measles encephalomyelitis—clinical and immunologic studies. N Engl J Med 1984;310:137–41.

63. Saitoh A, Sawyer MH, Leake JA. Acute disseminated encephalomyelitis associated with enteroviral infection. Pediatr Infect Dis J 2004;23:1174–5.

64. El Ouni F, Hassayoun S, Gaha M, et al. Acute disseminated encephalomyelitis following herpes simplex encephalitis. Acta Neurol Belg 2010;110:340–4.

65. Tullu MS, Patil DP, Muranjan MN, et al. Human immunodeficiency virus (HIV) infection in a child presenting as acute disseminated encephalomyelitis. J Child Neurol 2011;26:99–102.

66. Narciso P, Galgani S, Del Grosso B, et al. Acute disseminated encephalomyelitis as manifestation of primary HIV infection. Neurology 2001;57:1493–6.

67. Sawanyawisuth K, Phuttharak W, Tiamkao S, et al. MRI findings in acute disseminated encephalomyelitis following varicella infection in an adult. J Clin Neurosci 2007;14:1230–3.

68. Wang GF, Li W, Li K. Acute encephalopathy and encephalitis caused by influenza virus infection. Curr Opin Neurol 2010;23:305–11.

69. Revel-Vilk S, Hurvitz H, Klar A, et al. Recurrent acute disseminated encephalomyelitis associated with acute cytomegalovirus and Epstein-Barr virus infection. J Child Neurol 2000;15:421–4.

70. Igarashi K, Kajino M, Shirai M, et al. A case of acute disseminated encephalomyelitis associated with Epstein-Barr virus infection. No To Hattatsu 2011;43:59–61 [in Japanese].

71. Tselis AC, Lisak RP. Acute disseminated encephalomyelitis. In: Antel JP, Birnbaum G, Hartung HP, et al, editors. Clinical neuroimmunology. 2nd edition. New York, NY, USA: Oxford University Press; 2005. p. 147–71.

72. Hall MC, Barton LL, Johnson MI. Acute disseminated encephalomyelitis-like syndrome following group A beta-hemolytic streptococcal infection. J Child Neurol 1998;13:354–6.

73. Ning MM, Smirnakis S, Furie KL, et al. Adult acute disseminated encephalomyelitis associated with poststreptococcal infection. J Clin Neurosci 2005;12:298–300.

74. Budan B, Ekici B, Tatli B, et al. Acute disseminated encephalomyelitis (ADEM) after pertussis infection. Ann Trop Paediatr 2011;31:269–72.

75. Easterbrook PJ, Smyth EG. Post-infectious encephalomyelitis associated with Mycoplasma pneumoniae and Legionella pneumophila infection. Postgrad Med J 1992;68:124–8.

76. Hagiwara H, Sakamoto S, Katsumata T, et al. Acute disseminated encephalomyelitis developed after Mycoplasma pneumoniae infection complicating subclinical measles infection. Intern Med 2009;48:479–83.

77. van Assen S, Bosma F, Staals LM, et al. Acute disseminated encephalomyelitis associated with Borrelia burgdorferi. J Neurol 2004;251:626–9.

78. de Lau LM, Siepman DA, Remmers MJ, et al. Acute disseminating encephalomyelitis following Legionnaires disease. Arch Neurol 2010;67:623–6.

79. Wei TY, Baumann RJ. Acute disseminated encephalomyelitis after Rocky Mountain spotted fever. Pediatr Neurol 1999;21:503–5.

80. van der Wal G, Verhagen WI, Dofferhoff AS. Neurological complications following Plasmodium falciparum infection. Neth J Med 2005;63:180–3.

81. Hemachudha T, Griffin DE, Giffels JJ, et al. Myelin basic protein as an encephalitogen in encephalomyelitis and polyneuritis following rabies vaccination. N Engl J Med 1987;316:369–74.

82. Hemachudha T, Griffin DE, Johnson RT, et al. Immunologic studies of patients with chronic encephalitis induced by post-exposure Semple rabies vaccine. Neurology 1988;38:42–4.

83. Sejvar JJ, Labutta RJ, Chapman LE, et al. Neurologic adverse events associated with smallpox vaccination in the United States, 2002-2004. JAMA 2005;294:2744–50.

84. Bomprezzi R, Wildemann B. Acute disseminated encephalomyelitis following vaccination against human papilloma virus. Neurology 2010;74:864 [author reply: 864–5].

85. Shoamanesh A, Traboulsee A. Acute disseminated encephalomyelitis following influenza vaccination. Vaccine 2011;29:8182–5.

86. Denholm JT, Neal A, Yan B, et al. Acute encephalomyelitis syndromes associated with H1N1 09 influenza vaccination. Neurology 2010;75:2246–8.

87. Takahashi H, Pool V, Tsai TF, et al. Adverse events after Japanese encephalitis vaccination: review of post-marketing surveillance data from Japan and the United States. The VAERS Working Group. Vaccine 2000;18:2963–9.

88. Ozawa H, Noma S, Yoshida Y, et al. Acute disseminated encephalomyelitis associated with poliomyelitis vaccine. Pediatr Neurol 2000;23:177–9.

89. Tourbah A, Gout O, Liblau R, et al. Encephalitis after hepatitis B vaccination: recurrent disseminated encephalitis or MS? Neurology 1999;53:396–401.

90. Karaali-Savrun F, Altintas A, Saip S, et al. Hepatitis B vaccine related-myelitis? Eur J Neurol 2001;8:711–5.

91. Py MO, Andre C. Acute disseminated encephalomyelitis and meningococcal A and C vaccine: case report. Arq Neuropsiquiatr 1997;55:632–5 [in Portuguese].

92. Murphy J, Austin J. Spontaneous infection or vaccination as cause of acute disseminated encephalomyelitis. Neuroepidemiology 1985;4:138–45.

93. Tenembaum S, Chitnis T, Ness J, et al. Acute disseminated encephalomyelitis. Neurology 2007;68:S23–36.

94. Fenichel GM. Neurological complications of immunization. Ann Neurol 1982;12:119–28.

95. Garg RK. Acute disseminated encephalomyelitis. Postgrad Med J 2003;79:11–7.

96. Horowitz MB, Comey C, Hirsch W, et al. Acute disseminated encephalomyelitis (ADEM) or ADEM-like inflammatory changes in a heart-lung transplant recipient: a case report. Neuroradiology 1995;37:434–7.

97. Re A, Giachetti R. Acute disseminated encephalomyelitis (ADEM) after autologous peripheral blood stem cell transplant for non-Hodgkin's lymphoma. Bone Marrow Transplant 1999;24:1351–4.

98. Oh HH, Kwon SH, Kim CW, et al. Molecular analysis of HLA class II-associated susceptibility to neuroinflammatory diseases in Korean children. J Korean Med Sci 2004;19:426–30.

99. Alves-Leon SV, Veluttini-Pimentel ML, Gouveia ME, et al. Acute disseminated encephalomyelitis: clinical features, HLA DRB1*1501, HLA DRB1*1503, HLA DQA1*0102, HLA DQB1*0602, and HLA DPA1*0301 allelic association study. Arq Neuropsiquiatr 2009;67:643–51.

100. Pohl D, Rostasy K, Reiber H, et al. CSF characteristics in early-onset multiple sclerosis. Neurology 2004;63:1966–7.

101. Franciotta D, Columba-Cabezas S, Andreoni L, et al. Oligoclonal IgG band patterns in inflammatory demyelinating human and mouse diseases. J Neuroimmunol 2008;200:125–8.

102. Baum PA, Barkovich AJ, Koch TK, et al. Deep gray matter involvement in children with acute disseminated encephalomyelitis. AJNR Am J Neuroradiol 1994;15:1275–83.

103. Balasubramanya KS, Kovoor JM, Jayakumar PN, et al. Diffusion-weighted imaging and proton MR spectroscopy in the characterization of acute disseminated encephalomyelitis. Neuroradiology 2007;49:177–83.

104. Brinar VV, Habek M. Monophasic acute, recurrent, and multiphasic disseminated encephalomyelitis and multiple sclerosis. Arch Neurol 2008;65:675–6 [author reply: 676].

105. Brinar VV, Habek M. Diagnostic imaging in acute disseminated encephalomyelitis. Expert Rev Neurother 2010;10:459–67.

106. Kesselring J, Miller DH, Robb SA, et al. Acute disseminated encephalomyelitis. MRI findings and the distinction from multiple sclerosis. Brain 1990;113(Pt 2):291–302.

107. Mader I, Stock KW, Ettlin T, et al. Acute disseminated encephalomyelitis: MR and CT features. AJNR Am J Neuroradiol 1996;17:104–9.

108. Panicker JN, Nagaraja D, Kovoor JM, et al. Descriptive study of acute disseminated encephalomyelitis and evaluation of functional outcome predictors. J Postgrad Med 2010;56:12–6.

109. Singh S, Alexander M, Korah IP. Acute disseminated encephalomyelitis: MR imaging features. AJR Am J Roentgenol 1999;173:1101–7.

110. Singh S, Prabhakar S, Korah IP, et al. Acute disseminated encephalomyelitis and multiple sclerosis: magnetic resonance imaging differentiation. Australas Radiol 2000;44:404–11.

111. Verhey LH, Branson HM, Shroff MM, et al. MRI parameters for prediction of multiple sclerosis diagnosis in children with acute CNS demyelination: a prospective national cohort study. Lancet Neurol 2011;10(12):1065–73.

112. Filippi M, Tortorella C, Rovaris M, et al. Changes in the normal appearing brain tissue and cognitive impairment in multiple sclerosis. J Neurol Neurosurg Psychiatry 2000;68:157–61.

113. Inglese M, Salvi F, Iannucci G, et al. Magnetization transfer and diffusion tensor MR imaging of acute disseminated encephalomyelitis. AJNR Am J Neuroradiol 2002;23:267–72.

114. Harada M, Hisaoka S, Mori K, et al. Differences in water diffusion and lactate production in two different types of postinfectious encephalopathy. J Magn Reson Imaging 2000;11:559–63.

115. Chen CI, Mar S, Brown S, et al. Neuropathologic correlates for diffusion tensor imaging in postinfectious encephalopathy. Pediatr Neurol 2011;44:389–93.

116. Bizzi A, Ulug AM, Crawford TO, et al. Quantitative proton MR spectroscopic imaging in acute disseminated encephalomyelitis. AJNR Am J Neuroradiol 2001;22:1125–30.

117. Ben Sira L, Miller E, Artzi M, et al. ^{1}H-MRS for the diagnosis of acute disseminated encephalomyelitis: insight into the acute-disease stage. Pediatr Radiol 2010;40:106–13.

118. Rovira A, Pericot I, Alonso J, et al. Serial diffusion-weighted MR imaging and proton MR spectroscopy of acute large demyelinating brain lesions: case report. AJNR Am J Neuroradiol 2002;23:989–94.

119. Tabata K, Shishido F, Uemura K, et al. Positron emission tomography in acute disseminated encephalomyelitis: a case report. Kaku Igaku 1990;27:261–5 [in Japanese].

120. Broich K, Horwich D, Alavi A. HMPAO-SPECT and MRI in acute disseminated encephalomyelitis. J Nucl Med 1991;32:1897–900.

121. San Pedro EC, Mountz JM, Liu HG, et al. Postinfectious cerebellitis: clinical significance of Tc-99m HMPAO brain SPECT compared with MRI. Clin Nucl Med 1998;23:212–6.

122. Itti E, Huff K, Cornford ME, et al. Postinfectious encephalitis: a coregistered SPECT and magnetic resonance imaging study. Clin Nucl Med 2002;27:129–30.

123. Okamoto M, Ashida KI, Imaizumi M. Hypoperfusion following encephalitis: SPECT with acetazolamide. Eur J Neurol 2001;8:471–4.

124. Poser CM, Goutieres F, Carpentier MA, et al. Schilder's myelinoclastic diffuse sclerosis. Pediatrics 1986;77:107–12.

125. Susac JO, Daroff RB. Magnetic resonance images on Marburg variant. J Neuroimaging 2005;15:206 [author reply: 206].

126. Malhotra HS, Jain KK, Agarwal A, et al. Characterization of tumefactive demyelinating lesions using MR imaging and in-vivo proton MR spectroscopy. Mult Scler 2009;15:193–203.

127. Ohtaki E, Murakami Y, Komori H, et al. Acute disseminated encephalomyelitis after Japanese B encephalitis vaccination. Pediatr Neurol 1992;8:137–9.

128. Wang HS, Huang SC. Acute necrotizing encephalopathy of childhood. Chang Gung Med J 2001; 24:1–10.

129. Wong AM, Simon EM, Zimmerman RA, et al. Acute necrotizing encephalopathy of childhood: correlation of MR findings and clinical outcome. AJNR Am J Neuroradiol 2006;27:1919–23.

130. Dale RC, Church AJ, Cardoso F, et al. Poststreptococcal acute disseminated encephalomyelitis with basal ganglia involvement and auto-reactive anti-basal ganglia antibodies. Ann Neurol 2001;50: 588–95.

131. Lim KE, Hsu YY, Hsu WC, et al. Multiple complete ring-shaped enhanced MRI lesions in acute disseminated encephalomyelitis. Clin Imaging 2003;27:281–4.

132. Alexander M, Murthy JM. Acute disseminated encephalomyelitis: treatment guidelines. Ann Indian Acad Neurol 2011;14:S60–4.

133. Shahar E, Andraus J, Savitzki D, et al. Outcome of severe encephalomyelitis in children: effect of high-dose methylprednisolone and immunoglobulins. J Child Neurol 2002;17:810–4.

134. Nishikawa M, Ichiyama T, Hayashi T, et al. Intravenous immunoglobulin therapy in acute disseminated encephalomyelitis. Pediatr Neurol 1999;21:583–6.

135. Kleiman M, Brunquell P. Acute disseminated encephalomyelitis: response to intravenous immunoglobulin. J Child Neurol 1995;10:481–3.

136. Straussberg R, Schonfeld T, Weitz R, et al. Improvement of atypical acute disseminated encephalomyelitis with steroids and intravenous immunoglobulins. Pediatr Neurol 2001;24:139–43.

137. Sahlas DJ, Miller SP, Guerin M, et al. Treatment of acute disseminated encephalomyelitis with intravenous immunoglobulin. Neurology 2000;54:1370–2.

138. Pradhan S, Gupta RP, Shashank S, et al. Intravenous immunoglobulin therapy in acute disseminated encephalomyelitis. J Neurol Sci 1999;165:56–61.

139. Marchioni E, Marinou-Aktipi K, Uggetti C, et al. Effectiveness of intravenous immunoglobulin treatment in adult patients with steroid-resistant monophasic or recurrent acute disseminated encephalomyelitis. J Neurol 2002;249:100–4.

140. Hahn JS, Siegler DJ, Enzmann D. Intravenous gammaglobulin therapy in recurrent acute disseminated encephalomyelitis. Neurology 1996;46:1173–4.

141. Stricker RB, Miller RG, Kiprov DD. Role of plasmapheresis in acute disseminated (postinfectious) encephalomyelitis. J Clin Apher 1992;7:173–9.

142. RamachandranNair R, Rafeequ M, Girija AS. Plasmapheresis in childhood acute disseminated encephalomyelitis. Indian Pediatr 2005;42:479–82.

143. Miyazawa R, Hikima A, Takano Y, et al. Plasmapheresis in fulminant acute disseminated encephalomyelitis. Brain Dev 2001;23:424–6.

144. Keegan M, Pineda AA, McClelland RL, et al. Plasma exchange for severe attacks of CNS demyelination: predictors of response. Neurology 2002;58:143–6.

145. Lin CH, Jeng JS, Yip PK. Plasmapheresis in acute disseminated encephalomyelitis. J Clin Apher 2004;19:154–9.

146. Refai D, Lee MC, Goldenberg FD, et al. Decompressive hemicraniectomy for acute disseminated encephalomyelitis: case report. Neurosurgery 2005; 56:E872 [discussion: E871].

147. von Stuckrad-Barre S, Klippel E, Foerch C, et al. Hemicraniectomy as a successful treatment of mass effect in acute disseminated encephalomyelitis. Neurology 2003;61:420–1.

148. Tsai ML, Hung KL. Multiphasic disseminated encephalomyelitis mimicking multiple sclerosis. Brain Dev 1996;18:412–4.

149. Rust RS. Multiple sclerosis, acute disseminated encephalomyelitis, and related conditions. Semin Pediatr Neurol 2000;7:66–90.

150. Suwa K, Yamagata T, Momoi MY, et al. Acute relapsing encephalopathy mimicking acute necrotizing encephalopathy in a 4-year-old boy. Brain Dev 1999;21:554–8.

151. Khan S, Yaqub BA, Poser CM, et al. Multiphasic disseminated encephalomyelitis presenting as alternating hemiplegia. J Neurol Neurosurg Psychiatry 1995;58:467–70.

152. Hung KL, Liao HT, Tsai ML. Postinfectious encephalomyelitis: etiologic and diagnostic trends. J Child Neurol 2000;15:666–70.

153. van der Knaap MS, Valk J. Acute disseminated encephalomyelitis and acute hemorrhagic encephalomyelitis. In: van der Knaap MS, Valk J, editors. Magnetic resonance of myelin, myelination and myelin disorders. 2nd edition. Berlin, Heidelberg (Germany): Springer-Verlag; 1995. p. 320–6.

154. Epperson LW, Whitaker JN, Kapila A. Cranial MRI in acute disseminated encephalomyelitis. Neurology 1988;38:332–3.

155. Jacobs RK, Anderson VA, Neale JL, et al. Neuropsychological outcome after acute disseminated encephalomyelitis: impact of age at illness onset. Pediatr Neurol 2004;31:191–7.

156. Hahn CD, Miles BS, MacGregor DL, et al. Neurocognitive outcome after acute disseminated encephalomyelitis. Pediatr Neurol 2003;29:117–23.

157. Bala B, Banwell B, Till C. Cognitive and behavioural outcomes in individuals with a history of childhood

acute disseminated encephalomyelitis (ADEM). In: American Academy of Neurology, 62nd AAN Annual Meeting 2010. Honolulu, April 10-17, 2010.

158. Kuperan S, Ostrow P, Landi MK, et al. Acute hemorrhagic leukoencephalitis vs ADEM: FLAIR MRI and neuropathology findings. Neurology 2003;60:721–2.

159. Mader I, Wolff M, Niemann G, et al. Acute haemorrhagic encephalomyelitis (AHEM): MRI findings. Neuropediatrics 2004;35:143–6.

160. Seales D, Greer M. Acute hemorrhagic leukoencephalitis. A successful recovery. Arch Neurol 1991; 48:1086–8.

161. Rosman NP, Gottlieb SM, Bernstein CA. Acute hemorrhagic leukoencephalitis: recovery and reversal of magnetic resonance imaging findings in a child. J Child Neurol 1997;12:448–54.

162. Klein CJ, Wijdicks EF, Earnest FT. Full recovery after acute hemorrhagic leukoencephalitis (Hurst's disease). J Neurol 2000;247:977–9.

Childhood Transverse Myelitis and Its Mimics

Terrence Thomas, MD, MRCPCH[a],*,
Helen M. Branson, BSc, MBBS, FRACR[b]

KEYWORDS

- Transverse myelitis • Children • Spinal cord • Demyelination • Magnetic resonance imaging

KEY POINTS

- Transverse myelitis presents with acute motor weakness or sensory deficits, usually accompanied by bladder or bowel incontinence. These symptoms evolve over hours to days.
- Determining a clinical "spinal cord level" aids the planning of spinal cord imaging.
- Adequate spinal cord imaging requires good-quality magnetic resonance imaging with a minimum of T2-weighted sequences in 2 planes.
- Mimics such as tumors, epidural abscess, arteriovenous malformation, and compressive bone disease may require urgent intervention.

INTRODUCTION

Transverse myelitis (TM) is a monophasic, likely postinfectious, inflammatory disorder of the spinal cord. In some children, TM may represent the first clinical event of a chronic demyelinating disorder such as multiple sclerosis (MS) or neuromyelitis optica (NMO). Diagnostic criteria requires signs and symptoms attributable to the spinal cord, that is, sensory, motor, or bladder and bowel dysfunction, with progression to nadir in less than 21 days from onset, and cerebrospinal fluid (CSF) or neuroimaging evidence of spinal cord inflammation.[1]

A variety of extra-axial and spinal cord disorders gives rise to acute and subacute signs and symptoms in the spinal cord. This article describes the clinical and radiologic features of TM and its mimics (Box 1).

Acute deficits constitute a medical emergency requiring urgent spinal imaging, as vascular disorders and spinal cord compression have a time-sensitive relationship of treatment to outcome.[2,3] In TM, a rapid evolution of symptoms usually signifies more severe disease.[4]

ANATOMIC CONSIDERATIONS IN SPINAL CORD DISORDERS

The spinal cord consists of 31 segments: 8 cervical, 12 thoracic, 5 lumbar, 5 sacral, and 1 vestigial coccygeal segment. These segments map to respective clinical myotomes and dermatomes, and are named according to their level of supply, thus the 8 pairs of spinal nerves arising from the cervical segment are called C1 to C8. The anatomic location of the spinal cord segments do not correspond to the vertebral bodies that make up the vertebral canal. Almost all of the spinal cord itself rests in the cervical and thoracic regions of the vertebral column; only the sacral segments reside in the upper 2 lumbar vertebrae. As there are only 7 cervical vertebrae, the first 7 cervical nerve roots exit in the intervertebral foramina above their respective vertical bodies, and the C8 nerve exits below the seventh cervical vertebra. The thoracic (T1–T12), lumbar (L1–L5), and sacral (S1–S5) nerves exit below their respective vertebrae (Fig. 1).

The descending corticospinal and ascending sensory tracts in the spinal cord are arranged in

Financial disclosures and Conflicts of interest: The authors have nothing to disclose.
[a] Neurology Service, Department of Paediatrics, KK Women's and Children's Hospital, 100 Bukit Timah Road, Singapore 229899, Singapore; [b] Department of Neuroradiology, The Hospital for Sick Children, University of Toronto, 555 University Avenue, Toronto, Ontario M5G 1X8, Canada
* Corresponding author.
E-mail address: Terrence.Thomas@kkh.com.sg

neuroimaging.theclinics.com

Box 1
Clinical and radiologic mimics of transverse myelitis

Extra-axial Compression, Disease

1. Vertebral spine disorders
   a. Trauma
   b. Atlantoaxial subluxation
      i. Trisomy 21
      ii. Mucopolysaccharidosis type IV
      iii. Grisel syndrome
   c. Destructive lesions
      i. Tuberculosis
      ii. Lymphoma
      iii. Langerhans cell histiocytosis
   d. Scheuermann disease
2. Epidural disease
   a. Tumor
      i. Neuroblastoma
      ii. Wilms tumor
   b. Abscess
      i. Associated dermal sinus, vertebral body infection
3. Arachnoiditis
   a. Tuberculosis
   b. Cryptococcosis
   c. Carcinomatous infiltration
4. Spinal nerve root inflammation
   a. Guillain-Barré syndrome

Spinal Cord Disorders

1. Congenital malformation
   a. Neurenteric cysts
   b. Spinal cord tethering
2. Infection
   a. Nonpolio enteroviruses
   b. West Nile virus
   c. Human T-lymphocyte virus 1
   d. Neurocysticercosis
3. Vascular disorders
   a. Arteriovenous malformation
   b. Cavernomas
   c. Cobb syndrome
   d. Fibrocartilaginous embolization
   e. Spinal cord infarction

4. Vasculitis
   a. Systemic lupus erythematosus
   b. Behçet disease
5. Nutritional disorders
   a. Vitamin B12 deficiency
      (Subacute combined degeneration)
6. Toxic injury
   a. Chemotherapy (eg, methotrexate)

longitudinal bundles and are oriented with the lower body and leg regions situated medially. These considerations are important in planning spinal cord imaging, especially in hospitals in resource-limited regions, or when imaging of the entire spinal cord may not be possible. A patient with motor and sensory deficits mapping to the lower lumbar and sacral spinal cord segments will first require careful imaging of the spinal cord residing in the lower thoracic–lumbar vertebral region. A negative study will then prompt the evaluation of the cervical and upper thoracic regions.

TECHNICAL ASPECTS OF SPINAL CORD IMAGING

Acute spinal cord neurologic signs and symptoms that trigger an MR imaging request should have sequences targeted to assess the spinal cord. For this reason the authors image with standard spin-echo or fast spin-echo (FSE) T1-weighted and T2-weighted sequences, usually in 2 planes. The standard imaging protocol would include sagittal and axial T2-weighted sequences throughout the spinal column followed by sagittal T1-weighted sequences precontrast in most circumstances. If a lesion is seen in the cord, post-gadolinium sequences in the sagittal and axial plane will be applied. Extra sequences include thin-section axial T2-weighted sequences (targeted usually to a clinically suspected abnormal level) as well as sagittal diffusion and gradient-echo sequences to assess for cord ischemia and hemorrhage (**Table 1**).

It is important to discuss with the referring neurologist the clinical presentation. If the presentation is more consistent, for example with Guillain-Barré syndrome, sequences targeting the enhancement of the nerve roots such as axial and sagittal T1-weighted scans are used.

Scanning on a 1.5-T machine has been preferred to avoid multiple artifacts that occur in spinal cord imaging and which are magnified because of the higher signal-to-noise ratio with higher field magnets. However, improved pulse-sequence

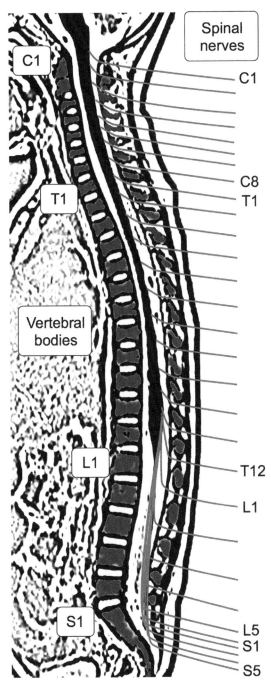

Spinal nerves

C1

C8
T1

T12

L1

L5
S1

S5

C1

T1

Vertebral bodies

L1

S1

Fig. 1. Spinal cord anatomy and relation of spinal root levels to vertebral body segments.

design has led to an increase in the use of 3 T,[5] and advanced imaging such as diffusion tensor imaging can also be reliably obtained. Marked CSF pulsation artifact, which can obscure the cord signal from flow-related artifact,[6] is an important artifact to consider. The body's mean daily CSF production is 500 mL, and it has a pulsatile motion caused by the expansion and contraction of the brain and intracranial vessels associated with the cardiac cycle. This pump effect causes the CSF flow in the cervical spaces to be 40% as fast as in the carotid arteries, resulting in multiple artifacts that may appear hypointense on T2-weighted images, particularly posterior to the spinal cord, where they can be very impressive (Fig. 2). Such artifacts are much more pronounced in children than in adults. Another artifact that can be a challenge is the "Gibbs or truncation artifact." These bright or dark lines are seen parallel to edges of abrupt intensity changes, sometimes described as "ringing" artifacts following signal-intensity borders. This pattern occurs when the number of phase-encoding steps at high spatial resolution is undersampled and, hence, is unable to faithfully reproduce the true anatomic details of the original image. In addition, these artifacts may occur when the number of peripheral Fourier lines in the k-space is small or insufficient. Such artifacts are observed particularly at 3 T, as a consequence of the improved signal-to-noise ratio in comparison with 1.5-T MR imaging. Their occurrence can be reduced by either increasing the spatial resolution or applying reconstruction filters, to smoothen the signal at the edges of k-space.

There has been variable success with diffusion-weighted sequences in spinal cord imaging, because of a combination of relatively long scan times, CSF pulsation, respiration, and sometimes cardiac artifact as well as magnetic field inhomogeneities, among others. Manara and colleagues[7] reported good success in differentiating cytotoxic edema caused by cord infarction from vasogenic edema caused by inflammation. Bammer and colleagues[8] also had success with using a phase-navigated spin-echo diffusion-weighted interleaved echo-planar sequence, which used increased k-space velocity to lead to a reduction in artifacts as well as reduced acquisition times.

Short-T1 inversion recovery (STIR) sequences are also used is spine imaging. Chen and colleagues[9] described an improved resolution obtained with this technique for intramedullary lesions. This technique suppresses fat, based on the differences in the T1 of tissues. The T1 of fat is shorter than that of water, thus allowing fat to be suppressed while water is not. The STIR sequences allow for additive T1 and T2 signal in comparison with conventional FSE sequences. Other studies have also demonstrated improved visibility of cord lesions with STIR. Philpott and Brotchie[10] found that a traditional STIR sequence was 8 times more likely to show superior lesion/cord contrast ratios when compared with the FSE T2 sequence within the cervical cord at 3 T. Other studies have shown similar results; Campi

Table 1								
MR imaging parameters								
Sequence	Flip Angle (°)	TR (ms)	TE (ms)	NSA	BW (Hz)	Slice/Gap (mm)	FOV (mm)	Pixel (mm)
Sag T2 TSE	90	2500	130	4	180	3/0.5	280	0.5 × 1
Sag T1 TSE	90	525	10	4	280	3/0.5	280	0.5 × 1.25
Ax T2 TSE	90	4775	130	4	186	3/0.5	150	0.5 × 0.5
Ax T1 TSE	90	603	13	4	322	5/7.5	150	0.8 × 0.9
Ax T2 FFE (MPGR)	20	720	23	2	108	4/0.5	150	0.6 × 0.6

Abbreviations: Ax, axial; BW, band width; FFE, fast field echo; FOV, field of view; MPGR, multiplanar gradient recalled; NSA, number of signal averages; Sag, sagittal; TE, time of echo; TR, time of repetition; TSE, turbo (fast) spin echo.

and colleagues[11] found that the contrast-to-noise ratio of 17 demyelinating lesions was significantly higher with STIR sequences than with any other sequence.

RADIOLOGIC FEATURES OF TRANSVERSE MYELITIS

The central gray complex and surrounding white matter of the spinal cord are isointense and indistinguishable on MR imaging. Inflammatory lesions in both gray and white matter show low and high signal intensity on T1-weighted and T2-weighted imaging, respectively, and may enhance with gadolinium. Edema in and around the affected region is often seen. Severe demyelinating lesions may be hemorrhagic,[12,13] drawing parallels to severe acute disseminated encephalomyelitis with hemorrhagic leukoencephalitis. This hemorrhage is best depicted on T1-weighted and T2-weighted sequences, and confirmed on a gradient-echo sequence.

Discrete and contiguous lesions are seen on spinal imaging in idiopathic TM (**Fig. 3**).[12,14] Contiguous lesions spanning 3 or more vertebral bodies, termed longitudinally extensive transverse myelitis (LETM), are often more extensive in children than in adults (mean length in vertebral bodies: children, 6.4 [±6.1] to 6.6 [±7.0][12,14] vs adults, 4.7 ± 2.9[15]).

On axial images, a variety of lesion topography is observed: involvement of the gray matter alone with either a central gray complex lesion or discrete involvement of the anterior horn cells, discrete lesions involving lateral white matter tracts or the posterior column, or diffuse lesions involving the entire transverse extent of the cord. Some patients have LETM extending the entire length of the cord; often these patients show a varying extent of transversal cord involvement when studied in axial sections (see **Fig. 3**).

Spinal cord imaging may be normal in some patients with TM.[12,16] These patients have acute

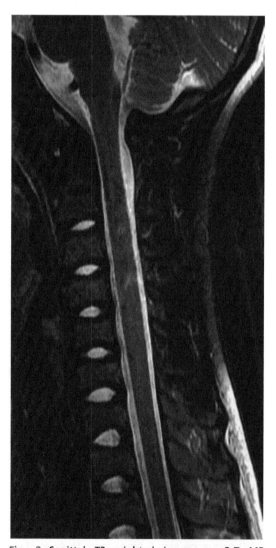

Fig. 2. Sagittal T2-weighted image on 3-T MR imaging. Sagittal T2-weighted image of the cervical spine demonstrates patchy hyperintense cord signal from prominent cerebrospinal fluid pulsation artifact.

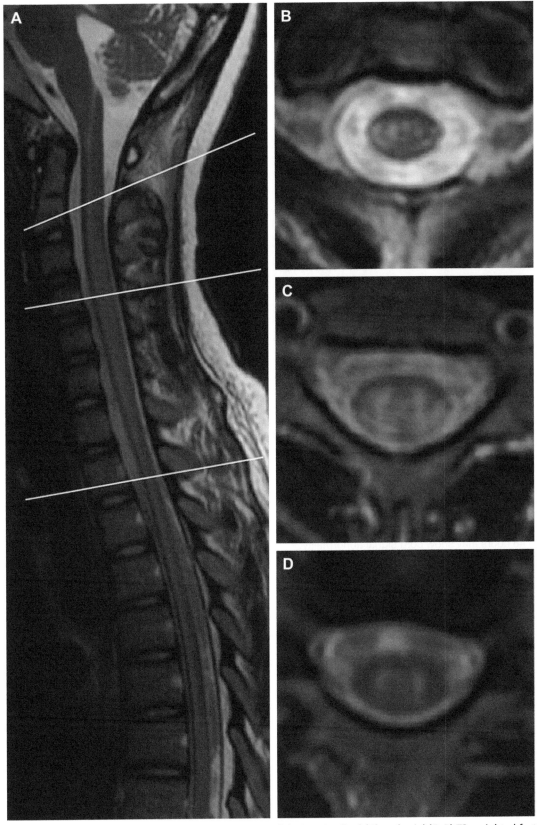

Fig. 3. Spinal cord lesions in children with transverse myelitis. Longitudinal (*A*) and axial (*B–D*) T2-weighted fast-spin echo (FSE) images. (*A*) Longitudinal lesion involving the entire spinal cord, with different transversal involvement throughout the lesion. (*B*) Predominantly anterior horn cell involvement. (*C*) Complete transverse cord involvement with edema. (*D*) Central gray matter complex.

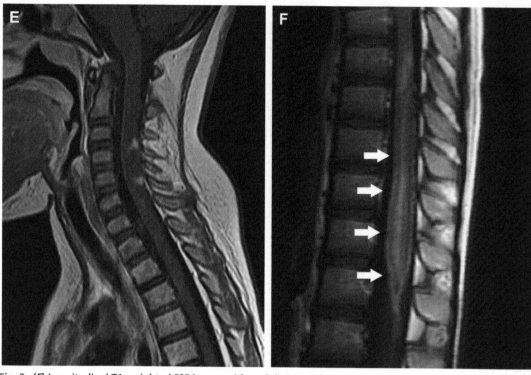

Fig. 3. (*E*) Longitudinal T1-weighted FSE image with gadolinium enhancement. (*F*) Longitudinal T1-weighted FSE image. (*E*) Intense contrast enhancement surrounding a T1-hypointense lesion. (*F*) Hyperintense signal from acute hemorrhage (*arrows*) involving the lower thoracic cord and conus medullaris.

neurologic symptoms referable to the spinal cord, CSF evidence of inflammation, and a favorable response to immunomodulatory therapy. In the authors' experience, when initial imaging is negative a short-interval follow-up MR imaging after 24 to 48 hours may show cord signal abnormality.

It is important to consider findings seen on diffusion-weighted imaging in the spinal cord, as improvements in technology and pulse-sequence design have led to increased use of this sequence for the cord. Traditionally, diffusion restriction has been thought to favor the diagnosis of an ischemic lesion; however, one must use such findings with caution, and experience has shown that there is overlap and that demyelinating lesions can also show diffusion restriction. Zecca and colleagues[17] showed a homogeneous diffusion restriction pattern in 6 patients with demyelinating cord lesion (3 of whom had relapsing MS).

MIMICS

A careful physical examination, demonstrating motor, sensory, and urinary or bowel sphincter involvement, will help to accurately localize the site of the spinal cord lesion. Additional attention should be paid to the vertebral spine, looking for abnormal curvature, gibbus, cutaneous lesions, or the presence of a dermal sinus.

The following conditions are important to consider when evaluating children with probable TM (**Fig. 4**). MR imaging helps considerably in further management, particularly in differentiating surgical from nonsurgical disease (eg, differentiating extra-axial causes and space-occupying lesions that may need surgery from intramedullary diseases such as demyelination, and ischemic and nutritional deficiencies).

Extra-Axial Cord Compression

The structures surrounding the spinal cord, namely spinal continuity, vertebral bodies, intervertebral disc, intervertebral foramina, and paravertebral spaces, should be inspected for abnormalities that may contribute to external cord compression.

Atlantoaxial subluxation resulting in cord compression is known to occur in mucopolysaccharidosis type IV, trisomy 21, and Grisel syndrome, a postinfectious disorder causing cervical spinal ligament laxity.[18–20] Disc herniation and spinal cord injury is a recognized complication of Scheuermann disease, a progressive skeletal disorder in adolescents; thoracic kyphosis and Schmorl nodes in the vertebral body are diagnostic clues.[21]

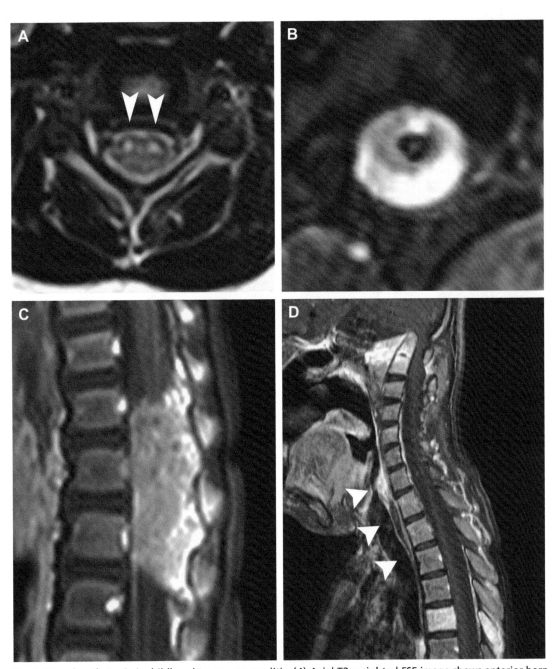

Fig. 4. Disorders that mimic childhood transverse myelitis. (*A*) Axial T2-weighted FSE image shows anterior horn cell involvement in the cervical cord from nonpolio enteroviral myelitis (*arrowheads*). (*B*) Intramedullary hemorrhage on axial gradient-echo T2*-weighted image. This gradient-echo sequence demonstrates marked blooming of hypointense signal within the center of the cord consistent with hemosiderin deposition. The presumed cause of such a focal lesion in the correct clinical context could be a cavernoma. (*C*) Sagittal T1-weighted FSE image with gadolinium contrast shows large contrast-enhancing neuroblastoma occupying the entire lumbar spinal canal, obliterating the spinal cord. (*D*) Sagittal T1-weighted fat-suppression image with gadolinium contrast shows spinal tuberculosis resulting in spinal cord compression at the craniocervical junction. There is enhancement in the C1 and C2 vertebral bodies with resultant basilar invagination, narrowing the craniocervical junction and causing severe spinal cord compression. A large paravertebral abscess tracks downward beneath the anterior spinal ligament (*arrowheads*). The T5 vertebral body is also involved.

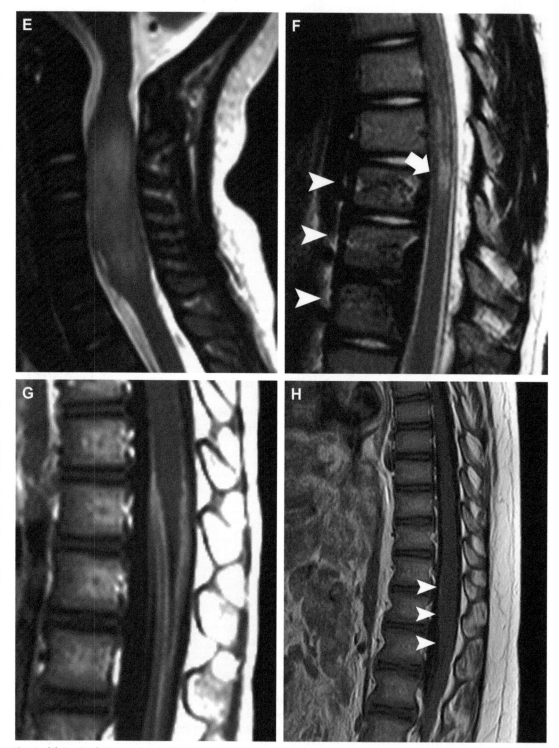

Fig. 4. (*E*) Sagittal T2-weighted FSE image shows intramedullary spinal cord astrocytoma. There is a large, well-demarcated, expansile, relatively homogeneous hyperintense lesion in the cervical spinal cord. (*F*) Sagittal T2-weighted FSE image shows arteriovenous malformation and spinal cord ischemia. Hypointense flow voids in the lower thoracic vertebral bodies (*arrowheads*) of an arteriovenous malformation are seen adjacent to a focal hyperintense lesion in the spinal cord (*arrow*), signifying ischemic injury. (*G*) Sagittal T1-weighted FSE image with gadolinium contrast shows spinal nerve root enhancement in the cauda equina in Guillain-Barré syndrome. (*H*) Sagittal T1-weighted FSE image with gadolinium contrast shows thin rim of gadolinium enhancement surrounding the lumbar cord, suggesting an arachnoiditis (*arrowheads*). This patient, who had a stable cranio-pharyngioma, developed tuberculous meningitis. Leakage of the contents of the craniopharyngioma may also cause a chemical arachnoiditis, which can mimic this appearance.

Cord Compression in Skeletal Disorders

Primary bone tumors, neuroblastoma, lymphoma, Wilms tumor, Langerhans cell histiocytosis, and soft-tissue sarcomas may infiltrate the vertebral body or extend through the paravertebral space via the intervertebral foramina, leading to vertebral body collapse, spinal deformity, and cord compression (see **Fig. 4**).[22,23] Rarely, vertebral hemangiomas may mimic a vertebral body tumor.[24]

Infections, usually from *Mycobacterium tuberculosis* or *Salmonella*, destroy the vertebral body but may also involve the intervertebral disc or have pus tracking under the adjacent posterior spinal ligament (see **Fig. 4**).[25,26] Spinal epidural abscess is uncommon unless associated with a congenital malformation, dermal sinus, or vertebral body infection.[27,28]

Inflammatory Disorders Surrounding the Spinal Cord

Gadolinium enhancement on the surface of the spinal cord, in the absence of intramedullary spinal cord abnormality, should raise the suspicion of arachnoiditis, which can be seen in tuberculosis, cryptococcal meningitis, or following intrathecal administration of chemotherapy.[29–31] Enhancement of the spinal nerve roots or cauda equina is seen in children with postinfectious acute immune demyelinating polyradiculopathy (Guillain-Barré syndrome).[32]

Intramedullary Spinal Cord Disorders

The nonpolio enteroviruses and West Nile virus are well-recognized causes of viral myelitis.[33,34] Pathologic studies in West Nile virus myelitis reveal involvement of both anterior and posterior horn cells, although spinal imaging demonstrates predominantly anterior horn cell involvement.[35] In endemic regions, spinal cord neurocysticercosis[36] and human T-lymphotropic virus 1–associated myelitis should be considered.[37] In the former, cystic lesions containing a parasitic scolex, similar to brain lesions, may be demonstrated.

Astrocytomas, ependymomas, and hemangioblastomas are the most common intramedullary spinal cord tumors.[38] Tumors have solid and/or cystic components, with cystic contents having signals different from CSF. Aggressive, infiltrating lesions have irregular margins. Ependymomas enhance better and more homogeneously than astrocytomas.[38] Hemorrhage may precipitate acute symptoms of spinal cord deficits.[39] Hemangioblastomas may be single or multiple; they have abundant vascular components, extensive perilesional edema, and may be associated with cerebellar, brainstem, and retinal hemangiomas (von Hippel–Lindau disease).[38,40]

Neurenteric cysts are congenital endodermal cysts that may resemble tumors, and present with acute spinal cord symptoms. MR imaging typically shows a well-circumscribed cystic lesion, usually of CSF density, with no contrast enhancement or surrounding edema.[41,42]

Nutritional deficiencies can also cause appearances in the spinal cord that could mimic findings similar to those of TM. The characteristic clinical triad of subacute combined degeneration caused by vitamin B_{12} deficiency includes symmetric diminished vibration sense, pyramidal signs, and peripheral neuropathy. Symmetric hyperintense signal in lateral columns and posterior columns on T2-weighted imaging has been reported to be the characteristic neuroimaging finding. In cases not suspected clinically, such MR imaging findings should lead to further workup of Vitamin B_{12} deficiency. The typical neurologic findings, a low serum cobalamin level along with macrocytic anemia, usually help the clinical diagnosis.[43]

Vascular Disorders of the Spinal Cord

Vascular disorders of the spinal cord, though rare, give rise to a rapid evolution of symptoms in the spinal cord. Glomerular and juvenile arteriovenous malformations (AVMs) and cavernomas have been described in children.[2] Cobb syndrome describes the association of a cutaneous vascular lesion and spinal cord vascular malformation occurring in the dermatomal territory mapped by the affected spinal cord segment.[44] Intramedullary spinal cord AVMs appear as a mass of dilated vascular structures, with mixed signal intensity on T1-weighted imaging and flow voids on T2-weighted imaging.[2]

Cavernomas have an irregular mulberry-like appearance with mixed T2 signal intensity surrounded by a rim of hypointensity, often with susceptibility artifact from previous bleeding evident on T2*-weighted gradient-echo sequences.[45] Perilesional edema may follow acute bleeding. Dilated perimedullary vessels accompany intramedullary lesions, with central hyperintensity and a hypointense rim on T2-weighted sequences in a dural AVM.[2]

Fibrocartilaginous Embolization

The typical history in patients with fibrocartilaginous embolization is the rapid onset and evolution of spinal cord deficits following trivial falls or trauma. The first reported case was of a 15-year-old boy who developed rapid tetraplegia and eventual death after falling on his coccyx during a basketball game.[46] Autopsy shows ischemic infarction in the acellular matrix of the nucleus pulposus in occluded feeding arterioles and draining veins.[47] Spinal imaging reveals vertebral body disease, loss of T2 signal hyperintensity in the adjacent nucleus pulposus, or the presence of Schmorl nodes.[7,47,48] In the cord itself there is ischemic injury in the anterior spinal artery territory. In some patients, only bilateral lesions involving anterior gray matter complex are evident, producing an "Owl's eyes sign" on T2-weighted sequences, similar to that seen in viral myelitis.[7]

TRIVIAL TRAUMA AND TRANSVERSE MYELITIS

Trivial trauma, as defined by minor falls or back pain that does not involve bone or joint injuries following physical or noncompetitive sporting activity, has been observed preceding the development of symptoms in up to 20% of children with TM.[12,16,49] Some of these children have minor abnormalities in the vertebral structures adjacent to the cord lesion, such as displacement of the posterior spinal ligament, narrowing or protrusion of the intervertebral disc, and loss of T2 signal intensity in the nucleus pulposus.[12] The outcome is generally good[12,16,49] in these children as opposed to those with cord infarction from fibrocartilaginous embolization.[47,48]

BRAIN LESIONS IN ACUTE TRANSVERSE MYELITIS

Discrete single or multiple T2-weighted hyperintense white matter lesions may be seen on acute MR imaging in up to 65% of patients with monophasic TM; 20% of these may fulfill McDonald criteria for dissemination in space.[12,49,50] In some patients with LETM, the contiguous lesion extends across the craniocervical junction to involve the brainstem.[12,14]

Symmetric T2 hyperintense white matter brain lesions together with a longitudinally extensive posterior-column spinal cord lesion may be seen in leukoencephalopathy with brainstem and spinal cord involvement and high lactate, a rare mitochondrial disorder.[51] Affected patients have a progressive disease with cognitive, pyramidal, cerebellar, and dorsal-column symptoms.

FOLLOW-UP MR IMAGING STUDIES

In a recent Canadian study, 11 of 25 children (44%) with TM had evidence of spinal cord atrophy (**Fig. 5**) in follow-up studies at a mean of 7 months

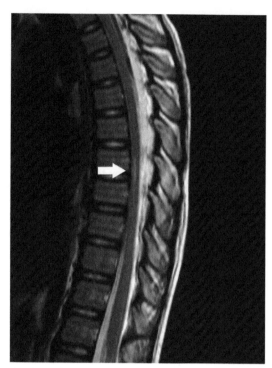

Fig. 5. Sagittal T2-weighted FSE image shows Wallerian degeneration and spinal cord atrophy following previous transverse myelitis. There is focal spinal cord atrophy with central high signal intensity at the T8-T9 region (*arrow*).

after illness; 3 of these patients had cord hemorrhage.[12] Wallerian degeneration (WD), as evidenced by high signal intensity on T1-weighted and T2-weighted sequences, in adults with traumatic spinal cord injury have been shown only to appear 7 weeks after the insult, although autopsy examination may document histologic evidence of WD as early as 8 to 12 days after insult.[52]

RISK OF MULTIPLE SCLEROSIS FOLLOWING TRANSVERSE MYELITIS

Children and adults who present with TM as the sentinel event of eventual MS share a propensity for cervical cord location and an incomplete transversal extent of lesions.[53,54] However, brain white matter lesions and LETM occur in children with both monophasic TM and TM with eventual multiple sclerosis, and do not help in prognosticating the diagnostic risk for MS.[12,55]

SUMMARY

Children with acute spinal cord symptoms require urgent and appropriate imaging to ascertain the cause. As treatments and interventions are often time sensitive, the radiologist needs to be reasonably certain as to the radiologic diagnosis. TM presents with a range of abnormalities and severity. Careful considerations of spinal cord pathology and the structures adjacent to the spinal cord are important in differentiating radiologic and clinical mimics of TM.

ACKNOWLEDGMENTS

The authors thank Manoj Singh, MRT, for preparing the table on MR imaging parameters.

REFERENCES

1. Transverse Myelitis Consortium Working Group. Proposed diagnostic criteria and nosology of acute transverse myelitis. Neurology 2002;59:499–505.
2. Krings T, Mull M, Gilsbach JM, et al. Spinal vascular malformations. Eur Radiol 2005;15:267–78.
3. Prasad D, Schiff D. Malignant spinal-cord compression. Lancet Oncol 2005;6:15–24.
4. Wilmshurst JM, Walker MC, Pohl KR. Rapid onset transverse myelitis in adolescence: implications for pathogenesis and prognosis. Arch Dis Child 1999; 80:137–42.
5. Shapiro MD. MR Imaging of the Spine at 3T. Magn Reson Imaging Clin N Am 2006;14:97–108.
6. Vargas M, Delavelle J, Kohler R, et al. Brain and spine MRI artifacts at 3Tesla. J Neuroradiol 2009; 36:74–81.
7. Manara R, Calderone M, Severino MS, et al. Spinal cord infarction due to fibrocartilaginous embolization: the role of diffusion weighted imaging and short-tau inversion recovery sequences. J Child Neurol 2010;25:1024–8.
8. Bammer R, Fazekas F, Augustin M, et al. Diffusion-weighted MR imaging of the spinal cord. AJNR Am J Neuroradiol 2000;21:587–91.
9. Chen E, Huang J, Hathout G. "STIR"ing the pot: the underutilized technique for evaluation of spinal cord lesions in multiple sclerosis. Paper presented at: 97th Scientific Assembly and Annual Meeting of the Radiological Society of North America; 2011 of Conference; Chicago. Available at: http://rsna2011.rsna.org/search/event_display.cfm?printmode=n&em_id=11002344. Accessed July 1, 2012.
10. Philpott C, Brotchie P. Comparison of MRI sequences for evaluation of multiple sclerosis of the cervical spinal cord at 3T. Eur J Radiol 2011; 80:780–5.
11. Campi A, Pontesilli S, Gerevini S, et al. Comparison of MRI pulse sequences for investigation of lesions of the cervical spinal cord. Neuroradiology 2000; 42:669–75.
12. Thomas T, Branson HM, Verhey LH, et al. The demographic, clinical, and magnetic resonance imaging (MRI) features of transverse myelitis in children. J Child Neurol 2012;27:11–21.
13. Parmar RC, Bavdekar SB, Sira P, et al. Necrotizing myelitis in an immunocompetent child: a case report with review of literature. Indian J Med Sci 2003;57: 556–8.
14. Alper G, Petropoulou KA, Fitz CR, et al. Idiopathic acute transverse myelitis in children: an analysis and discussion of MRI findings. Mult Scler 2011;17:74–80.
15. Tartaglino LM, Croul SE, Flanders AE, et al. Idiopathic acute transverse myelitis: MR imaging findings. Radiology 1996;201:661–9.
16. Pidcock FS, Krishnan C, Crawford TO, et al. Acute transverse myelitis in childhood: center-based analysis of 47 cases. Neurology 2007;68:1474–80.
17. Zecca C, Cereda C, Wetzel S, et al. Diffusion-weighted imaging in acute demyelinating myelopathy. Neuroradiology 2012;54:573–8.
18. Horovitz DD, Magalhaes TD, Pena e Costa A, et al. Spinal cord compression in young children with type VI mucopolysaccharidosis. Mol Genet Metab 2011;104:295–300.
19. Hankinson TC, Anderson RC. Craniovertebral junction abnormalities in Down syndrome. Neurosurgery 2010;66:32–8.
20. Mathern GW, Batzdorf U. Grisel's syndrome. Cervical spine clinical, pathologic, and neurologic manifestations. Clin Orthop Relat Res 1989;(244): 131–46.
21. Kapetanos G, Hantzidis P, Anagnostidis K, et al. Thoracic cord compression caused by disk herniation in Scheuermann's disease. Eur Spine J 2006; 15:553–8.
22. Gunes D, Uysal KM, Cetinkaya H, et al. Paravertebral malignant tumors of childhood: analysis of 28 pediatric patients. Childs Nerv Syst 2009;25:63–9.
23. Loh JK, Lin CK, Hwang YF, et al. Primary spinal tumors in children. J Clin Neurosci 2005;12:246–8.
24. Cheung N, Doorenbosch X, Christie J. Rapid onset aggressive vertebral haemangioma. Childs Nerv Syst 2011;27:469–72.
25. Andronikou S, Jadwat S, Douis H. Patterns of disease on MRI in 53 children with tuberculous spondylitis and the role of gadolinium. Pediatr Radiol 2002;32:798–805.
26. Schmit P, Glorion C. Osteomyelitis in infants and children. Eur Radiol 2004;14(Suppl 4):L44–54.
27. Tsiodras S, Falagas ME. Clinical assessment and medical treatment of spine infections. Clin Orthop Relat Res 2006;444:38–50.
28. Chan CT, Gold WL. Intramedullary abscess of the spinal cord in the antibiotic era: clinical features, microbial etiologies, trends in pathogenesis, and outcomes. Clin Infect Dis 1998;27:619–26.
29. Srivastava T, Kochar DK. Asymptomatic spinal arachnoiditis in patients with tuberculous meningitis. Neuroradiology 2003;45:727–9.

30. Woodall WC 3rd, Bertorini TE, Bakhtian BJ, et al. Spinal arachnoiditis with Cryptococcus neoformans in a nonimmunocompromised child. Pediatr Neurol 1990;6:206–8.

31. Bay A, Oner AF, Etlik O, et al. Myelopathy due to intrathecal chemotherapy: report of six cases. J Pediatr Hematol Oncol 2005;27:270–2.

32. Yikilmaz A, Doganay S, Gumus H, et al. Magnetic resonance imaging of childhood Guillain-Barre syndrome. Childs Nerv Syst 2010;26:1103–8.

33. Kelly H, Brussen KA, Lawrence A, et al. Polioviruses and other enteroviruses isolated from faecal samples of patients with acute flaccid paralysis in Australia, 1996-2004. J Paediatr Child Health 2006;42:370–6.

34. Hussain IH, Ali S, Sinniah M, et al. Five-year surveillance of acute flaccid paralysis in Malaysia. J Paediatr Child Health 2004;40:127–30.

35. Guarner J, Shieh WJ, Hunter S, et al. Clinicopathologic study and laboratory diagnosis of 23 cases with West Nile virus encephalomyelitis. Hum Pathol 2004;35:983–90.

36. Homans J, Khoo L, Chen T, et al. Spinal intramedullary cysticercosis in a five-year-old child: case report and review of the literature. Pediatr Infect Dis J 2001; 20:904–8.

37. Verdonck K, Gonzalez E, Van Dooren S, et al. Human T-lymphotropic virus 1: recent knowledge about an ancient infection. Lancet Infect Dis 2007;7:266–81.

38. Baleriaux DL. Spinal cord tumors. Eur Radiol 1999;9: 1252–8.

39. Scheinemann K, Bartels U, Huang A, et al. Survival and functional outcome of childhood spinal cord low-grade gliomas. Clinical article. J Neurosurg Pediatr 2009;4:254–61.

40. Kanno H, Yamamoto I, Nishikawa R, et al. Spinal cord hemangioblastomas in von Hippel-Lindau disease. Spinal Cord 2009;47:447–52.

41. Rizk T, Lahoud GA, Maarrawi J, et al. Acute paraplegia revealing an intraspinal neurenteric cyst in a child. Childs Nerv Syst 2001;17:754–7.

42. Muzumdar D, Bhatt Y, Sheth J. Intramedullary cervical neurenteric cyst mimicking an abscess. Pediatr Neurosurg 2008;44:55–61.

43. Maamar M, Mezalek ZT, Harmouche H, et al. Contribution of spinal MRI for unsuspected cobalamin deficiency in isolated sub-acute combined degeneration. Eur J Intern Med 2008;19:143–5.

44. Clark MT, Brooks EL, Chong W, et al. Cobb syndrome: a case report and systematic review of the literature. Pediatr Neurol 2008;39:423–5.

45. Weinzierl MR, Krings T, Korinth MC, et al. MRI and intraoperative findings in cavernous haemangiomas of the spinal cord. Neuroradiology 2004;46:65–71.

46. Naiman JL, Donohue WL, Prichard JS. Fatal nucleus pulposus embolism of spinal cord after trauma. Neurology 1961;11:83–7.

47. Toro G, Roman GC, Navarro-Roman L, et al. Natural history of spinal cord infarction caused by nucleus pulposus embolism. Spine 1994;19:360–6.

48. Duprez TP, Danvoye L, Hernalsteen D, et al. Fibrocartilaginous embolization to the spinal cord: serial MR imaging monitoring and pathologic study. AJNR Am J Neuroradiol 2005;26:496–501.

49. De Goede CG, Holmes EM, Pike MG. Acquired transverse myelopathy in children in the United Kingdom–a 2 year prospective study. Eur J Paediatr Neurol 2010;14:479–87.

50. Polman CH, Reingold SC, Edan G, et al. Diagnostic criteria for multiple sclerosis: 2005 revisions to the "McDonald Criteria". Ann Neurol 2005;58:840–6.

51. Van Der Knaap MS, Van Der Voorn P, Barkhof F, et al. A new leukoencephalopathy with brainstem and spinal cord involvement and high lactate. Ann Neurol 2003; 53:252–8.

52. Becerra J, Puckett W, Hiester E, et al. MR-pathologic comparisons of Wallerian degeneration in spinal cord injury. AJNR Am J Neuroradiol 1995; 16:125–33.

53. Verhey LH, Branson HM, Makhija M, et al. Magnetic resonance imaging features of the spinal cord in pediatric multiple sclerosis: a preliminary study. Neuroradiology 2010;52:1153–62.

54. Cordonnier C, de Seze J, Breteau G, et al. Prospective study of patients presenting with acute partial transverse myelopathy. J Neurol 2003;250:1447–52.

55. Banwell B, Bar-Or A, Arnold DL, et al. Clinical, environmental, and genetic determinants of multiple sclerosis in children with acute demyelination: a prospective national cohort study. Lancet Neurol 2011;10:436–45.

Diagnosing Neuromyelitis Optica

Naila Makhani, MD, MPH, FRCPC[a],*, Sandra Bigi, MD[a],
Brenda Banwell, MD, FRCPC[a],
Manohar Shroff, MD, DABR, FRCPC[b]

KEYWORDS

• Neuromyelitis optica • Optic neuritis • Transverse myelitis

KEY POINTS

• Neuromyelitis optica (NMO) is typically characterized by recurrent attacks of optic neuritis and transverse myelitis.
• NMO is most common in individuals of female sex and non-Caucasian ethnicity.
• NMO IgG is directed against the water channel aquaporin 4 and its presence in serum is 73% sensitive and 91% specific in distinguishing adult-onset NMO from multiple sclerosis.
• Increased T2 signal of the optic nerve and/or optic nerve enhancement characterize MR imaging in acute optic neuritis. Longitudinally extensive lesions (>3 spinal segments) are the hallmark spinal imaging finding of NMO. Brain lesions typically follow the distribution of aquaporin 4 expression and may be symptomatic.
• Spinal fluid analysis in NMO typically reveals a moderate lymphocytic or neutrophilic pleocytosis. Oligoclonal bands are detected in <10% of children with NMO.

INTRODUCTION

Neuromyelitis optica (NMO) is a severe, inflammatory demyelinating disorder of the central nervous system (CNS) that was first described by Devic in 1894. NMO is characterized by recurrent inflammatory demyelination typically restricted to the optic nerve and spinal cord. Historically there has been considerable debate about the relationship between NMO and multiple sclerosis (MS), but NMO is now generally considered a distinct disease with unique clinical, laboratory, and magnetic resonance (MR) imaging features (Table 1). The recent identification of NMO immunoglobin G (IgG) directed against the aquaporin 4 water channel has aided in the recognition of the broad spectrum of aquaporin 4–related autoimmunity and has improved diagnostic certainty.[1]

DEMOGRAPHICS AND EPIDEMIOLOGY

Due to its rarity, the precise incidence of pediatric-onset NMO remains unknown. Although generally considered a disease of adulthood, several

Financial Disclosures: Sandra Bigi has nothing to disclose. Naila Makhani has received speaker's honoraria from EMD Serono and Teva Neuroscience. Brenda Banwell has received speaker's honoraria from Merck-Serono, Biogen-IDEC, Bayer Healthcare, and Teva Neuroscience. Brenda Banwell serves as an advisor on pediatric therapies for Biogen-IDEC, Merk-Serono, and Genzyme. Brenda Banwell is supported by the Multiple Sclerosis Society of Canada (MSSC), the Canadian Multiple Sclerosis Scientific Research Foundation, and a New Emerging Team Grant in Autoimmunity supported by the CIHR and MSSC. Manohar Shroff has no financial disclosures.

[a] Division of Neurology, Department of Pediatrics, Hospital for Sick Children, University of Toronto, 555 University Avenue, Toronto, Ontario M5G 1X8, Canada; [b] Division of Neuroradiology, Department of Diagnostic Imaging, Hospital for Sick Children, University of Toronto, 555 University Avenue, Toronto, Ontario M5G 1X8, Canada
* Corresponding author.
E-mail address: naila.makhani@sickkids.ca

Table 1
Comparison of typical features of childhood neuromyelitis optica and multiple sclerosis

	Neuromyelitis Optica	Multiple Sclersosis
Female:male ratio	Up to 7:1	2:1
Relapsing course	53%–100%	96%
Secondary progression	Rare	Common
CSF characteristics	Marked pleocytosis (often >50 cells/μL) Lymphocytes or neutrophils	Mild pleocytosis (typically <30 cells/μL) Lymphocytes
CSF oligoclonal bands	90%	<10%
MR imaging brain	Normal, nonspecific white matter changes, or characteristic diencephalic and brainstem lesions	Perventricular, juxtacortical, callosal, with T1 "black holes" indicating chronicity
MR imaging spine	≥3 segments with central/holocordinvolvement	Short-segment and partial cord involvement

pediatric case series have now published.[2–6] In adult-onset NMO, there is a marked female predominance with female-to-male ratio reported as high as 9:1.[7–11] This striking female predilection is also present in childhood-onset NMO with a female-to-male ratio in pediatric case series reported to be between 2:1 and 7:1.[2–6] Gender may play a role in influencing NMO disease course; female gender was predictive of a relapsing (as opposed to monophasic) course in 1 large study of adult-onset NMO patients.[12]

Although NMO has been reported in many countries worldwide, its prevalence seems to be the highest in countries with predominantly non-Caucasian populations.[13–18] In childhood NMO, there is a reported overrepresentation of non-Caucasian ethnicity when compared with other demyelinating diseases such as MS.[3–6,19,20] In a US study of 88 pediatric NMO IgG-seropositive patients, 42 of 58 patients for whom ethnicity was known (73%) were non-Caucasian.[5]

IMMUNOPATHOGENESIS

The recently discovered NMO IgG biomarker is 73% sensitive and 91% specific in distinguishing adult-onset NMO from MS[1] and has similar sensitivity and specificity in children.[4] NMO IgG is directed toward aquaporin 4, a water channel that is expressed on the astrocyte end feet that are a component of the blood-brain barrier.[21] The CNS areas enriched in aquaporin 4 coincide with areas of clinical disease activity (typically optic nerves, spinal cord, brainstem, and diencephalon).

The exact role that NMO IgG plays in disease development has yet to be fully elucidated.

Aquaporin 4 is highly expressed in other organs outside of the CNS, including the gut and the kidney, but these organs are generally not clinically affected in NMO patients. Aquaporin 4 is also expressed within the CNS in areas that are often uninvolved (either clinically or radiologically), including the hippocampus, cerebellar granule cells, cerebral cortex, hippocampus, lateral septal nuclei, and the substantia nigra.[22]

However, the high specificity for NMO IgG for a diagnosis of NMO,[1] the association of higher NMO IgG titers during relapses as opposed to remission,[23,24] and the correlation between antibody titers and cerebral or spinal lesion size[25] all suggest a direct role in disease pathogenesis. Peripherally injected NMO IgG causes exacerbation of disease activity in experimental autoimmune encephalitis, resulting in typical NMO pathologic abnormalities.[26,27] NMO IgG may be pathogenic by causing internalization of aquaporin 4, complement deposition, altered excitatory neurotransmission, and increased blood-brain barrier permeability.[28,29]

CLINICAL COURSE

NMO is typically characterized by the simultaneous or rapidly sequential occurrence of optic neuritis (ON) and transverse myelitis. ON is typically characterized by subacute onset of visual loss (unilateral or bilateral), pain with eye movements, and red color desaturation. Reduced visual acuity (typically 20/200 or worse in NMO), a relative afferent pupillary defect, and optic disc swelling may be detected on physical examination. Transverse myelitis is typically characterized by subacute onset of motor weakness and sensory changes with or without bowel or bladder dysfunction. L'Hermitte symptom (pain with forward neck flexion) may be present with cervical cord involvement. A spinal sensory level is usually detected on physical examination. Myelitis may extend into the brainstem causing hiccups, nausea or vomiting, and respiratory distress.

The clinical course in NMO may be either monophasic (a single attack of ON and transverse myelitis) or relapsing (multiple episodes of ON, myelitis, or attacks involving the brain). In relapsing disease, attacks may be separated by months or years.[7,8] In children, a relapsing course has been reported in 53% to 100% of patients, although some of these studies had limited follow-up duration.[2–6] Predictors of a relapsing course in 1 large adult-onset NMO study included female sex, older age at onset, and evidence of systemic autoimmunity.[8] The presence of NMO IgG in serum also seems to be a biomarker for relapsing disease[30–32] and NMO IgG titer may correlate with disease severity.[25]

NMO is typically characterized by severe attacks and poor recovery, leading to rapid accrual of disability. In 1 large adult-onset NMO cohort study, 47% (31/66) of patients were functionally blind (visually acuity of 20/200 or poorer) in at least 1 eye and 45% (32/71) of patients experienced permanent monoplegia or paraplegia after a mean follow-up time of 16.9 years in the relapsing patients and 7.7 years in the monophasic patients. Respiratory failure was observed in one-third of relapsing NMO patients in this study.[8] In 1 study of childhood NMO, residual motor impairment occurred in 44% (21/44) of patients and persistent visual deficits occurred in 54% (26/48) of patients after a median follow-up time of 12 months.[5]

The identification of the relatively specific NMO IgG biomarker has led to increasing recognition of the broad clinical spectrum of aquaporin 4–related autoimmunity (Box 1). NMO IgG has been found in the serum of patients with recurrent ON and transverse myelitis,[1,8,33–41] which suggests that there may be a continuum of NMO-related disorders ranging from monophasic ON or transverse myelitis to relapsing NMO.

SYMPTOMATIC BRAIN INVOLVEMENT

As discussed later in this article, brain MR imaging lesions in NMO typically follow the distribution of aquaporin 4 water channel expression (Fig. 1). Brainstem involvement may present as hiccups, nausea or vomiting, and in severe cases, respiratory failure and death.[8,42–48] Diencephalic

Box 1
Neuromyelitis optica spectrum disorders

- Neuromyelitis optica
- Incomplete/partial forms of neuromyelitis optica
  - Single or recurrent longitudinally extensive transverse myelitis
  - Recurrent or simultaneous bilateral optic neuritis
- Asian opticospinal multiple sclerosis
- Optic neuritis or longitudinally extensive transverse myelitis with systemic autoimmune disease
- Optic neuritis or longitudinally extensive transverse myelitis with brain lesions typical for neuromyelitis optica (eg, diencephalon or brainstem)

Adapted from Wingerchuk DM, Lennon VA, Lucchinetti CF, et al. The spectrum of neuromyelitis optica. Lancet Neurol 2007;6:805–15.

involvement may manifest as hypersomnolence, narcolepsy, syndrome of inappropriate antidiuretic hormone secretion, or menstrual irregularities.[49–52] Rarely, coma and death may result from diffuse multifocal cerebral demyelination.[53] Symptomatic brain lesions are thought to occur in less than 15% of adult-onset NMO patients. Symptomatic brain lesions may be more common in childhood-onset disease as demonstrated in 1 study of 42 pediatric NMO patients in which 26 children (45%) had symptoms attributable to brain involvement, including ophthalmoplegia, encephalopathy, seizures, intractable vomiting or hiccups, syndrome of inappropriate antidiuretic

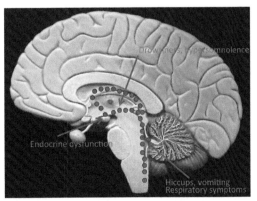

Fig. 1. Schematic diagram of brain aquaporin 4 distribution (*circles*) with localization of associated symptoms (*arrows*).

hormone secretion, and menstrual dysfunction.[5] In some children, clinical features (polyfocal neurologic deficits and encephalopathy) and MR imaging findings (see later discussion) may resemble acute disseminated encephalomyelitis (ADEM).

DIAGNOSTIC CRITERIA

Revised consensus criteria for adult-onset NMO have incorporated the presence of brain lesions and include NMO IgG as a supportive laboratory test. These criteria require the presence of ON, transverse myelitis, and at least 2 of the following supportive criteria: MR imaging evidence of a spinal cord lesion $\geq$3 segments in length, brain MR images nondiagnostic for MS, or NMO-IgG seropositivity. The presence of 2 of 3 of these supportive criteria confers 99% sensitivity and 90% specificity in distinguishing NMO from MS.[54]

Pediatric consensus criteria for NMO similarly require the presence of ON and transverse myelitis with evidence of either a longitudinally extensive spinal cord lesion or NMO IgG seropositivity (Box 2).[55] Although NMO IgG was present in 78% of children with relapsing NMO in 1 case series,[4] the sensitivity and specificity of the full diagnostic criteria have not yet been formally evaluated in childhood NMO.

SYSTEMIC AUTOIMMUNITY

There is considerable debate about the precise relationship between NMO and other systemic autoimmune disorders. There is a high frequency of coexisting autoimmune conditions in NMO patients.[8,56–68] Associated autoimmune conditions, including systemic lupus erythematosus, Sjogren syndrome, juvenile rheumatoid arthritis, Graves disease, and autoimmune hepatitis, were

---

observed in 42% (16/38) of children in 1 pediatric NMO case series.[3] Additionally, up to 76% of pediatric NMO patients may demonstrate evidence of serum autoantibodies typically present in other y production even in the absence of a clinical diagnosis of another autoimmune disease.[3,5] Evidence of systemic autoimmunity may be more commonly found in individuals with relapsing (as opposed to monophasic) disease.[8] Because many patients harbor autoantibodies for other autoimmune conditions apart from NMO without meeting formal diagnostic criteria, the presence of these antibodies may suggest heightened generalized systemic autoantibody production in NMO patients.

MAGNETIC RESONANCE IMAGING

MR imaging is an important tool in the diagnostic workup of patients suspected of having NMO and in monitoring disease activity.

MR Imaging Features of Optic Neuropathy in NMO

Patients with ON due to NMO often have bilateral ON and visual acuity typically 20/200 or worse. To date, no MR imaging features have been described that allow differentiation of ON in NMO from ON in MS or other inflammatory causes.[3,69,70]

Inflammation and demyelination lead to blood-optic barrier breakdown and nerve tissue edema that can be visualized on MR imaging.[69,70] In acute ON, fat-suppressed T2-weighted images and short tau-inversion recovery sequences show a hyperintense signal of the affected optic nerve. Fat-suppressed T1-weighted sequences with gadolinium show contrast media enhancement in 94% of patients.[69] Optic nerve enhancement helps to distinguish ON from acute nonarteritic anterior ischemic optic neuropathy, but enhancement alone, however, is not diagnostic for a demyelinating cause. Optic nerve enhancement also occurs in other inflammatory, infectious, or neoplastic diseases.[69] Typical MR imaging features of acute ON are shown in Fig. 2.

Following acute ON, optic nerve atrophy may occur and may be detected even in patients who have recovered normal visual acuity. MR images in these patients may show persistent abnormalities in short tau-inversion recovery sequences in the absence of contrast media enhancement.[69,71]

The location and the length of the enhancing optic nerve segment may correlate with the degree of visual loss but is not a predictor of final visual outcome.[69,70] In a study of 107 patients with acute ON, enhancement >10 mm correlated with more constricted visual fields,

---

Box 2

Diagnostic criteria for pediatric neuromyelitis optica

- Optic neuritis
- Transverse myelitis
- One of the following:
  - Longitudinally extensive spinal lesion ($\geq$3 spinal segments)
  - NMO IgG seropositivity

Adapted from Krupp LB, Banwell B, Tenembaum S. Consensus definitions proposed for pediatric multiple sclerosis and related disorders. Neurology 2007;68:S7–12.

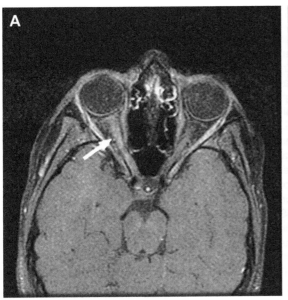
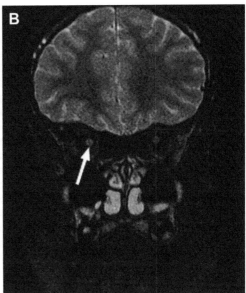

Fig. 2. Typical MR imaging features of optic neuritis as seen in an NMO patient include (*A*) optic nerve thickening and enhancement (*arrow*) on T1 postcontrast images and (*B*) increased signal (*arrow*) on coronal T2 fat-saturated image through the orbit.

and enhancement >17 mm was also associated with significant reduction of visual acuity and color vision at baseline. Visual outcome at 6 months was not correlated with initial enhancement location or length.[69]

MR Imaging Features of Transverse Myelitis in NMO

Longitudinally extensive transverse myelitis (LETM) is the characteristic spinal cord lesion in patients with NMO.[72] Lesions usually extend over more than 3 segments (on average 5.5 segments), but shorter lesions may be observed and do not rule out a diagnosis of NMO.[3,73] Lesions are usually localized to the cervical and upper thoracic cord in children as well as in adults.[3,73] In the acute stage, the lesions usually show high signal intensity on T2-weighted images, affecting white and gray matter, and exhibit diffuse uptake of contrast media mainly in the central component of the lesion. The T2 hyperintensive signal surrounds the enhancing part of the lesion, usually interpreted as perifocal edema. Other signal changes including an "eyelike" appearance of the anterior horns mimicking acute ischemia of the anterior spinal artery can occur in patients with NMO (**Fig. 3**). Contrast media enhancement and diffusion restriction can be seen in both ischemic and inflammatory lesions, although breakdown of the blood-brain barrier in ischemic lesions leading to contrast media enhancement is usually seen after days rather than immediately, as in NMO.

In ischemic myelopathy, but not in NMO, edema within the vertebral bodies is expected.[74,75]

In the chronic stage, the spinal cord shows a variable degree of atrophy at the site of the original lesion. Long-term outcome does not seem to be correlated to the initial size, extent, or diameter of the lesion, but the presence of atrophy is usually associated with more severe disability.[3,73]

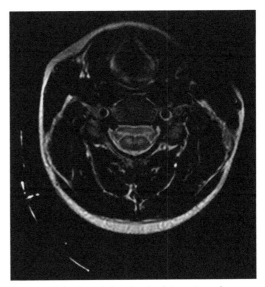

Fig. 3. Axial T2-weighted spinal imaging shows an "eyelike" appearance of the anterior horn cells typical of NMO.

In patients with LETM, NMO is the most probable underlying cause. However, LETM occurs in some patients with MS, and in multisystemic autoimmune inflammatory diseases (Sjogren syndrome, systemic lupus erythematosus, sarcoidosis, and Behcet disease), and thus investigations should exclude these disorders.[76] Although LETM can occur, spinal cord lesions in MS typically do not exceed more than 1 or 2 segments, and lesions are often well circumscribed and located in the dorsal or lateral part of the spinal cord or in the central spinal gray matter rather than traversing the entire spine. Ring-shaped or patchy enhancement after gadolinium application is usually seen in the acute stage of spinal MS lesions. In adults, LETM is seen most often in patients with secondary progressive MS, whereas 27% of pediatric patients with MS have LETM at their first or serial scan.[76,77] Comparative MR images of the spine of 2 patients with NMO and MS, respectively, are shown in **Fig. 4**.

Brain MR Imaging in Patients with NMO

Previously thought to be an almost pure opticospinal disease, brain involvement in patients with NMO is increasingly recognized, aided by the availability of serum NMO IgG evaluation.[78,79] Brain lesions "not compatible with multiple sclerosis" are now 1 of the 3 supportive criteria in the diagnosis of NMO in adults, but neuroradiologic criteria to distinguish NMO from MS reliably are still lacking.[54]

Brain lesions in NMO are hyperintense on T2-weighted images and may show contrast media enhancement acutely. In the large case series described by Pittock and colleagues,[79] 60% of patients with NMO had brain lesions. Lesions were scored as MS-like or non-MS-like according to the evaluation of lesion location, size, configuration, enhancement, and presence of mass effect. The non-MS-like lesions were subsequently classified as "atypical" or "nonspecific". Most of the patients (42%) had "nonspecific" lesions; 10% had "MS-like" lesions, and 8% had "atypical" lesions. Comparative brain MR images of 2 patients with NMO and MS, respectively, are shown in **Fig. 5**.

In a further study, Pittock and colleagues correlated brain lesions in NMO patients to areas of high aquaporin 4 expression.[80] Areas of high aquaporin 4 expression are shown in **Fig. 1**. Lesions in the distribution of high aquaporin 4 expression are shown in **Fig. 6**. "Typical NMO lesions" are usually observed around the third and fourth ventricle (hypothalamus, area postrema; see **Fig. 7**) and in the centrodorsal medulla.[78–80] Tumefactive brainstem lesions, linear lesions along the ependyma, lesions with cloudlike enhancement, or fulminant demyelinating lesions are not uncommon in patients with NMO, especially if they are NMO-IgG positive.[2,5,6,46,53,78,79,81]

Similar to adult NMO patients, brain lesions also occur in 50% to 100% of children with NMO.[2–4,6,82] As in adults, most of the lesions

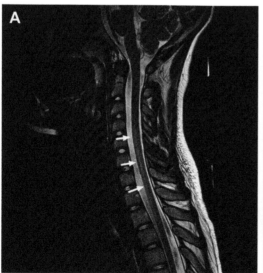
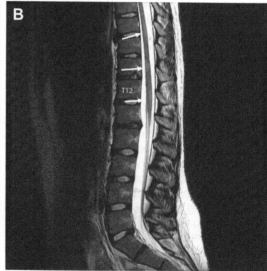

Fig. 4. Sagittal-weighted spine imaging shows (*A*) longitudinally extensive abnormal T2 signal (*arrows*) suggestive of transverse myelitis typical for NMO and (*B*) short segmental lesions seen as hyperintense areas (*arrows*) more typical of MS.

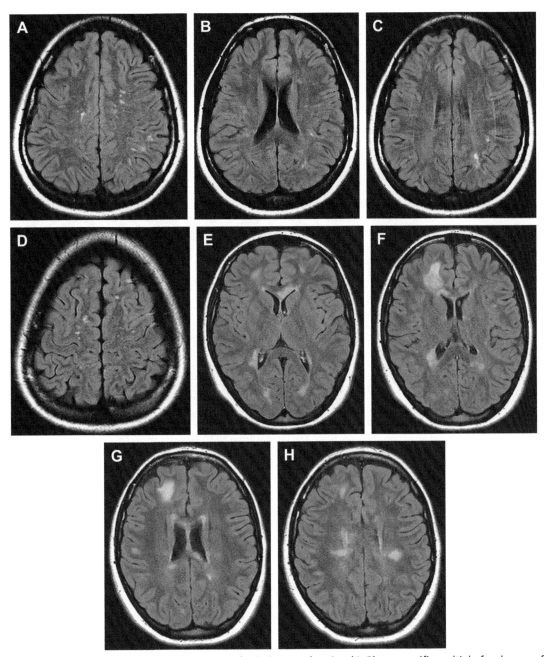

Fig. 5. Axial fluid attenuated inversion recovery brain images showing (*A–D*) nonspecific multiple focal areas of increased T2 signal in the brain, involving the subcortical and deep white matter of the brain in an NMO patient and (*E–H*) characteristic brain lesions involving the corpus callosum and periventricular white matter in MS.

are nonspecific. Large and tumefactive lesions can be observed in pediatric NMO and may resemble those seen in ADEM. Distinguishing the 2 entities has important implications for management. The following MR imaging features are typical for ADEM but unusual for NMO: symmetric involvement of the central gray matter (basal ganglia, thalami); supratentorial and

infratentorial bilateral but asymmetrical involvement of the gray-white matter junction; sparing of the periventricular white matter.[83,84]

LABORATORY

Laboratory investigations are helpful in distinguishing NMO from other disorders that present

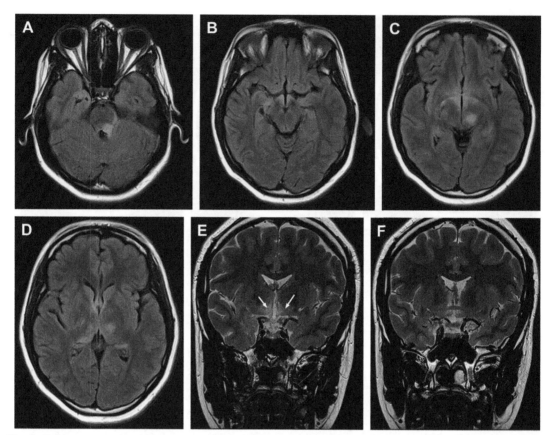

Fig. 6. Fluid attenuated inversion recovery brain MR images from NMO patients show (*A–D*) diencephalic lesions including lesions in the pons, midbrain, along floor of the third ventricle, hypothalamus, and in the thalami; (*E–F*) coronal T2 images show lesions along the floor of the third ventricle and hypothalamus (*arrows*).

in a similar manner, including MS. The most common cerebrospinal fluid (CSF) abnormality in NMO is a pleocytosis (often ≥50 leukocytes/μL) with either a neutrophilic or a lymphocytic predominance.[2,5,7,8,85] This is in contrast to the moderate lymphocytic pleocytosis (typically ≤25 leukocytes/μL) characteristic of pediatric MS.[86] In 1 series of 211 adult-onset and pediatric-onset NMO patients, pleocytosis (white blood cell count >5 leukocytes/μL) was observed in 50% of spinal fluid samples with a median cell count of 19 leukocytes/μL (range, 6–380).[87] In this case series, CSF white blood cell counts were higher in samples obtained from patients experiencing relapses as compared with those who were clinically stable.

The presence of oligoclonal bands in CSF that are absent in serum is characteristic of MS, but may occur in up to 10% of children with NMO[2,4,5] as compared with greater than 90% of children with MS.[86] Visual-evoked potential responses are frequently abnormal in NMO, just as they are in MS patients (with optic nerve involvement) with a characteristic delay or absence of the P100 response, reflecting involvement of the anterior visual pathway. In adults with NMO, abnormal visual-evoked responses at baseline have been correlated with more severe visual outcome.[88]

Optical coherence tomography is a noninvasive technique that allows measurement of the retinal nerve fiber layer thickness. Studies using optical coherence tomography have shown that retinal nerve fiber layer thinning is frequently seen in NMO and that the nerve fiber layer is significantly thinner after an episode of ON associated with NMO as opposed to MS, although such quantitative differences are not diagnostic.[89–92]

PATHOLOGIC ABNORMALITIES

NMO lesions demonstrate distinct pathologic characteristics. Spinal lesions demonstrate extensive demyelination associated with cavitary necrosis, axonal changes (eg, spheroids), and

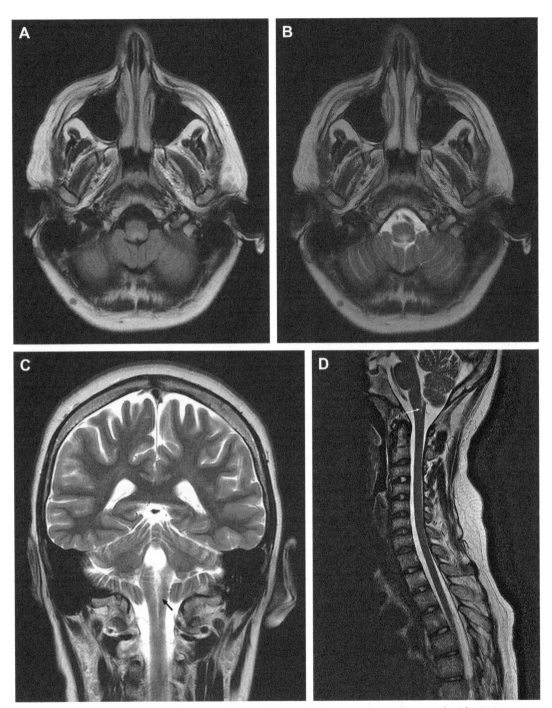

Fig. 7. This teenager presented with intractable vomiting and hiccups and was diagnosed with NMO spectrum disorder. Axial fluid attenuated inversion recovery (*A*) and T2 images (*B*) through the medulla show increased signal in the region of the area postrema. Coronal T2 (*black arrow*) (*C*) and sagittal T2 (*white arrow*) (*D*) also confirm the focal lesion in the region of the area postrema. The area postrema is located on the dorsal surface of the medulla oblongata at the caudal end of the fourth ventricle.

oligodendrocyte loss in both gray and white matter.[93] Astrocyte loss is observed in both acute and chronic NMO lesions, suggesting that astrocyte damage occurs early in the disease.[94,95]

Active lesions demonstrate inflammatory infiltration by macrophages, neutrophils, and eosinophils with rare T lymphocytes in a typical "rim and rosette" pattern.[93,96] NMO lesions demonstrate a distinct lack of aquaporin 4 at all stages.[96] Blood vessels are often hyalinized and fibrotic within both active and chronic NMO lesions.[93,96] Autopsy studies suggest that brain lesions exhibit the same histopathologic characteristics as spinal cord lesions.[94,97]

Immunoglobulins and complement are deposited in a characteristic vasocentric pattern within active lesions further supporting a presumed autoantibody-mediated disease process.[93] The vasocentric distribution of NMO pathologic abnormalities corresponds to the location of aquaporin 4 expression within astrocyte end feet at the blood-brain barrier.

A unique pattern of perivascular inflammation in the absence of demyelination has been described in the floor of the fourth ventricle and area postrema.[96] In addition, when NMO IgG was intravenously administered in mice, NMO IgG binding was observed in the area postrema, but not elsewhere in the brain, or within the spinal cord or optic nerves,[98] which suggests that the area postrema may potentially be a site at which NMO IgG accesses the CNS.

SUMMARY

NMO is a severe inflammatory demyelinating disorder that is increasingly being diagnosed in children. Advances in MR imaging techniques and the discovery of the NMO IgG biomarker have led to improved diagnostic accuracy and greater recognition of the broad clinical spectrum of aquaporin 4–related autoimmunity. Early recognition of NMO spectrum disorders has important therapeutic implications given the high risk of recurrent attacks and consequent severe disability in the very youngest NMO patients.

REFERENCES

1. Lennon VA, Wingerchuk DM, Kryzer TJ, et al. A serum autoantibody marker of neuromyelitis optica: distinction from multiple sclerosis. Lancet 2004;364:2106–12.
2. Huppke P, Bluthner M, Bauer O, et al. Neuromyelitis optica and NMO-IgG in European pediatric patients. Neurology 2010;75:1740–4.
3. Lotze TE, Northrop JL, Hutton GJ, et al. Spectrum of pediatric neuromyelitis optica. Pediatrics 2008;122: e1039–47.
4. Banwell B, Tenembaum S, Lennon VA, et al. Neuromyelitis optica-IgG in childhood inflammatory demyelinating CNS disorders. Neurology 2008;70:344–52.
5. McKeon A, Lennon VA, Lotze T, et al. CNS aquaporin-4 autoimmunity in children. Neurology 2008;71:93–100.
6. Pena JA, Ravelo ME, Mora-La Cruz E, et al. NMO in pediatric patients: brain involvement and clinical expression. Arq Neuropsiquatr 2011;69:34–8.
7. O'Riordan JI, Gallagher HL, Thompson AJ, et al. Clinical, CSF, and MRI findings in Devic's neuromyelitis optica. J Neurol Neurosurg Psychiatry 1996;60: 382–7.
8. Wingerchuk DM, Hogancamp WF, O'Brien PC, et al. The clinical course of neuromyelitis optica (Devic's syndrome). Neurology 1999;53:1107–14.
9. de Seze J, Stojkovic T, Ferriby D, et al. Devic's neuromyelitis optica: clinical, laboratory, MRI and outcome profile. J Neurol Sci 2002;197:57–61.
10. Ghezzi A, Bergamaschi R, Martinelli V, et al. Clinical characteristics, course and prognosis of relapsing Devic's Neuromyelitis Optica. J Neurol 2004;251: 47–52.
11. Wingerchuk DM. Neuromyelitis optica: effect of gender. J Neurol Sci 2009;286:18–23.
12. Wingerchuk DM, Weinshenker BG. Neuromyelitis optica: clinical predictors of a relapsing course and survival. Neurology 2003;60:848–53.
13. Papais-Alvarenga RM, Miranda-Santos CM, Puccioni-Sohler M, et al. Optic neuromyelitis syndrome in Brazilian patients. J Neurol Neurosurg Psychiatry 2002;73:429–35.
14. Kira J. Multiple sclerosis in the Japanese population. Lancet Neurol 2003;2:117–27.
15. Cabre P, Heinzlef O, Merle H, et al. MS and neuromyelitis optica in Martinique (French West Indies). Neurology 2001;56:507–14.
16. Chopra JS, Radhakrishnan K, Sawhney BB, et al. Multiple sclerosis in North-West India. Acta Neurol Scand 1980;62:312–21.
17. Bizzoco E, Lolli F, Repice AM, et al. Prevalence of neuromyelitis optica spectrum disorder and phenotype distribution. J Neurol 2009;256: 1891–8.
18. Benamer HT, Ahmed ES, Al-Din AS, et al. Frequency and clinical patterns of multiple sclerosis in Arab countries: a systematic review. J Neurol Sci 2009; 278:1–4.
19. Banwell B, Krupp L, Kennedy J, et al. Clinical features and viral serologies in children with multiple sclerosis: a multinational observational study. Lancet Neurol 2007;6:773–81.
20. Yeh EA, Chitnis T, Krupp L, et al. Pediatric multiple sclerosis. Nat Rev Neurol 2009;5:621–31.
21. Lennon VA, Kryzer TJ, Pittock SJ, et al. IgG marker of optic-spinal multiple sclerosis binds to the aquaporin-4 water channel. J Exp Med 2005;202: 473–7.
22. Costa C, Tortosa R, Domenech A, et al. Mapping of aggrecan, hyaluronic acid, heparan sulphate proteoglycans and aquaporin 4 in the central nervous system of the mouse. J Chem Neuroanat 2007;33:111–23.

23. Jarius S, Aboul-Enein F, Waters P, et al. Antibody to aquaporin-4 in the long-term course of neuromyelitis optica. Brain 2008;131:3072–80.

24. Weinstock-Guttman B, Miller C, Yeh E, et al. Neuromyelitis optica immunoglobulins as a marker of disease activity and response to therapy in patients with neuromyelitis optica. Mult Scler 2008; 14:1061–7.

25. Takahashi T, Fujihara K, Nakashima I, et al. Anti-aquaporin-4 antibody is involved in the pathogenesis of NMO: a study on antibody titre. Brain 2007; 130:1235–43.

26. Bennett JL, Lam C, Kalluri SR, et al. Intrathecal pathogenic anti-aquaporin-4 antibodies in early neuromyelitis optica. Ann Neurol 2009;66:617–29.

27. Bradl M, Misu T, Takahashi T, et al. Neuromyelitis optica: pathogenicity of patient immunoglobulin in vivo. Ann Neurol 2009;66:630–43.

28. Vincent T, Saikali P, Cayrol R, et al. Functional consequences of neuromyelitis optica-IgG astrocyte interactions on blood-brain barrier permeability and granulocyte recruitment. J Immunol 2008;181: 5730–7.

29. Hinson SR, Roemer SF, Lucchinetti CF, et al. Aquaporin-4-binding autoantibodies in patients with neuromyelitis optica impair glutamate transport by down-regulating EAAT2. J Exp Med 2008;205: 2473–81.

30. Matiello M, Lennon VA, Jacob A, et al. NMO-IgG predicts the outcome of recurrent optic neuritis. Neurology 2008;70:2197–200.

31. Weinshenker BG, Wingerchuk DM, Vukusic S, et al. Neuromyelitis optica IgG predicts relapse after longitudinally extensive transverse myelitis. Ann Neurol 2006;59:566–9.

32. Akman-Demir G, Tuzun E, Waters P, et al. Prognostic implications of aquaporin-4 antibody status in neuromyelitis optica patients. J Neurol 2011; 258:464–70.

33. Pirko I, Blauwet LA, Lesnick TG, et al. The natural history of recurrent optic neuritis. Arch Neurol 2004;61:1401–5.

34. Chan KH, Tsang KL, Fong GC, et al. Idiopathic severe recurrent transverse myelitis: a restricted variant of neuromyelitis optica. Clin Neurol Neurosurg 2005;107:132–5.

35. Zuliani L, Lopez de Munain A, Ruiz Martinez J, et al. NMO-IgG antibodies in neuromyelitis optica: a report of 2 cases. Neurologia 2006;21:314–7 [in Spanish].

36. Nakashima I, Fujihara K, Miyazawa I, et al. Clinical and MRI features of Japanese patients with multiple sclerosis positive for NMO-IgG. J Neurol Neurosurg Psychiatry 2006;77:1073–5.

37. Marignier R, De Seze J, Vukusic S, et al. NMO-IgG and Devic's neuromyelitis optica: a French experience. Mult Scler 2008;14:440–5.

38. Matsumoto H, Shimizu T, Okabe S, et al. Recurrent spinal cord attacks in a patient with a limited form of neuromyelitis optica. Intern Med 2011;50: 509–13.

39. Petzold A, Pittock S, Lennon V, et al. Neuromyelitis optica-IgG (aquaporin-4) autoantibodies in immune mediated optic neuritis. J Neurol Neurosurg Psychiatry 2010;81:109–11.

40. Chan KH, Ramsden DB, Yu YL, et al. Neuromyelitis optica-IgG in idiopathic inflammatory demyelinating disorders amongst Hong Kong Chinese. Eur J Neurol 2009;16:310–6.

41. Dinkin MJ, Cestari DM, Stein MC, et al. NMO antibody-positive recurrent optic neuritis without clear evidence of transverse myelitis. Arch Ophthalmol 2008;126:566–70.

42. Rison RA, Berkovich R. Teaching neuroimages: hiccoughs and vomiting in neuromyelitis optica. Neurology 2010;75:e70.

43. Popescu BF, Lennon VA, Parisi JE, et al. Neuromyelitis optica unique area postrema lesions: nausea, vomiting, and pathogenic implications. Neurology 2011;76:1229–37.

44. Wang KC, Lee CL, Chen SY, et al. Prominent brainstem symptoms/signs in patients with neuromyelitis optica in a Taiwanese population. J Clin Neurosci 2011;18:1197–200.

45. Sato D, Fujihara K. Atypical presentations of neuromyelitis optica. Arq Neuropsiquiatr 2011;69: 824–8.

46. Kim W, Kim SH, Lee SH, et al. Brain abnormalities as an initial manifestation of neuromyelitis optica spectrum disorder. Mult Scler 2011;17:1107–12.

47. Takahashi T, Miyazawa I, Misu T, et al. Intractable hiccup and nausea in neuromyelitis optica with anti-aquaporin-4 antibody: a herald of acute exacerbations. J Neurol Neurosurg Psychiatry 2008;79: 1075–8.

48. Misu T, Fujihara K, Nakashima I, et al. Intractable hiccup and nausea with periaqueductal lesions in neuromyelitis optica. Neurology 2005;65:1479–82.

49. Kanbayashi T, Shimohata T, Nakashima I, et al. Symptomatic narcolepsy in patients with neuromyelitis optica and multiple sclerosis: new neurochemical and immunological implications. Arch Neurol 2009;66:1563–6.

50. Baba T, Nakashima I, Kanbayashi T, et al. Narcolepsy as an initial manifestation of neuromyelitis optica with anti-aquaporin-4 antibody. J Neurol 2009; 256:287–8.

51. You XF, Qin W, Hu WL. Aquaporin-4 antibody positive neuromyelitis optica with syndrome of inappropriate antidiuretic hormone secretion. Neurosciences (Riyadh) 2011;16:68–71.

52. Vernant JC, Cabre P, Smadja D, et al. Recurrent optic neuromyelitis with endocrinopathies: a new syndrome. Neurology 1997;48:58–64.

53. Newey CR, Bermel RA. Fulminant cerebral demyelination in neuromyelitis optica. Neurology 2011; 77:193.

54. Wingerchuk DM, Lennon VA, Pittock SJ, et al. Revised diagnostic criteria for neuromyelitis optica. Neurology 2006;66:1485–9.

55. Krupp LB, Banwell B, Tenembaum S. Consensus definitions proposed for pediatric multiple sclerosis and related disorders. Neurology 2007;68: S7–12.

56. Pittock SJ, Lennon VA, de Seze J, et al. Neuromyelitis optica and non organ-specific autoimmunity. Arch Neurol 2008;65:78–83.

57. Adoni T, Lino AM, da Gama PD, et al. Recurrent neuromyelitis optica in Brazilian patients: clinical, immunological, and neuroimaging characteristics. Mult Scler 2010;16:81–6.

58. McKeon A, Lennon VA, Jacob A, et al. Coexistence of myasthenia gravis and serological markers of neurological autoimmunity in neuromyelitis optica. Muscle Nerve 2009;39:87–90.

59. Jarius S, Jacobi C, de Seze J, et al. Frequency and syndrome specificity of antibodies to aquaporin-4 in neurological patients with rheumatic disorders. Mult Scler 2011;17:1067–73.

60. Matijaca M, Pavelin S, Kaliterna DM, et al. Pathogenic role of aquaporin antibodies in the development of neuromyelitis optica in a woman with celiac disease. Isr Med Assoc J 2011;13:182–4.

61. Bergamaschi R, Jarius S, Robotti M, et al. Two cases of benign neuromyelitis optica in patients with celiac disease. J Neurol 2009;256:2097–9.

62. Uzawa A, Mori M, Iwai Y, et al. Association of anti-aquaporin-4 antibody-positive neuromyelitis optica with myasthenia gravis. J Neurol Sci 2009;287: 105–7.

63. Furukawa Y, Yoshikawa H, Yachie A, et al. Neuromyelitis optica associated with myasthenia gravis: characteristic phenotype in Japanese population. Eur J Neurol 2006;13:655–8.

64. Bichuetti DB, Barros TM, Oliveira EM, et al. Demyelinating disease in patients with myasthenia gravis. Arq Neuropsiquiatr 2008;66:5–7.

65. Mehta LR, Samuelsson MK, Kleiner AK, et al. Neuromyelitis optica spectrum disorder in a patient with systemic lupus erythematosus and anti-phospholipid antibody syndrome. Mult Scler 2008; 14:425–7.

66. Kahlenberg JM. Neuromyelitis optica spectrum disorder as an initial presentation of primary Sjogren's syndrome. Semin Arthritis Rheum 2011;40: 343–8.

67. Squatrito D, Colagrande S, Emmi L. Devic's syndrome and primary APS: a new immunological overlap. Lupus 2010;19:1337–9.

68. Sergio P, Mariana B, Alberto O, et al. Association of neuromyelitis optic (NMO) with autoimmune disorders: report of two cases and review of the literature. Clin Rheumatol 2010;29:1335–8.

69. Kupersmith MJ, Alban T, Zeiffer B, et al. Contrast-enhanced MRI in acute optic neuritis: relationship to visual performance. Brain 2002;125: 812–22.

70. Pau D, Al Zubidi N, Yalamanchili S, et al. Optic neuritis. Eye (Lond) 2011;25:833–42.

71. Kapoor R, Miller DH, Jones SJ, et al. Effects of intravenous methylprednisolone on outcome in MRI-based prognostic subgroups in acute optic neuritis. Neurology 1998;50:230–7.

72. Mata S, Lolli F. Neuromyelitis optica: an update. J Neurol Sci 2011;303:13–21.

73. Krampla W, Aboul-Enein F, Jecel J, et al. Spinal cord lesions in patients with neuromyelitis optica: a retrospective long-term MRI follow-up study. Eur Radiol 2009;19:2535–43.

74. Suzuki T, Kawaguchi S, Takebayashi T, et al. Vertebral body ischemia in the posterior spinal artery syndrome: case report and review of the literature. Spine (Phila Pa 1976) 2003;28:E260–4.

75. Faig J, Busse O, Salbeck R. Vertebral body infarction as a confirmatory sign of spinal cord ischemic stroke: report of three cases and review of the literature. Stroke 1998;29:239–43.

76. Trebst C, Raab P, Voss EV, et al. Longitudinal extensive transverse myelitis-it's not all neuromyelitis optica. Nat Rev Neurol 2011;7(12):688–98.

77. Verhey LH, Branson HM, Makhija M, et al. Magnetic resonance imaging features of the spinal cord in pediatric multiple sclerosis: a preliminary study. Neuroradiology 2010;52:1153–62.

78. Cabrera-Gomez JA, Kister I. Conventional brain MRI in neuromyelitis optica. Eur J Neurol 2011;19(6): 812–9.

79. Pittock SJ, Lennon VA, Krecke K, et al. Brain abnormalities in neuromyelitis optica. Arch Neurol 2006; 63:390–6.

80. Pittock SJ, Weinshenker BG, Lucchinetti CF, et al. Neuromyelitis optica brain lesions localized at sites of high aquaporin 4 expression. Arch Neurol 2006; 63:964–8.

81. Ito S, Mori M, Makino T, et al. "Cloud-like enhancement" is a magnetic resonance imaging abnormality specific to neuromyelitis optica. Ann Neurol 2009; 66:425–8.

82. Collongues N, Marignier R, Zephir H, et al. Long-term follow-up of neuromyelitis optica with a pediatric onset. Neurology 2010;75:1084–8.

83. Lee YJ. Acute disseminated encephalomyelitis in children: differential diagnosis from multiple sclerosis on the basis of clinical course. Korean J Pediatr 2011;54:234–40.

84. Tenembaum S, Chitnis T, Ness J, et al. Acute disseminated encephalomyelitis. Neurology 2007; 68:S23–36.

85. Milano E, Di Sapio A, Malucchi S, et al. Neuromyelitis optica: importance of cerebrospinal fluid examination during relapse. Neurol Sci 2003;24: 130–3.

86. Pohl D, Rostasy K, Reiber H, et al. CSF characteristics in early-onset multiple sclerosis. Neurology 2004;63:1966–7.

87. Jarius S, Paul F, Franciotta D, et al. Cerebrospinal fluid findings in aquaporin-4 antibody positive neuromyelitis optica: results from 211 lumbar punctures. J Neurol Sci 2011;306:82–90.

88. Watanabe A, Matsushita T, Doi H, et al. Multimodality-evoked potential study of anti-aquaporin-4 antibody-positive and -negative multiple sclerosis patients. J Neurol Sci 2009;281:34–40.

89. Merle H, Olindo S, Donnio A, et al. Retinal peripapillary nerve fiber layer thickness in neuromyelitis optica. Invest Ophthalmol Vis Sci 2008;49: 4412–7.

90. Naismith RT, Tutlam NT, Xu J, et al. Optical coherence tomography differs in neuromyelitis optica compared with multiple sclerosis. Neurology 2009; 72:1077–82.

91. Ratchford JN, Quigg ME, Conger A, et al. Optical coherence tomography helps differentiate neuromyelitis optica and MS optic neuropathies. Neurology 2009;73:302–8.

92. de Seze J, Blanc F, Jeanjean L, et al. Optical coherence tomography in neuromyelitis optica. Arch Neurol 2008;65:920–3.

93. Lucchinetti CF, Mandler RN, McGavern D, et al. A role for humoral mechanisms in the pathogenesis of Devic's neuromyelitis optica. Brain 2002;125: 1450–61.

94. Almekhlafi MA, Clark AW, Lucchinetti CF, et al. Neuromyelitis optica with extensive active brain involvement: an autopsy study. Arch Neurol 2011; 68:508–12.

95. Parratt JD, Prineas JW. Neuromyelitis optica: a demyelinating disease characterized by acute destruction and regeneration of perivascular astrocytes. Mult Scler 2010;16:1156–72.

96. Roemer SF, Parisi JE, Lennon VA, et al. Pattern-specific loss of aquaporin-4 immunoreactivity distinguishes neuromyelitis optica from multiple sclerosis. Brain 2007;130:1194–205.

97. Hengstman GJ, Wesseling P, Frenken CW, et al. Neuromyelitis optica with clinical and histopathological involvement of the brain. Mult Scler 2007;13: 679–82.

98. Ratelade J, Bennett JL, Verkman AS. Intravenous neuromyelitis optica autoantibody in mice targets aquaporin-4 in peripheral organs and area postrema. PLoS One 2011;6:e27412.

Childhood Central Nervous System Vasculitis

Mahendranath Moharir, MD, MSc, FRACP[a],
Manohar Shroff, MD, DABR, FRCPC[b],
Susanne M. Benseler, MD, PhD[c],*

KEYWORDS

- Vasculitis • Neuroinflammation • Angiitis • Stroke • MRI • Angiography • Treatment
- Immunosuppression

KEY POINTS

- Inflammation has to be considered as the underlying pathomechanism in children presenting with newly acquired neurological and/or psychiatric deficit. Inflammation of the cerebral blood vessel walls can solely target the brain and spinal cord and is then termed primary CNS vasculitis. Several underlying conditions have been found to be associated with a secondary CNS vasculitis; a careful diagnostic evaluation for these conditions is mandatory.
- Neuroimaging is crucial in guiding the diagnostic evaluation in childhood CNS vasculitis. It identifies characteristic features of distinct CNS vasculitis subtypes. Children with angiography positive CNS vasculitis commonly present with stroke features, have vascular stenoses or other abnormalities and may have evidence of contrast in the thickened, inflamed cerebral vessel wall. In contrast, neuroimaging may demonstrate multiple T2/Flair positive lesions in non-large vessel territories in children with angiography-negative small vessel vasculitis, which is confirmed on brain biopsy. Neuroimaging has a high sensitivity, but lacks specificity for distinct subtypes of childhood inflammatory brain diseases.
- Early recognition, rapid diagnostic evaluation including novel imaging strategies such as contrast wall enhancement and timely initiation of targeted immunosuppressive therapy have dramatically improved the outcome of children with primary and secondary CNS vasculitis.

INTRODUCTION

Inflammation is an increasingly recognized underlying pathologic condition in children presenting with acquired neurologic deficits. All the individual components of the central nervous system (CNS) and peripheral nervous system can be targets of a dysregulated innate or adaptive immune system.[1,2] The interaction between the target structure and the specific antibodies or cellular response will determine the clinical phenotype of the disease, including the mode of onset, severity, and long-term evolution. A typical clinical presentation of inflammatory brain disease in children is subacute, often multifocal, with a fluctuating but rapid progressive course, either idiopathic or less frequently in the context of a systemic illness or paraneoplastic process.[3–6]

Primary inflammatory brain diseases solely affect the brain and/or spinal cord and encompass vasculitis and nonvasculitic diseases, such as demyelination, neuronal antibody mediated inflammation, T-cell mediated diseases, and granulomatous inflammatory brain diseases.[3,6,7] Secondary

[a] Division of Neurology, Department of Pediatrics, The Hospital for Sick Children, University of Toronto, 555 University Avenue, Toronto, Ontario M5G 1X8, Canada; [b] Department of Diagnostic Imaging, The Hospital for Sick Children, University of Toronto, 555 University Avenue, Toronto, Ontario M5G 1X8, Canada; [c] Division of Rheumatology, Department of Pediatrics, The Hospital for Sick Children, University of Toronto, 555 University Avenue, Toronto, Ontario M5G 1X8, Canada
* Corresponding author.
E-mail address: Susanne.benseler@sickkids.ca

Neuroimag Clin N Am 23 (2013) 293–308
http://dx.doi.org/10.1016/j.nic.2012.12.008
1052-5149/13/$ – see front matter © 2013 Elsevier Inc. All rights reserved.

inflammatory brain diseases result when brain inflammation occurs in the context of a systemic disease, such as infections, rheumatic diseases, systemic inflammatory diseases, and other systemic illness or exposures.[4,8–29] The diagnosis of inflammatory brain disease is based on a thorough clinical evaluation, including features of systemic inflammatory illnesses; blood and cerebrospinal fluid (CSF) analysis; neuroimaging studies; supportive testing, such as electromyography/nerve conduction studies and electroencephalography; and targeted tests, such as specific antibodies or brain biopsies.[30]

Every child with a newly acquired neurologic deficit (focal or systemic) should be investigated for an underlying inflammatory cause. The differential diagnosis for neuro-inflammatory conditions is very wide and rapidly expanding. This article focuses on childhood CNS vasculitis, whereby the target of inflammation is the blood vessels, and its resultant effects on neurologic functioning.

PRIMARY CNS VASCULITIS

Primary angiitis of the central nervous system (PACNS) is the most common cause of severe, acquired neurologic deficits in previously healthy children.[15,31,32] PACNS was first described in adults in 1959.[33] Initial cases were almost exclusively diagnosed at autopsy, demonstrating granulomatous inflammation of the cerebral arteries.[34] In 1988, Calabrese and Mallek[31] described 8 new cases and summarized the available literature of PACNS in adults. He coined the term PACNS and proposed diagnostic criteria for adults. These criteria mandate (1) a newly acquired neurologic deficit, (2) angiographic and/or histologic evidence of CNS vasculitis, and (3) the absence of a systemic condition that could explain these findings.[31] The Calabrese criteria were adopted and modified for childhood PACNS (cPACNS), requiring a newly acquired neurologic deficit and/or psychiatric symptom in patients aged 18 years or younger.[15] In the authors' tertiary care center, cPACNS was the most frequently diagnosed inflammatory brain disease over the past 5 years. The current classification of cPACNS is based on affected cerebral vessel size and disease presentation and natural history.[15,35] Three subtypes are currently recognized: (1) nonprogressive (NP) large-medium vessel cPACNS (angiography positive), (2) progressive (P), large-medium vessel cPACNS (angiography positive), and (3) small vessel (SV) cPACNS (angiography negative, biopsy positive).[15,35] The 3 subtypes display distinct presenting symptoms, laboratory findings, disease course, and treatment outcome.[15,35]

Angiography-Positive NP-cPACNS

Clinical features
Children with NP-cPACNS typically present with sudden-onset focal neurologic deficits and are frequently diagnosed with arterial ischemic stroke.[15] This subtype affects boys more commonly than girls, corresponding to the gender predilection in stroke overall.[36] Focal deficits can include abrupt onset of aphasia, visual disturbance, ataxia, hemiparesis, hemifacial weakness, hemisensory loss, and fine motor skill loss.[15] The presentation can either be hyperacute and acute or sometimes of a stutteringtype.[37] The latter refers to recurrent focal deficits lasting few minutes/hours, eventually progressing to a complete irreversible deficit either within one or multiple vascular territories depending on the extent of the vasculitis. Approximately 10% of children present with additional diffuse focal deficits, such as decreased cognition or behavior change. Overall, headaches are present in 40% of the children with NP-cPACNS.[15] Seizures are not a frequent feature but can be present, particularly in younger children.

Laboratory tests
Systemic inflammatory markers, including C-reactive protein and erythrocyte sedimentation rate (ESR), are frequently normal. The endothelial cell marker von Willebrand Factor antigen has been documented to be elevated in some patients but remains to be studied systematically in this population. In NP-cPACNS, less than 50% of the patients have an elevated protein level or evidence of leukocytosis on CSF analysis.[15,38] The role of the opening pressure remains uncertain. Thus, the value of seeking inflammatory markers either in blood and CSF seems limited from the diagnostic point of view. The presence of inflammatory abnormalities can certainly help in diagnosis, but their absence does not rule out CNS vessel wall inflammation. Thus, there is a clear need for other diagnostic markers, which could be potentially used to reliably detect CNS inflammation in the absence of systemic signs of inflammation. One such marker, CSF neopterin, which is released by CNS macrophages, appears[39] and merits further research because it has been demonstrated to be elevated in a variety of inflammatory disorders affecting the CNS, although it is not clear whether the elevated levels represent a primary inflammation in the CNS or a secondary inflammatory response to non–immune-mediated brain damage.

The evaluation of potential prothrombotic abnormalities is mandatory in most patients. But the role of thrombophilia testing has not been carefully studied in this specific population, although testing can be potentially beneficial in terms of ascertaining stroke recurrence risk because it is becoming increasingly clear that stroke in children results from a disturbance of multiple risk factors.[40] Abnormal tests do require repeat testing in 10 to 12 weeks to check for persistence of the abnormality.

Neuroimaging features

The mainstay of diagnosis of NP-cPACNS is neuroimaging. Plain and contrast head computed tomography (CT) have limited diagnostic value in children who present with an acute focal neurologic deficit because the differential diagnosis is wide in children in addition to stroke caused by NP-cPACNS. This circumstance necessitates the use of magnetic resonance (MR) imaging for a rapid and accurate diagnosis of NP-cPACNS. Diffusion-weighted imaging (DWI) and apparent diffusion coefficient maps are vital for the diagnosis of acute ischemic stroke, which is essentially the sole presenting feature of NP-cPACNS. Based on the duration of symptoms, other sequences, such as T1, T2, and fluid-attenuated inversion recovery (FLAIR), will show the evolution of radiographic changes. T2 or gradient echo or susceptibility-weighted imaging are important in the acute setting to detect hemorrhage because this can influence the decision to initiate thrombolytic or antithrombotic therapy for the acute stroke. The role of perfusion-weighted imaging, either with CT or with MR imaging, to detect "brain tissue at risk for further ischemia in the presence of a documented thrombus in a major cerebral blood vessel"[41] and inform decisions to initiate thrombolytic therapy has been established in adults but not yet in children.[41] This area of neuroimaging in pediatric stroke deserves further study.

The strokes in NP-cPACNS typically involve the basal ganglia for reasons mentioned later. Cortical and subcortical ischemic infarction can also be seen. The mechanism of stroke is either related to artery-to-artery embolism of hypoperfusion injury distal to an occluded artery. The anterior circulation is more frequently involved than the posterior circulation in terms of stroke location.

Intracranial vascular imaging is mandatory for demonstration of the vascular abnormalities. Time-of-flight MR angiography (TOF-MRA) is typically available in all centers now and is reasonably helpful in the demonstration of vascular abnormalities, but it has the potential to both underestimate as well as overestimate abnormalities in children.[42] Gadolinium-enhanced MRA (Auto-Triggered Elliptic Centric Ordered sequence [ATECO]-MRA) has been used in adults[43] for a much better demonstration of the intracranial blood vessels, although this technique has not been systematically studied in children, mainly because of technical difficulties. CT angiography (CTA) can overcome the artifact-related problems with TOF-MRA in children based on the authors' experience. However, radiation exposure is always a concern; hence, this technique should be used cautiously in children. Conventional catheter cerebral angiography (CCCA) is the gold standard for demonstrating vasculitis. The authors use this technique at their center in carefully selected cases of CNS vasculitis for diagnosis. The invasive nature of the technique and the lack of easily available skilled pediatric neuroangiographers remain big barriers to its wider applicability. Gadolinium-enhanced contrast study of the affected vascular wall segment is a promising new technique to detect large/medium vessel vasculitis and should be requested.[44,45] In NP-cPACNS, this sequence may reveal wall thickening and concentric contrast enhancement of the affected segment of the vessel wall. The mechanism of gadolinium uptake by the arterial wall in this condition is poorly understood and is speculated to be a result of wall inflammation, although this has not yet been proven. Vessel wall imaging is a potentially exciting area for prospective studies in CNS vasculitis imaging.

In NP-cPACNS, a variety of vascular abnormalities are seen. These abnormalities include narrowing/stenosis ranging from mild to complete occlusion, irregularity, concentric bands of narrowing (Fig. 1), and vasospasm. Sometimes intraluminal thrombus can be seen either partially or fully occluding the lumen of the affected vessel. The typical location of vasculitis is unilateral; the anterior circulation is predominantly involved, with posterior circulation being far less frequently affected. Isolated posterior circulation involvement is exceedingly rare. In the anterior circulation, selective involvement of the distal internal carotid artery (ICA), proximal segments of the anterior (ACA) and/or middle (MCA) cerebral arteries in varying combinations is seen, whereas involvement of the more smaller-sized arteries is rather uncommon.[15] The site of vascular involvement seems typical and explains the higher frequency of basal ganglia strokes in this condition because the lenticulostriate arteries, the sole source of blood supply for the basal ganglia, arise from the proximal segments of the MCA and ACA.

The radiological features of NP-cPACNS are quite typical; in the presence of concordant clinical features, the diagnosis is relatively easy. Similar vascular appearances, however, could potentially occur with other vasculopathies, such as intracranial vessel dissection (although extracranial dissection is more common in children), unilateral moyamoya, and a thrombus arising

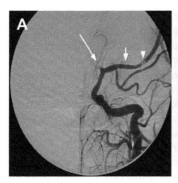
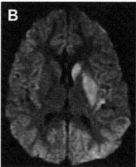
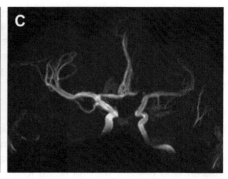

Fig. 1. Angiography-positive NP-cPACNS. (A) Conventional catheter cerebral angiography (Left internal carotid artery [ICA] injection) showing irregularity and narrowing of the distal ICA and middle cerebral artery (MCA) and complete occlusion of the anterior cerebral artery (*long arrow*). Note the concentric bands of narrowing in the MCA (*short arrow*) with a partially occlusive filling defect (*arrowhead*) suggestive of thrombus. This child presented with an acute right-sided hemiplegia caused by an acute ischemic stroke (B, C) involving the left caudate nucleus and putamen. There was a history of chicken pox about 7 to 8 months before the episode leading to a diagnosis of presumed postvaricella large vessel vasculitis.

from a downstream vessel or heart and lodging in the affected vessel. In the authors' experience, these seem to be rare and, when suspected, do need specific investigations for clarification. For instance, to rule out dissection, CCCA and T1 fat-saturated sequence on MR imaging (to screen for eccentric wall hematoma) and T1 wall imaging with contrast (concentric gadolinium uptake by the affected wall helps in the diagnosis) can be helpful (Fig. 2). For moyamoya, CCCA remains the gold standard for staging and, in particular, detecting hypertrophied basal ganglia perforators, the moyamoya vessels. For detecting thromboembolism from a downstream vascular structure, MRA of the neck vessels and cardiac echo can be helpful. In a small proportion of children at the authors' center, NP-cPACNS cases with normal MRA and CCCA at diagnosis have been encountered, which on serial follow-up imaging (4–6 weeks, 3 months) were found to have abnormalities, such as stenosis/narrowing of the expected large vessels in the anterior circulation. This finding shows that a child with acute basal ganglia stroke caused by NP-cPACNS may have no abnormalities on vascular imaging; therefore, close, careful follow-up is essential over the initial 6 months or so to prove or disprove the presence of NP-cPACNS.

Etiopathogenesis

The pathophysiology and cause of NP-cPACNS is still not well understood. NP-cPACNS in its current form has been labeled as *transient cerebral arteriopathy (TCA)* coined by Chabrier and colleagues[46] and more recently as "unilateral focal cerebral arteriopathy of childhood (FCA)" by Bernard and colleagues.[47] It is generally accepted that a subset of NP-cPACNS aka TCA aka FCA are related to

varicella (postvaricella angiopathy, PVA) because exactly similar clinicoradiological appearances have been reported in children with basal ganglia strokes following a varicella infection in the preceding 12 months of presentation. This finding raised the hypothesis that PVA is an inflammatory vasculopathy affecting the large vessels of the anterior circulation and mediated by either reactivation of the virus in the nerves (trigeminal system) innervating the circle of Willis causing invasion of the vessels by the virus or triggering a lymphocytic infiltration of the affected vessels.[48] There is some pathologic data to support this hypothesis. But whether all cases of TCA are postinfectious or inflammatory is still debated. Hence, Braun and colleagues[49] came up with the term focal unilateral intracranial vasculopathy because their argument, also supported by others, was that there could be some children in whom TCA might not necessarily have an inflammatory basis; hence, it would be more appropriate to simply give a descriptive term to the radiological picture of the typical involvement of the distal ICA and proximal ACA and MCA in these children. It is also argued that the term *TCA* is misleading because the progression of vascular abnormalities can occur after diagnosis, albeit over the short-term duration of 3 to 6 months. Thus, it is clear that several aspects of the pathophysiology, cause, and pathology of NP-cPACNS still have not been well elucidated, mainly because of the lack of consistent pathologic data because specimen of blood vessels are understandably difficult to acquire. However, as the current thinking stands, most centers consider NP-cPACNS as a monophasic vasculopathy of likely inflammatory origin that is progressive only in the short-term without evolution into chronicity.

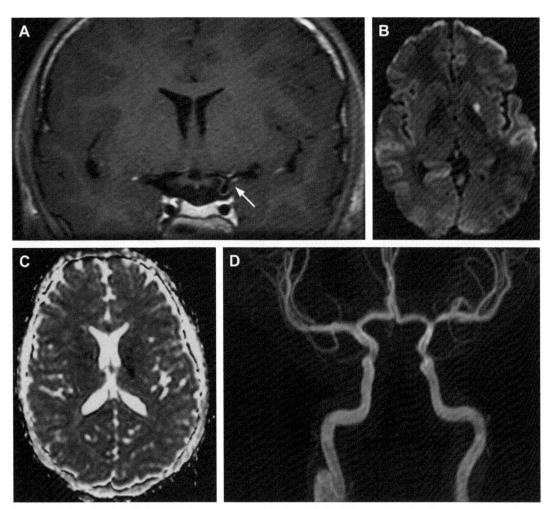

Fig. 2. Wall imaging in NP-cPACNS. Coronal postgadolinium T1 FLAIR image (*A*) showing concentric enhancement of the left distal internal carotid, proximal MCA (*arrow*) and proximal ACA in an 11-year-old girl presenting with acute right face, arm, and leg weakness. DWI (*B, C*) showed acute ischemic stroke involving left putamen and internal capsule. TOF-MRA (*D*) showed a questionable narrowing of the left distal ICA and proximal MCA.

Management

A 3-pronged approach is recommended for the treatment of NP-cPACNS: (1) neuroprotection for the acute ischemic stroke, (2) antithrombotic therapy to treat/prevent thrombus formation in the affected vessel, and (3) immunomodulation for vessel wall inflammation.

Neuroprotection for any child with acute ischemic stroke caused by NP-cPACNS is mandatory. Maintenance of normothermia, normovolemia, normotension, and normoglycemia is vital to protect the "brain tissue at risk" beyond the infracted core of the stroke. The prevention of increases in intracranial pressure, particularly with large MCA strokes, is important. Decompressive craniectomy may need consideration in some children if malignant cerebral edema is imminent.

Prompt management of seizures is also recommended because they can increase the cerebral metabolic demand and have the potential to recruit larger areas of the brain in the infracted zone. Prophylactic anticonvulsants are, however, controversial. A low threshold to electroencephalogram (EEG) and, in selected cases, continuous EEG monitoring does need consideration. Overall, the management of children in the intensive care unit can be beneficial.

Children with NP-cPACNS are typically commenced on antithrombotic therapy at diagnosis, although regimens vary between centers. The rationale behind starting antithrombotics in the presence of a preexisting thrombus in the affected vessel wall is to prevent clot propagation and allow the body's fibrinolytic system to dissolve the clot. In certain instances, thrombolytic therapy (tissue plasminogen activator [tPA]) has been potentially considered in teenagers with NP-cPACNS who have a confirmed stroke with documented intraluminal thrombus, provided they are within the time window and there are no contraindications to give tPA.[50] It must, however, be remembered that safety of tPA in the pediatric age group has not yet been well established.[51] In the absence of a documented luminal thrombus, the rationale behind giving antithrombotic agents is to prevent clot formation in the inflamed vessel because inflammation causes narrowing of vessel lumen and triggers both the coagulation cascade as well as activates platelets increasing the risk of thrombosis. The choice between anticoagulants and antiplatelets is a matter of debate because there are no head-to-head comparative trials in pediatric stroke. Consensus-based treatment guidelines have still not adopted a completely unified approach to antithrombotic therapy in childhood stroke.[52] As a result, treatment is usually based on the preferences of individual centers and physicians. Frequently, anticoagulants, mainly heparin derivatives, are started in the acute setting, particularly in children with a high degree of vascular stenosis followed by long-term, low-dose aspirin for secondary stroke prevention. However, the duration of the treatment for heparin and aspirin, both in the short term and/or long term, varies considerably between centers and reflects the lack of prospective clinical studies in pediatric stroke. Most centers will, however, continue children on some form of antithrombotic therapy for at least 1 to 2 years after the initial stroke provided all risk factors, including vascular risk factors, are no longer active. In the presence of persisting risk factors of recurrent events and significant vascular stenosis, children with NP-cPACNS commonly receive antithrombotic agents, particularly aspirin, for several years.

Immunomodulation therapy with corticosteroids for 3 months remains controversial.[38]

Outcome

Nonprogression of vascular changes is usually confirmed on repeat vascular imaging at 3 months, establishing no evidence of involvement of new vascular beds and resolution of contrast enhancement in the vascular wall in steroid-treated patients. Recurrent ischemic events are seen in 30% to 60% of children.[38] The long-term outcome remains to be systematically studied; it seems to be closely related to the location and extent of the ischemic lesion, stroke recurrence, and possibly the use of corticosteroids. Early comprehensive rehabilitation, as practiced in adult stroke care models, has not been systematically performed or studied in this population; however, it seems to have striking benefits.

Angiography-Positive P-cPACNS

Children with P-cPACNS can commonly present with both focal and diffuse neurologic deficits.[15,53] Interestingly, both angiography-positive CNS vasculitis subtypes, NP-cPACNS and P-cPACNS, predominately affect boys. Children with P-cPACNS are commonly diagnosed when they develop focal deficits, including hemisensory loss or fine motor skill deficits.[15] In addition, difficulty in concentration, cognitive dysfunction, and mood and personality changes are present in these patients.[15] These diffuse deficits develop insidiously. Correspondingly, the time from onset of any symptoms to diagnosis is frequently longer in patients with P-cPACNS compared with patients with NP-cPACNS. Headaches are the leading clinical symptom and present in 95% of patients with P-cPACNS.[15] Systemic underlying conditions have to be carefully looked for and excluded because the clinical and imaging pattern of P-cPACNS is frequently found in angiography-positive, secondary CNS vasculitis of childhood (see later discussion).

Children with P-cPACNS may have mild to moderately increased inflammatory markers; however, inflammatory markers and CSF analysis are not discriminative.[15] A normal CSF cell count or a normal ESR does not exclude an angiography-positive CNS vasculitis. Required MR imaging sequences are identical to those performed in suspected NP-cPACNS. In P-cPACNS, parenchymal lesions on MR imaging can be ischemic and/or inflammatory and are commonly present in more than one vascular territory. One in 4 children has bilateral MR imaging lesions, which are more frequently asymmetric in appearance.[54] The angiography characteristically demonstrates vasculitis of proximal and distal segments of the cerebral arteries (Fig. 3), typically involving multiple vascular beds.[54] Different degrees of gadolinium contrast enhancement can be found in affected vessel wall segments. The anterior circulation is more commonly affected; isolated posterior circulation vasculitis is less common. Conventional angiography provides additional information about the length and degree of stenosis potentially impacting in antithrombotic treatment choices.[55] It also visualizes collateral blood flow into the affected brain tissue identifying additional brain at risk.

Children with P-cPACNS require combination immunosuppressive therapy in addition to antithrombotic therapy. At the time of diagnosis, once-daily intravenous methylprednisolone pulses

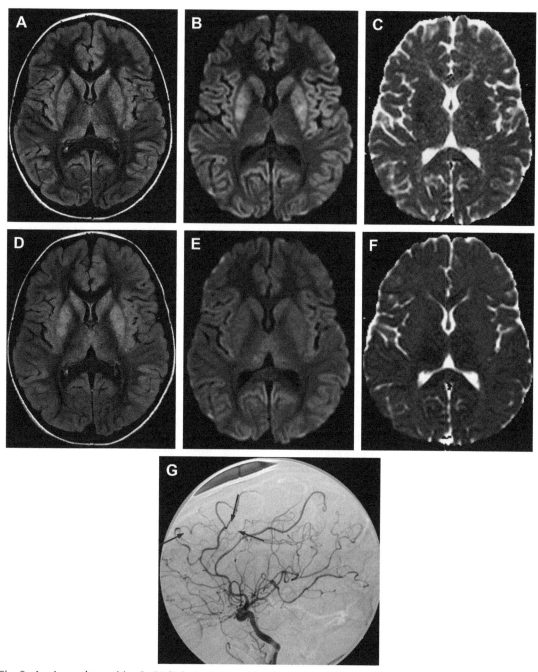

Fig. 3. Angiography-positive P-cPACNS. An 8-year-old girl presented with acute fever, confusion, hallucinations, and generalized tonic-clonic seizures. Physical examination revealed an encephalopathic child with nonfocal neurologic examination without signs of raised intracranial pressure. Brain MR imaging revealed a mildly increased signal in both putamina on FLAIR (*A*), which was mildly restricted in diffusion (*B, C*). There was no gadolinium enhancement, MRA was not done. First follow-up MR imaging, following clinical deterioration and an unrewarding infectious/inflammatory/metabolic workup including CSF, in a week revealed some progression of signal to involve both thalami and insular region (*D–F*). TOF-MRA was normal. Conventional catheter cerebral angiography (*G*) the next day revealed multifocal scattered areas of medium-sized branch irregularity (*arrows*) with narrowing and widening throughout the right and left ICA systems suggesting CNS angiitis.

(30 mg/kg/d) are given at many centers for 3 to 7 days. Subsequently, corticosteroid therapy is switched to daily oral prednisone (2 mg/kg/d, maximum of 60–80 mg), with significant variation between centers. Barron and colleagues[56] first documented the efficacy of cyclophosphamide in cPACNS. In 2001, Gallagher and colleagues[53] reported cyclophosphamide efficacy in 5 children with P-cPACNS. Intravenous monthly cyclophosphamide pulses are commonly given for 6 months, followed by oral maintenance immunosuppression while tapering the child off corticosteroids. The long-term outcome of children with P-cPACNS has not been systematically studied. Residual focal neurologic deficits are often seen in this subtype.[15]

Angiography-Negative, SV-cPACNS

SV-cPACNS is increasingly recognized in intensive care units around the world (Fig. 4). Children present with severe encephalopathy, extensive focal deficits, and/or seizure status and require a rapid, invasive evaluation, including an elective brain biopsy. The differential diagnosis is equally challenging and includes demyelinating diseases, neuronal antibody-mediated inflammatory brain disease, and other less common conditions (Table 1). In contrast to angiography-positive disease, SV-cPACNS has a female predominance.[35,57,58] The mode of onset varies significantly from child to child. Some patients develop significant cognitive deficits over weeks and months, complain of constant headaches, or are diagnosed with focal seizures.[57] Inflammation associated cognitive decline is particularly difficult to detect in children with an underlying learning disability or autism. In contrast, some children have a rapidly progressive disease onset and present with a meningitislike illness. Systemic features, including fever and fatigue, can be present.[44] Seizures are common at diagnosis of SV-cPACNS. All seizure types are seen. Status epilepticus or refractory status epilepticus in previously healthy children mandates an evaluation for an underlying inflammatory brain disease, particularly for SV-cPACNS. In 1990, Matsell and colleagues,[45] were the first to report a case of a child with refractory status epilepticus in whom the diagnosis of cPACNS was made, unfortunately only on autopsy.

Inflammatory markers are frequently abnormal in children with SV-cPACNS; however, the degree of abnormality varies between patients. Hutchinson and colleagues[44] documented that 3 out of 4 children with SV-cPACNS had at least one abnormal inflammatory marker in the blood at diagnosis. More importantly, more than 90% had an abnormal CSF analysis, including increased CSF protein and/or cell count.[57] Mild to moderate CSF lymphocytosis is most commonly seen.

MR imaging abnormalities are present in most patients with SV-cPACNS at diagnosis.[54] Serial studies may be required. MR imaging lesions are best viewed on T2/FLAIR sequences (see Fig. 4). Ischemic lesions are very uncommon.[59] Lesional gadolinium contrast enhancement is present in less than 50% of children with active disease at diagnosis. Meningeal contrast enhancement is equally infrequently seen; however, it is one of the few specific MR imaging finding of SV-cPACNS after infectious meningitis is excluded.[60] It is not present in other inflammatory brain diseases,[61–63] including demyelinating diseases.[64] Inflammatory lesions are most commonly found in the subcortical white matter and cortical gray matter[44]; however, any MR imaging pattern can be seen in SV-cPACNS because of the ubiquitous presence of small blood vessels in the brain and spinal cord. Autopsies have established the generalized character of small vessel vasculitis in contrast to the focal nature of disease suggested by detectable MR imaging lesions. Children presenting in status epilepticus may even have repeatedly normal MR imaging studies and brain biopsy evidence of SV-cPACNS (Senq Lee, 2012, personal communication).

By definition, all patients with SV-cPACNS have normal MRA and conventional angiography studies. Other neuroimaging techniques have so far not provided additional diagnostic certainty in SV-cPACNS. The next step in the diagnostic evaluation is an elective brain biopsy, which should be completed within 10 days from starting immunosuppressive therapy. The brain biopsy should preferably target lesions identified on MR imaging.[64] However, these may either not be accessible or in functionally important areas. In these children, nonlesional biopsies should be performed targeting the nondominant frontal lobe. The diagnostic yield of elective brain biopsies performed for suspected inflammatory brain disease and other treatable conditions other than tumors in children was found to be 69% (1996–20 030).[30,34] The yield is, therefore, significantly higher than in adults.[30,34] The review of brain biopsies in children with SV-cPACNS reveals intramural, inflammatory infiltrates consisting predominantly of lymphocytes. These can also be detected in the perivascular space (see Fig. 1).[35,57,64–66] Childhood CNS vasculitis is a lymphocytic vasculitis that is histologically not characterized by vessel wall destruction, fibrinoid necroses, or evidence of necrosis or granulomas as seen in other types of vasculitis. Granulomatous infiltrates, which are frequently described in adult

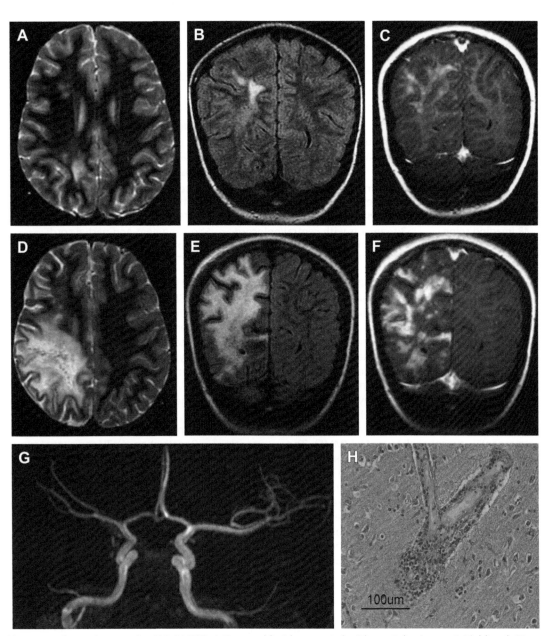

Fig. 4. Angiography-negative SV-cPACNS. A 5-year-old girl presented with partial seizures. Initial head CT was normal. EEG revealed right-sided epileptiform abnormalities. Initial MR imaging revealed multifocal, ill-defined, enhancing areas of T2 and FLAIR hyperintensity scattered throughout the deep white matter of the right cerebral hemisphere, including the right temporal lobe (A–C). There was partial response to anticonvulsant medications. She then developed a slowly progressive left-sided hemiparesis with noticeable cognitive decline. MR imaging 6 months later showed significant interval progression of the white matter abnormalities along with cerebral volume loss (D–F). MRA (G) showed paucity of vessels in the affected region; but conventional catheter cerebral angiography failed to demonstrate angiitis. Right temporal lobe brain and leptomeningeal biopsy revealed nongranulomatous, non-necrotizing small-vessel vasculitis selectively involving the veins, venules, and microvasculature (H, Hematoxylin & Eosin stain, magnification ×400).

PACNS, have so far not been reported in children with cPACNS.[32,35,57,65]

Children with SV-cPACNS require combination immunosuppressive therapy in addition to the mandatory therapy for seizures, abnormal movements, or psychiatric symptoms. Treatment should be initiated rapidly to control the devastating brain inflammation and the resulting clinical features and prevent disease-related damage. Hutchinson and colleagues[57] reported an open-label treatment

Table 1
Comparison of characteristic features of neuromyelitis optic and multiple sclerosis

	Neuromyelitis Optica	Multiple Sclerosis
Female/male ratio	Up to 7:1	2:1
Relapsing course	53%–100%	96%
Secondary progression	Rare	Common
CSF characteristics	Marked pleocytosis (often >50 cells/μL) Lymphocytes or neutrophils	Mild pleocytosis (typically <30 cells/μL) Lymphocytes
CSF oligoclonal bands	90%	<10%
MR imaging brain	Normal, nonspecific white matter changes or characteristic diencephalic and brainstem lesions	Periventricular, juxtacortical, callosal, with T1 black holes indicating chronicity
MR imaging spine	≥3 segments with central/holocord involvement	Short-segment and partial cord involvement

study of children with SV-cPACNS receiving a 6-month induction protocol consisting of corticosteroids (initial methylprednisolone pulses 30 mg/kg/d, with a maximum of 1000 mg for 3–5 days followed by oral prednisone 2 mg/kg, with a maximum of 60 mg/d with defined monthly taper) plus monthly intravenous cyclophosphamide pulses (500–750 mg/m^2, plus sodium-2-mercaptoethane sulfonate [MESNA] and hyperhydration). After 6 months, children were switched to maintenance treatment initially with azathioprine but more recently mycophenolate mofetil (MMF). The treatment was found to be effective and safe. After 24 months, 70% of the children had no evidence of any functional neurologic deficit as measured by the pediatric stroke outcome measure.[57] Case series from other centers supported the efficacy of cyclophosphamide and MMF.[67,68] Most series document good recovery of neurologic deficits. At many centers, children continue the anticonvulsive medication beyond 24 months.

SECONDARY CNS VASCULITIS
Infection-Associated Secondary CNS Vasculitis

The most common cause for a secondary inflammatory brain disease is infection.[69] Infections can cause a true infectious CNS vasculitis with bacteria infecting the vessel wall as seen, for example, with streptococcus pneumonia or mycobacterium tuberculosis meningitis. Infections can lead to a postinfectious inflammatory vasculitis; finally, infections can cause MR imaging lesions mimicking those seen with vasculitis. A comprehensive infectious workup is mandatory in all children with suspected vasculitic or nonvasculitic inflammatory brain disease. Standardized approaches, such as encephalitis registries, are helpful.[69] Most infections can be identified in

cultures and/or by polymerase chain reaction of serum and CSF.[69] However, specific circumstances, including travel history, have to be considered when testing.

Varicella zoster virus (VZV) can infect a wide variety of cell types in the central and peripheral nervous system and cause severe infective encephalitis.[19] VZV infection can lead to latency of the virus in the nerve root ganglia, including the trigeminal nerve, which is located in close proximity to the branching of the major cerebral blood vessels.[19,55] Reactivation of VZV and axonal migration causes a focal, unilateral inflammation of the vascular wall of the adjacent proximal segments of the large CNS vessels virtually indistinguishable from NP-cPACNS apart from evidence of VZV infection.[19,53,55] This condition is referred to as postvaricella angiopathy (PVA) or transient cerebral angiopathy. The proposed treatment regime includes antiviral therapy plus immunosuppression with high-dose corticosteroids. Many physicians consider the different diseases PVA, transient cerebral angiopathy, and NP-cPACNS to be widely overlapping and primarily inflammatory in nature.

Human immunodeficiency virus (HIV) (Fig. 5) can cause a secondary CNS vasculitis in children and adults, which closely resembles P-cPACNS.[55] The initiation of antiviral therapy frequently causes an immune reconstitution inflammatory syndrome with worsening vascular disease. Immunosuppressive therapy has to be considered. Many other viruses, bacteria, and fungal infections can cause secondary CNS vasculitis.

Secondary CNS Vasculitis in Rheumatic and Systemic Inflammatory Diseases

Secondary CNS vasculitis can be the presenting symptom in childhood rheumatic diseases or develop in the course of illness.[54] CNS vasculitis is

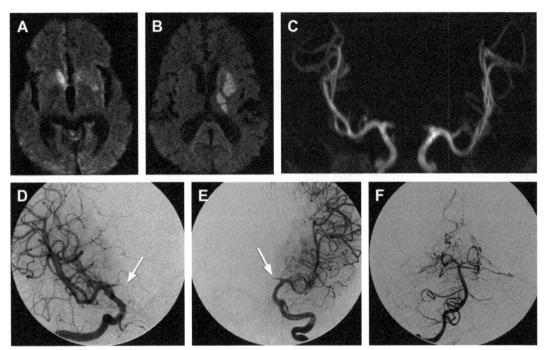

Fig. 5. Infection-related secondary CNS vasculitis in a child. An 8-year-old boy who was HIV seropositive presented who was admitted to the hospital for Salmonella bacteremia developed sudden-onset new right-sided hemiparesis involving face, arm, and leg. DWI (*A, B*) confirmed acute ischemic infarction of the left putamen, left caudate nucleus, left corona radiata, as well as the head of the right caudate nucleus. MRA (*C*) revealed occlusion of both anterior cerebral arteries, which was subsequently confirmed on the conventional angiography (*D, E, arrows*) that revealed additional posterior circulation involvement in the form of left posterior cerebral artery narrowing (*F*).

seen in children with systemic lupus erythematosus; anti-neutrophil cytoplasmic antibody–associated systemic vasculitis, including granulomatosis with polyangiitis (previously known as Wegener granulomatosis) and microscopic polyangitis (MPA); in polyarteritis nodosa (PAN); and Takayasu arteritis.[23,26,28,54,70] The treatment of secondary CNS vasculitis in rheumatic diseases commonly includes high-dose corticosteroids and cyclophosphamide. Inflammatory conditions, such as hemophagocytic lymphohistiocytosis (HLH) (**Fig. 6**), Kawasaki disease, and inflammatory bowel disease, can be complicated with secondary CNS vasculitis.[71,72]

HLH is a rare, potentially fatal disease of activated histiocytes and macrophages clinically presenting as fever, hepatosplenomegaly, pancytopenia, low fibrinogen level, organ dysfunction, elevation of liver enzymes, ferritin and lactate dehydrogenase, and hypertriglyceridemia.[73] The pathology relates to the dysfunction of activated CD8+ T lymphocytes and natural killer cells and their inability to kill targets, such as virus-infected cells. Subsequently, macrophage is activated and hemophagocytosis is present in multiple organs causing organ dysfunction. CNS involvement is frequently present. The neuropathological hallmarks of HLH consist of

a diffuse infiltration by monocytes and activated lymphocytes of leptomeninges and brain parenchyma along penetrating vessels. Infiltration is associated with focal and confluent areas of myelin pallor as well as neuronal loss, tissue necrosis, and cavitation.[8,74] The presenting symptoms reflect the CNS localization of the lesions. They can be present only in the white matter of the cortex and cerebellum but often involve the cortical structures or the brainstem. Moshous and colleagues[72] describe a 4-year-old girl with CNS vasculitis and perforin deficiency without classic laboratory or clinical signs of active HLH at the time of her CNS manifestations. Therefore, a new neurologic deficit in children with systemic inflammatory diseases should lead to prompt further investigations, such as MRI; MRA; angiography; and, if required, a brain biopsy.

The primary form, the familial HLH (FHLH), typically seen during infancy and early childhood, is thought to be fatal, with a median survival without therapy of 2 months after onset if not rescued by bone marrow transplantation.[8,75] The known genetic causes involve genes that regulate proteins that are important in the secretory cytolytic pathway: perforin (*PRF*) in FHLH2, adaptor protein-3 β1 subunit (*AP3B1*) in Hermansky-Pudlak type 2, the

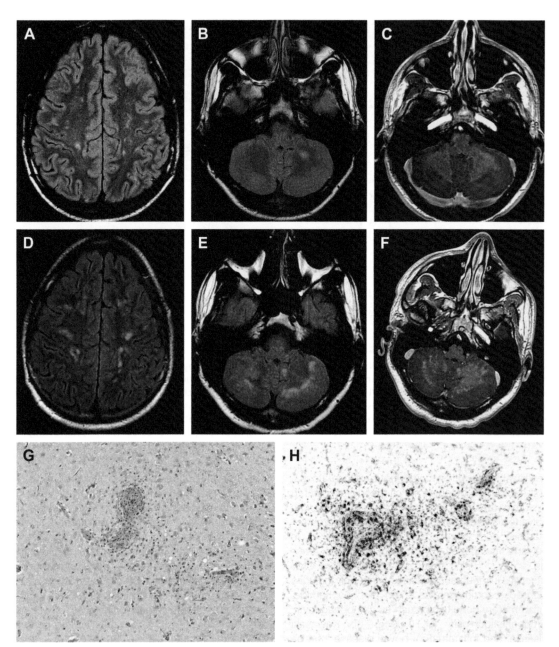

Fig. 6. Neoplasm-related secondary CNS vasculitis. A 14-year-old young man presented with a subacute history of weight loss, dizziness, transient lower limb paresthesias, and ataxia. Past history was remarkable for history of HLH in infancy, which remitted well on chemotherapy. He remained well all these years until the recent onset of neurologic symptoms. His brain MR imaging showed multiple small areas of high signal intensity on T2 and FLAIR images in the cerebral white matter (A) as well as the cerebellum (B). There was faint enhancement of some of the lesions (C). He also had a few lesions in the cervical and thoracic cord (not shown here). He was initially treated with corticosteroids that resulted in transient clinical and radiological improvement. However, after about 6 weeks, he re-presented with history of increasing ataxia and excessive lethargy progressing onto reduced level of consciousness. Repeat MR imaging showed marked progression of new lesions in the white matter (D) as well as the cerebellum (E) that enhanced on gadolinium (F). Vascular imaging (MRAs) all through this time was normal. He eventually had a brain biopsy and was confirmed to have lymphocytic small vessel vasculitis of the CNS (hematoxylin-eosin [G]; immunohistochemistry also showed macrophages [H]). At this time, he also had a bone marrow biopsy, which confirmed a systemic relapse of the HLH. Genetic testing confirmed Griscelli syndrome type-II, which had been suspected all along because of his striking blond hair, although hair pathology was not conclusive.

lysosomal trafficking regulator (*LYST*) in Chediak-Higashi syndrome, Rab27z (*RAB27A*) in Griscelli type 2, Munc13-4 (*UNC13D*) in FHLH3, and Stx-11 (*STX11*) in FHLH4.[75] Macrophage activation and hemophagocytosis also occur in association with severe infections, malignancies, or rheumatologic diseases. In 1994, the Histiocyte Society developed a common treatment protocol (HLH-94) in which immunotherapy with cyclosporine A (CSA) is combined with corticosteroids (CS) and VP-16. Intrathecal methotrexate is added in selected patients. The aim is first to achieve a clinically stable resolution and ultimately to cure by bone-marrow transplantation.

Kawasaki disease is a systemic vasculitis mainly involving the coronary arteries. However, it can be complicated with secondary CNS vasculitis.[10] Although MR imaging scans do not reveal abnormalities in the acute stage of the disease, in some patients single-photon emission CT imaging demonstrated localized cerebral hypoperfusion[76] and postmortem brain examinations may reveal leptomeningeal thickening, endarteritis, and periarteritis.[10] A different pathophysiological mechanism of CNS injury in Kawasaki is related to the macrophage activation syndrome (MAS). The clinical and laboratory similarities between HLH and MAS have led to the general acceptance of MAS as a form of secondary HLH.[69,77,78]

Secondary CNS Vasculitis in Other Systemic Diseases/Exposures

Secondary CNS vasculitis has been described in patients after radiation therapy.[11] Graft-versus-host disease can also cause CNS vasculitis in children who were treated for malignancies. Drugs, such as cocaine and amphetamines, can cause a secondary CNS vasculitis but are also capable of mimicking CNS vasculitis without an inflammatory component but a vasoconstrictive component.[79]

SUMMARY

Children with CNS vasculitis typically present with acquired new-onset, often focal neurologic deficits; however, symptoms and signs of diffuse involvement can also occur depending on the size of the blood vessels involved. The diagnosis of CNS vasculitis in children mandates a thorough search for confirmation of the diagnosis by a judicious use of laboratory inflammatory markers and a variety of neuroimaging techniques because the latter is the key for diagnosis. Pattern recognition of subtypes of CNS vasculitis is essential to decide more invasive diagnostic techniques, such as catheter cerebral angiography and brain biopsy in selected cases. The treatment of childhood CNS vasculitis entails the protection of the brain from the ill effects of vascular inflammation, and the most important among these being acute ischemic stroke and its resultant long-term as well as potential short-term deleterious effects. Neuroprotection, antithrombotic therapy, and anti-inflammatory therapy remain the cornerstones of the management of CNS vasculitis in varying proportions. Early diagnosis likely improves the outcome by early facilitation of specific treatment regimen. The outcome can be potentially improved by a multidisciplinary care with expertise from neurology, neuroradiology, rheumatology, hematology, intensive care, and rehabilitation services. Long-term prospective studies are, however, essential for optimal individualized care.

REFERENCES

1. Hajj-Ali RA, Calabrese LH. Central nervous system vasculitis. Curr Opin Rheumatol 2009;21:10–8.
2. Siva A. Vasculitis of the nervous system. J Neurol 2001;248:451–68.
3. Cellucci T, Benseler SM. Central nervous system vasculitis in children. Curr Opin Rheumatol 2010; 22:590–7.
4. Dalmau J, Gleichman AJ, Hughes EG, et al. Anti-NMDA-receptor encephalitis: case series and analysis of the effects of antibodies. Lancet Neurol 2008;7(12):1091–8.
5. Elbers J, Benseler SM. Central nervous system vasculitis in children. Curr Opin Rheumatol 2008; 20:47–54.
6. Dale RC, Brilot F, Banwell B. Pediatric central nervous system inflammatory demyelination: acute disseminated encephalomyelitis, clinically isolated syndromes, neuromyelitis optica, and multiple sclerosis. Curr Opin Neurol 2009;22:233–40.
7. Cellucci T, Benseler SM. Diagnosing central nervous system vasculitis in children. Curr Opin Pediatr 2010;22:731–8.
8. Akima M, Sumi SM. Neuropathology of familial erythrophagocytic lymphohistiocytosis: six cases and review of the literature. Hum Pathol 1984;15:161–8.
9. Alper G, Wang L. Demyelinating optic neuritis in children. J Child Neurol 2009;24:45–8.
10. Amano S, Hazama F. Neutral involvement in Kawasaki disease. Acta Pathol Jpn 1980;30:365–73.
11. Aoki S. Radiation-induced arteritis: thickened wall with prominent enhancement on cranial MR images report of five cases and comparison with 18 cases of Moyamoya disease. Radiology 2002; 223:683–8.
12. Begelman SM, Olin JW. Fibromuscular dysplasia. Curr Opin Rheumatol 2000;12:41–7.

13. Bien CG, Scheffer IE. Autoantibodies and epilepsy. Epilepsia 2011;52(Suppl 3):18–22.

14. Byg KE, Milman N, Hansen S. Sarcoidosis in Denmark 1980-1994. A registry-based incidence study comprising 5536 patients. Sarcoidosis Vasc Diffuse Lung Dis 2003;20:46–52.

15. Benseler SM. Primary central nervous system vasculitis in children. Arthritis Rheum 2006;54: 1291–7.

16. Covarrubias DJ, Luetmer PH, Campeau NG. Posterior reversible encephalopathy syndrome: prognostic utility of quantitative diffusion-weighted MR images. AJNR Am J Neuroradiol 2002;23:1038–48.

17. Cross AH, Golumbek PT. Neurologic manifestations of celiac disease: proven, or just a gut feeling? Neurology 2003;60:1566–8.

18. de Oliveira SK, Pelajo CF. Pediatric Autoimmune Neuropsychiatric Disorders Associated with Streptococcal Infection (PANDAS): a controversial diagnosis. Curr Infect Dis Rep 2010;12:103–9.

19. Gilden DH, Kleinschmidt-DeMasters BK, LaGuardia JJ, et al. Neurologic complications of the reactivation of varicella-zoster virus. N Engl J Med 2000;342:635–45.

20. Hoffmann AL, Milman N, Byg KE. Childhood sarcoidosis in Denmark 1979-1994: incidence, clinical features and laboratory results at presentation in 48 children. Acta Paediatr 2004;93:30–6.

21. Ibrahimi DM, Tamargo RJ, Ahn ES. Moyamoya disease in children. Childs Nerv Syst 2010;26: 1297–308.

22. Milman N, Hoffmann AL. Childhood sarcoidosis: long-term follow-up. Eur Respir J 2008;31:592–8.

23. Nishino H, Rubino FA, DeRemee RA, et al. Neurological involvement in Wegener's granulomatosis: an analysis of 324 consecutive patients at the Mayo Clinic. Ann Neurol 1993;33:4–9.

24. Pardo CA. The pathology of Rasmussen syndrome: stages of cortical involvement and neuropathological studies in 45 hemispherectomies. Epilepsia 2004;45:516–26.

25. Rafay MF. Craniocervical arterial dissection in children: clinical and radiographic presentation and outcome. J Child Neurol 2006;21:8–16.

26. Rossi CM, Di Comite G. The clinical spectrum of the neurological involvement in vasculitides. J Neurol Sci 2009;285:13–21.

27. Kramer U. Febrile infection-related epilepsy syndrome (FIRES): pathogenesis, treatment, and outcome: a multicenter study on 77 children. Epilepsia 2011; 52(11):1956–65.

28. von Scheven E, Lee C, Berg BO. Pediatric Wegener's granulomatosis complicated by central nervous system vasculitis. Pediatr Neurol 1998;19:317–9.

29. Wingerchuk DM, Hogancamp WF, O'Brien PC, et al. The clinical course of neuromyelitis optica (Devic's syndrome). Neurology 1999;53:1107–14.

30. Venkateswaran S, Hawkins C, Wassmer E. Diagnostic yield of brain biopsies in children presenting to neurology. J Child Neurol 2008;23:253–8.

31. Calabrese LH, Mallek JA. Primary angiitis of the central nervous system. Report of 8 new cases, review of the literature, and proposal for diagnostic criteria. Medicine (Baltimore) 1988;67:20–39.

32. Salvarani C. Primary central nervous system vasculitis: analysis of 101 patients. Ann Neurol 2007;62: 442–51.

33. Cravioto H, Feigin I. Noninfectious granulomatous angiitis with a predilection for the nervous system. Neurology 1959;9:599–609.

34. Lie JT. Primary (granulomatous) angiitis of the central nervous system: a clinicopathologic analysis of 15 new cases and a review of the literature. Hum Pathol 1992;23:164–71.

35. Benseler SM. Angiography-negative primary central nervous system vasculitis in children: a newly recognized inflammatory central nervous system disease. Arthritis Rheum 2005;52:2159–67.

36. Golomb MR, Fullerton HJ, Nowak-Gottl U, et al. Male predominance in childhood ischemic stroke: findings from the international pediatric stroke study. Stroke 2009;40:52–7.

37. Braun KPJ, Rafay MF, Uiterwaal CSPM, et al. Mode of onset predicts etiological diagnosis of arterial ischemic stroke in children. Stroke 2007; 38:298–302.

38. Soon GS. Non-progressive primary CNS vasculitis in children: immunosuppression reduces recurrent ischemic event risk. Arthritis Rheum 2008;9:S942.

39. Dale RC, Brilot F, Fagan E, et al. Cerebrospinal fluid neopterin in pediatric neurology: a marker of active central nervous system inflammation. Dev Med Child Neurol 2009;51(4):317–23.

40. Kenet G, Lutkhoff LK, Albisetti M, et al. Impact of thrombophilia on risk of arterial ischemic stroke or cerebral sinovenous thrombosis in neonates and children. A systematic review and meta-analysis of observational studies. Circulation 2010;121: 1838–47.

41. Schellinger P, Fiebach JC. Perfusion-weighted imaging/diffusion-weighted imaging mismatch on MRI can now be used to select patients for recombinant tissue plasminogen activator beyond 3 hours. Stroke 2005;36:1098–101.

42. Husson B, Rodesch G, Lasjaunias P, et al. Magnetic resonance angiography in childhood arterial brain infarcts: a comparative study with contrast angiography. Stroke 2002;33:1280–5.

43. Mikulis DJ, Roberts TPL. Neuro MR: protocols. J Magn Reson Imaging 2007;26(4):838–47.

44. Kuker W. Vessel wall contrast enhancement: a diagnostic sign of cerebral vasculitis. Cerebrovasc Dis 2008;26:23–9.

45. Matsell DG, Keene DL, Jimenez C, et al. Isolated angiitis of the central nervous system in childhood. Can J Neurol Sci 1990;17(2):151–4.

46. Chabrier S, Rodesch G, Lasjaunias P, et al. Transient cerebral arteriopathy: a disorder recognized by serial angiograms in children with stroke. J Child Neurol 1998;13:27–32.

47. Bernard TJ, Manco-Johnson MJ, Lo W, et al. Towards a consensus-based classification of childhood arterial ischemic stroke. Stroke 2012;43(2):371–7.

48. Askalan R, Laughlin S, Mayank S, et al. Chicken pox and stroke in childhood: a study of frequency and causation. Stroke 2001;32:1257–62.

49. Braun KP, Bulder MM, Chabrier S, et al. The course and outcome of unilateral intracranial arteriopathy in 79 children with ischemic stroke. Brain 2009;132: 544–57.

50. Amlie-Lefond C, Benedict S, Bernard T, et al, the International Paediatric Stroke Study Investigators. Thrombolysis in children with arterial ischemic stroke: initial results from the International Paediatric Stroke Study. Stroke 2007;38:485.

51. Amlie-lefond C, Chan AK, Kirton A, et al, The Thrombolysis in Pediatric Stroke (TIPS) Investigators. Thrombolysis in acute childhood stroke: design and challenges of the thrombolysis in pediatric stroke clinical trial. Neuroepidemiology 2009;32:279–86.

52. Roach ES, Golomb MR, Adams R, et al. Management of stroke in infants and children: a scientific statement from a Special Writing Group of the American Heart Association Stroke Council and the Council on Cardiovascular Disease in the Young. Stroke 2008;39:2644–91.

53. Ueno M, Oka A, Koeda T, et al. Unilateral occlusion of the middle cerebral artery after varicella-zoster virus infection. Brain Dev 2002;24:106–8.

54. Pomper MG, Miller TJ, Stone JH, et al. CNS vasculitis in autoimmune disease: MR imaging findings and correlation with angiography. AJNR Am J Neuroradiol 1999;20:75–85.

55. Nogueras C. Recurrent stroke as a manifestation of primary angiitis of the central nervous system in a patient infected with human immunodeficiency virus. Arch Neurol 2002;59:468–73.

56. Barron TF, Ostrov BE, Zimmerman RA, et al. Isolated angiitis of CNS: treatment with pulse cyclophosphamide. Pediatr Neurol 1993;9:73–5.

57. Hutchinson C. Treatment of small vessel primary CNS vasculitis in children: an open-label cohort study. Lancet Neurol 2010;9:1078–84.

58. Matsell DG, Keene DL, Jimenez C, et al. Isolated angiitis of the central nervous system in childhood. Can J Neurol Sci 1990;17:151–4.

59. Monagle P, Chalmers E, Chan A, et al. Antithrombotic therapy in neonates and children: American College of Chest Physicians evidence-based clinical practice guidelines (8th edition). Chest 2008;133: 887S–968S.

60. Aviv RI. MR imaging and angiography of primary CNS vasculitis of childhood. AJNR Am J Neuroradiol 2006;27:192–9.

61. Paediatric Stroke Working Group. Stroke in childhood: clinical guidelines for diagnosis, management and rehabilitation. Published by the Royal College of Physicians of London (UK) November 2004. Available at: http://www.rcplondon.ac.uk/pubs/books/childstroke/.

62. Gallagher KT. Primary angiitis of the central nervous system in children: 5 cases. J Rheumatol 2001;28: 616–23.

63. Aviv RI. Angiography of primary central nervous system angiitis of childhood: conventional angiography versus magnetic resonance angiography at presentation. AJNR Am J Neuroradiol 2007;28:9–15.

64. Elbers J, Halliday W, Hawkins C, et al. Brain biopsy in children with primary small-vessel central nervous system vasculitis. Ann Neurol 2010;68:602–10.

65. Lanthier S. Isolated angiitis of the CNS in children. Neurology 2001;56:837–42.

66. Yaari R. Childhood primary angiitis of the central nervous system: two biopsy-proven cases. J Pediatr 2004;145:693–7.

67. Sen ES. Treatment of primary angiitis of the central nervous system in childhood with mycophenolate mofetil. Rheumatology (Oxford) 2010;49:806–11.

68. Bitter KJ, Epstein LG, Melin-Aldana H, et al. Cyclophosphamide treatment of primary angiitis of the central nervous system in children: report of 2 cases. J Rheumatol 2006;33:2078–80.

69. Ford-Jones EL. Acute childhood encephalitis and meningoencephalitis: diagnosis and management. Paediatr Child Health 1998;3:33–40.

70. Seror R. Central nervous system involvement in Wegener granulomatosis. Medicine (Baltimore) 2006;85:54–65.

71. Nadeau SE. Neurologic manifestations of systemic vasculitis. Neurol Clin 2002;20:123–50, vi.

72. Moshous D. Primary necrotizing lymphocytic central nervous system vasculitis due to perforin deficiency in a four-year-old girl. Arthritis Rheum 2007;56: 995–9.

73. Perry MC, Harrison EG Jr, Burgert EO Jr, et al. Familial erythrophagocytic lymphohistiocytosis. Report of two cases and clinicopathologic review. Cancer 1976;38:209–18.

74. Goldberg J, Nezelof C. Lymphohistiocytosis: a multifactorial syndrome of macrophagic activation clinico-pathological study of 38 cases. Hematol Oncol 1986;4:275–89.

75. Gupta S, Weitzman S. Primary and secondary hemophagocytic lymphohistiocytosis: clinical features, pathogenesis and therapy. Expert Rev Clin Immunol 2010;6:137–54.

76. Ichiyama T. Cerebral hypoperfusion during acute Kawasaki disease. Stroke 1998;29:1320–1.

77. Grom AA. Macrophage activation syndrome and reactive hemophagocytic lymphohistiocytosis: the same entities? Curr Opin Rheumatol 2003;15: 587–90.

78. Ramanan AV, Schneider R. Macrophage activation syndrome–what's in a name! J Rheumatol 2003;30: 2513–6.

79. Singhal AB. Reversible cerebral vasoconstriction syndromes: analysis of 139 Cases. Arch Neurol 2011;68(8):1005–12.

Anti–NMDA Receptor Encephalitis

Kevin Charles Jones, MD[a], Susanne M. Benseler, MD, PhD[b],
Mahendranath Moharir, MD, MSc, FRACP[a],*

KEYWORDS

- Anti-NMDA receptor encephalitis • Pediatric age • Inflammatory brain disorder
- Paraneoplastic conditions

KEY POINTS

- Anti–N-methyl-D-aspartate (NMDA) receptor encephalitis is a severe but potentially reversible neurologic disorder that is clinically recognizable in children and adolescents.
- Prompt diagnosis and treatment are essential to facilitate recovery.
- The clinical syndrome is confirmed by the presence of NMDA receptor antibodies in cerebrospinal fluid or serum.
- Treatment consists of corticosteroids, intravenous immunoglobulin, or plasma exchange as first-line therapy followed by cyclophosphamide or rituximab, if necessary, as second-line immunotherapy. Patients with tumor-associated encephalitis benefit from tumor resection.
- More than 75% of patients make a substantial recovery, which occurs in the reverse order of symptom presentation associated with a decline in antibody titers.

INTRODUCTION

In 2005, 4 young women with a syndrome of acute psychiatric symptoms, seizures, memory loss, encephalopathy, and hypoventilation associated with an ovarian teratoma were reported. These women were found to have antibodies that reacted with neuronal cell-surface antigens.[1] These antibodies were subsequently found out to be auto-antibodies targeting the NR1 and NR2 N-methyl-D-aspartate (NMDA) glutamate receptors in another series of 12 women with a similar neuropsychiatric syndrome in the presence of ovarian teratoma.[2] These reports were just the beginning of what has now turned out to be an increasingly reported new immune-mediated neurologic syndrome, anti-NMDA receptor (NMDAR)-mediated encephalitis. A seminal publication in 2008 by Dalmau and

colleagues[3] described the syndrome in great detail and outlined its salient characteristics in a large cohort of 100 patients. The majority of reported subjects in the cohort were adult females who had an ovarian teratoma in the background. Since this article was published, however, it has become increasingly clear that the syndrome is not restricted to adult females but can also be seen in adult males and children of either sex in the absence of an associated systemic neoplasm.[4] It appears that this syndrome is still underrecognized as its existence is only being gradually appreciated. However, other previously reported disorders could perhaps have been anti-NMDAR encephalitis; these include idiopathic encephalitis with psychiatric manifestations or dyskinesias,[5] coma associated with intense bursts of abnormal

[a] Division of Neurology, Department of Pediatrics, The Hospital for Sick Children, 555 University Avenue, Toronto, Ontario M5G 1X8, Canada; [b] Division of Rheumatology, Department of Pediatrics, The Hospital for Sick Children, University of Toronto, 555 University Avenue, Toronto, Ontario M5G 1X8, Canada
* Corresponding author.
E-mail address: mahendranath.moharir@sickkids.ca

Neuroimag Clin N Am 23 (2013) 309–320
http://dx.doi.org/10.1016/j.nic.2012.12.009

movements and long-lasting cognitive and behavioral disturbances,[6] acquired reversible autistic syndrome in acute encephalopathic illness in children,[7] immune-mediated chorea encephalopathy syndrome in childhood,[8] juvenile acute nonherpetic encephalitis,[7] and encephalitis lethargica.[9] Moreover, with increasing literature the syndrome appears to encompass a far wider spectrum of clinical presentation than initially described. The discovery of anti-NMDAR encephalitis has led to the detection of a growing list of many other autoimmune synaptic receptor encephalitides, including those mediated by antibodies toward the 2-amino-3-(3-hydroxy-5-methyl-isoxazol-4-yl) propanoic acid (AMPA) receptor,[10] γ-aminobutyric acid (GABA) B receptor,[11] and leucine-rich, glioma-B inactivated 1 (LGI1) receptor. The LGI1 receptor is the antigen previously ascribed to voltage-gated potassium channel encephalitis.[12] These immune-mediated responses are now providing an understanding of the function of the neurotransmitter receptors affected by these antibodies.[4] This article focuses on anti-NMDAR encephalitis in the pediatric age group.

EPIDEMIOLOGY

The incidence of anti-NMDAR encephalitis in both children and adults is unknown at present. It appears to be more common than previously thought, given the increasing literature. A retrospective study of adults with encephalitis of unknown origin identified NMDAR antibodies in 1% of patients admitted to intensive care.[13] A multicenter, population-based prospective study of causes of encephalitis in adults and children in the United Kingdom showed that 4% of patients had anti-NMDAR encephalitis. The most common immune-mediated causes were acute disseminated encephalomyelitis, followed by anti-NMDAR encephalitis and other antibody-associated encephalitides.[14] The California Encephalitis project tested 20 patients and identified 10 as anti-NMDAR positive. All 10 patients had negative viral studies, but 4 were positive for serum *Mycoplasma* immunoglobulin M antibodies. The median age was 18.5 years, with a predilection for Asians and Pacific Islanders.[5] In a case series in children and adults in 2009, 40% were children younger than 18 years with the youngest child being only 23 months old.[4] In the Dalmau series of 100 patients, 22 were children younger than 18 years, 55% of whom had an underlying tumor.[3] A child as young as 20 months has been reported with symptoms and neuronal antibodies consistent with anti-NMDAR encephalitis.[15]

CLINICAL PRESENTATION

Anti-NMDAR encephalitis presents as a characteristic syndrome that develops in progressive stages of illness and recovery. The clinical syndrome was first defined in a series of 100 patients, which included adults and children.[3] This study was followed by a second series that concentrated on 32 children younger than 18 years who were compared with 49 adults identified at the same time.[4] Individual case reports and smaller case series have substantiated these findings.[16] The phenotype in adults and children is similar, except that autonomic dysfunction and hypoventilation are probably less common and less severe in children.[4]

Prodromal Features

At the onset of the syndrome, symptoms including fever, headache, rhinitis, vomiting, and diarrhea have been recorded in 48% of children.[4]

Psychiatric Features

Within 2 weeks, patients usually develop psychiatric symptoms, including anxiety, paranoia, fear, psychosis, mania, and insomnia. Social withdrawal and stereotypical behavior are also possible. In a series of mostly adult patients, 85% presented initially to a psychiatrist for anxiety, agitation, and visual or auditory hallucinations.[3] Of 32 children, 87% presented with changes in behavior or personality.[4] The recognition of psychosis in young children is challenging. The behavioral changes include increased tantrums, irritability, and hyperactivity. Behavior can be hypersexual or aggressive. Acute mania with psychosis and a catatonic state has been reported in an adolescent female with anti-NMDAR encephalitis.[17] As patients with psychosis are often treated initially with neuroleptic medications, neuroleptic malignant syndrome can compound the clinical picture because symptoms of rigidity, autonomic instability, and elevation of muscle enzymes, typically associated with this syndrome, can occur independently in anti-NMDAR encephalitis in the absence of neuroleptics.[18]

Neurologic Features

In children, the chief features include movement disorders, seizures and cognitive problems. Other features reported in adults appear to be less common in children such as autonomic instability and sleep disorders.[18]

Movement disorders

Movement disorders are a very frequent neurologic feature of this syndrome and have been reported in 84% of a case series in children with orofacial dyskinesias occurring in 45%, choreoathetosis in 32%, and dystonia in 32%. Oculogyric crisis, rigidity, and opisthotonic postures are also reported.[4] Orofacial dyskinesias are described as chewing, tongue thrusting, lip smacking, and facial grimacing movements. There are descriptions of more complex, stereotyped movements including pelvic thrusting, pseudo–piano-playing motions, and writhing of the extremities. Some movements, such as pelvic thrusting, have the potential to be considered as nonorganic phenomena. Limb movements mimicking epileptic seizures may also occur. Patients may develop episodic opisthotonus, dystonia, and oculogyric crises, associated with tachycardia and hypertension, which is suggestive of autonomic storming.[19] Opsoclonus-myoclonus has been reported in a woman with anti-NMDAR encephalitis.[20]

Seizures

Seizures are reported in about 77% of children,[4] and can be difficult to recognize and treat. Both partial and generalized seizures as well as status epilepticus can occur, although partial seizures seem to predominate.[4] Abnormal repetitive movements may mimic partial seizures, necessitating video electroencephalogram (VEEG) monitoring for definitive diagnosis of seizures in some cases.[21] The presentation of partial status epilepticus in anti-NMDAR encephalitis may lead to the consideration of a diagnosis of Rasmussen syndrome.[22] Unexplained new-onset epilepsy in young women and adolescents may be a feature of anti-NMDAR encephalitis.[23]

Cognitive problems

Short-term memory loss is underestimated, as the assessment of memory is affected by the psychiatric symptoms and speech problems.[3] Retrospectively, patients often report amnesia of the illness.[3,24] A rapid deterioration of language, ranging from reduced verbal output and echolalia with echopraxia to frank mutism, is common.[25] This symptom may be followed by a decreased level of consciousness and alternate periods of agitation and catatonia. Dissociative responses to stimuli are often noted.[26]

Autonomic Dysfunction

Tachycardia, hypertension, and hyperthermia occurred in 86% of a case series of 32 children.[4] Autonomic instability and hypoventilation are reported to be less severe, and dysrhythmias in children are less likely to require pacing than in adults.[4] Mechanical ventilation may sometimes be needed for central hypoventilation and airway protection.[4] Hyperthermia is common throughout the disease, frequently leading to extensive investigations to exclude infectious processes. Hypersalivation and urinary incontinence are some of the other frequently reported symptoms.

Miscellaneous Features

Insomnia is reported as an early presenting sign, at least in adults. Sleep-wake cycles are disrupted and patients arouse frequently. During recovery patients may have hypersomnia. Symptoms of hypothalamic dysfunction have been recognized in a few patients. Recurrent optic neuritis with transient cerebral lesions has been reported in one patient.[27]

Anti-NMDAR encephalitis has also been reported in an adolescent female, with recurrent relapses associated with extensive longitudinal myelitis and optic neuritis mimicking neuromyelitis optica.[28]

Physical Examination

Systemic and neurologic signs are nonspecific. There are no markers in the clinical examination that can suggest anti-NMDAR encephalitis. Hence, a low threshold of suspicion is warranted in patients with a constellation of movement disorder, seizures, and neuropsychiatric problems. Patients show signs of a diffuse encephalopathy, indicating that there is neurologic dysfunction of subcortical, limbic, and frontostriatal circuitry.[25] Various levels of altered consciousness are possible. Signs of increased intracranial pressure are usually uncommon, although they may be secondarily present in the wake of prolonged status epilepticus. Neurologic examination may reveal nonspecific signs of diffuse cerebral dysfunction such as exaggerated deep tendon reflexes, extensor plantar responses, and tone abnormalities, in addition to movement disorders. Soft neurologic signs such mild ataxia and difficulties with fine motor coordination can also be seen.

INVESTIGATIONS
Neuroimaging

Computed tomography (CT) of the head is not useful because of its poor sensitivity. Magnetic resonance (MR) imaging of the brain is unremarkable in 50% of cases. In the other 50%, MR imaging may show nonspecific T2 or fluid-attenuated inversion recovery (FLAIR) signal hyperintensity within the hippocampus; cerebellar, frontobasal, or insular cortex; basal ganglia; brainstem; and, occasionally, the spinal cord.[25] These changes are usually mild or transient, and have been associated with contrast enhancement in the hyperintense areas or the meninges.[3] Occasionally the MR imaging shows extensive T2 FLAIR abnormalities.[18] The radiologic differential diagnosis with these abnormalities remains broad. Follow-up brain MR imaging either remains normal or shows minimal change. Patients with refractory seizures have been reported to show brain atrophy. Lesions can be transient and nonenhancing, and may have a demyelinating appearance.[27,28] MR spectroscopy has not yet been documented to be of any proven value. In short, no clear patterns of brain involvement are evident in this condition (Figs. 1–3), which makes a diagnosis of anti-NMDAR encephalitis based solely on neuroimaging features rather difficult.

Functional Neuroimaging

Most of the literature on functional neuroimaging in anti-NMDAR encephalitis is case based and anecdotal. The utility of functional neuroimaging modalities has not been systematically studied. ^{18}F-Fluorodeoxyglucose positron emission tomography (FDG-PET) imaging showed cortical hypometabolism in 2 young girls aged 3 years and 7 years, with relapsing anti-NMDAR encephalitis; this included the frontal, parietal, temporal, and occipital cortex, and the thalamic nuclei.[29] PET was reportedly more sensitive than MR imaging in these patients. However, a previous report of acute anti-NMDAR encephalitis contrasted this with signs of cortical hypermetabolism.[4] An adolescent with anti-NMDAR encephalitis was found to have abnormal cerebral blood flow in on ^{99m}Tc-labeled D,L-hexamethylpropylene amine oxime single-photon emission CT (HMPAO SPECT). Images showed multiple focal areas of radiotracer uptake in a corticobasal hyperperfusion pattern, which suggested the possibility of frontobasal circuitry involvement. Repeated brain ^{99m}Tc-HMPAO SPECT showed almost complete normalization.[30]

Electroencephalography

Electroencephalograms (EEGs) are consistently abnormal in most patients, and show nonspecific slowing and disorganization of background activity. These findings may be associated with electrographic seizures, which are more common in the initial disease stage.[3] During the catatonic stage slow, continuous, delta, or theta, rhythmic activity predominates.[4,31] The slow rhythmic activity has not been associated with movement abnormalities and has not responded to antiepileptic medication. VEEG monitoring may be beneficial in diagnosing seizures appropriately.

Cerebrospinal Fluid and Serum

NMDARs form part of the ligand-gated cation channels, which play an important role in synaptic transmission and plasticity. The NMDARs are heteromers of NR1 subunits that bind to glycine and NR2 (A, B, C, or D) subunits, which bind to glutamate.[3] The presence of NMDAR antibodies was confirmed by serum or cerebrospinal fluid (CSF) reactivity with hippocampal rat brain, cell-surface labeling hippocampal neurons in culture, and reactive NR1- or NR2-transfected human embryonic kidney (HEK) cells.[3] Definitive diagnosis of anti-NMDAR encephalitis is established by demonstrating antibodies to the NR1 subunit in patients' serum or CSF.[4] In a series of children with anti-NMDAR encephalitis, all patients had CSF or

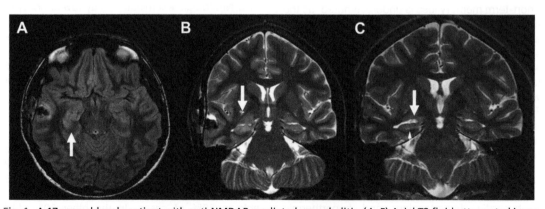

Fig. 1. A 17-year-old male patient with anti-NMDAR mediated encephalitis. (A, B) Axial T2 fluid-attenuated inversion recovery (FLAIR) and coronal T2 images, respectively, with subtle hyperintense signal of the right hippocampus without volume loss (arrow). A right temporal brain biopsy had been performed. (C) Coronal T2 image 3 months after discharge showing atrophy of the right hippocampus (arrow).

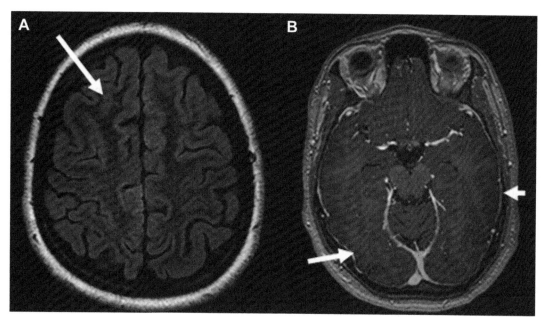

Fig. 2. A 13-year-old girl presented with a 2-week history of right-sided facial weakness, behavior changes, dysarthria, and new-onset focal seizures with secondary generalization. She was confirmed to have anti-NMDAR encephalitis. (*A*) Axial T2 FLAIR view with a tiny focus of abnormal high signal intensity in the subcortical white matter in the right frontal lobe (*arrow*). There was no mass effect or evidence of diffusion restriction. (*B*) Axial T1 view with gadolinium, showing diffuse dural enhancement without nodularity (*arrows*). There were no signs of leptomeningeal enhancement.

serum antibodies that reacted with extracellular epitopes of the NR1 subunit.[4] Paired CSF and serum samples from 21 patients showed stronger antibody reactivity in CSF. Patients with a teratoma had higher antibody CSF titers than those without a teratoma. Seven patients treated with empiric plasma exchange or intravenous immunoglobulins had positive antibodies in CSF, but not in serum.[4] Antibody titers may change over time. A patient who recovered showed a high serum antibody titer and absent or barely detectable CSF antibody titer at follow-up.[32] Although viral encephalitis, stroke, epilepsy, and systemic lupus erythematosus have been associated with NMDAR antibodies,

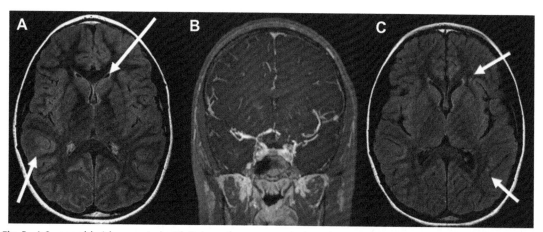

Fig. 3. A 9-year-old girl presented with 6 days of acute encephalopathy and had positive serum anti-NMDAR antibodies. (*A*) Axial T2 FLAIR view, showing bilateral cortical sulcal effacement with small lateral ventricles, reflecting brain swelling (*arrows*). (*B*) T1 coronal view postgadolinium, showing diffuse supratentorial leptomeningeal enhancement suggestive of pial congestion. There was also enhancement along the perforator arteries of the basal ganglia. (*C*) Repeat imaging performed 1 month later with axial T2 FLAIR view. There were multiple hyperintense foci involving the subcortical white matter, with frontal lobe predominance (*arrows*). Interval prominence of the ventricles caused by volume loss had also occurred.

the NR1 receptor region appears to associate uniquely with anti-NMDAR encephalitis.[5] This finding is consistent with an immune response, systemically triggered by a tumor or another unknown cause, which is reactivated and expanded in the central nervous system (CNS).[25]

CSF white blood cells are often increased, in the range of fewer than 200/mm^3, and pleocytosis was found in 87% of a series of children.[3,4] Protein concentration is normal or mildly increased, and CSF-specific oligoclonal bands are positive in 60%. The immunoglobulin G (IgG) index and oligoclonal band testing are clinically useful, as they can be abnormal in the setting of normal CSF cell counts and protein concentrations.

Tumor Association

Approximately 80% of patients with anti-NMDAR encephalitis have so far been women. The detection of a tumor is dependent on age, gender, and ethnicity.[3,4] Approximately 60% of patients have tumors proven to contain nervous tissue. In women, frequency of ovarian teratoma amounts to about 62%, whereas only 22% of men have associated tumors (testicular teratoma and small-cell lung cancer).[2,3] In adolescent females younger than 18 and children younger than 14 years, tumors were diagnosed in 31% and 9%, respectively.[4] The ovarian teratomas of 25 patients studied expressed NMDARs in each case.[33] There is one case report of a child with anti-NMDAR encephalitis and neuroblastoma.[26] Ovarian tumors were found in a few patients who had surgery with exploratory laparoscopies and blind oophorectomies, but in others no tumor was detected.[24]

Pelvic or testicular ultrasonography is an appropriate initial screen for ovarian or testicular teratomas. MR imaging has been used as a more sensitive test for small ovarian tumors. Yearly screening for a tumor, particularly if the patient has a recurrence or continues to be symptomatic, is recommended.[18]

PATHOGENESIS

The pathogenic role of antibodies in anti-NMDAR encephalitis can be established using the following in vivo and in vitro criteria: (1) if antigens are membrane proteins then antibodies should bind to extracellular antigenic epitopes in living cells and/or tissues; (2) the antibody's ability to recognize an antigen should be assessed by expressing the antigen in heterologous cells, which are assayed by immunostaining or immunoprecipitation and Western blot; (3) antibodies cause structural or functional changes of the target antigen that can be established in vitro in dissociated neuron cultures and in vivo after antibody infusion, and antibody treatment may alter the target antigen leading to secondary change in cellular or synaptic function; (4) the clinical syndrome associated with the antibody should resemble the phenotype of the pharmacologic or genetic manipulation of the antigen; (5) passive transfer of the antibodies to animals should recreate the effects of the antibodies on the antigen as well as the clinical features of the disorder; and (6) cellular and synaptic changes, in addition to clinical signs and symptoms, should improve as the antibody titer is reduced.[34]

The anti-NMDAR antibody fulfills these criteria. Antibodies of patients with anti-NMDAR encephalitis recognize the N-terminal extracellular domain of NR1 and bind, cap, cross-link, and internalize NMDARs.[35] The presence of NMDAR antibodies was confirmed by serum or CSF reactivity with hippocampal tissue of rat brain, cell-surface labeled cultures of hippocampal neurons, and reactivity with NR1- or NR2-transfected HEK cells.[3] This process caused a specific, titer-dependent, and reversible reduction of NMDAR surface and total cluster density, resulting in NMDAR-mediated synaptic dysfunction.[35] Patients' antibodies decreased NMDAR synaptic currents on whole-cell patch-clamp recordings of miniature excitatory postsynaptic currents in rat hippocampal neuron cultures, but did not change the localization or expression of synaptic proteins, other glutamate receptors, synapse number, dendritic spine complexity, or cell survival.[35] The effects of NMDAR antibodies resemble those of the NMDAR antagonists phencyclidine and ketamine.

The various stages of the syndrome probably arise from an antibody-mediated progressive reduction of NMDAR clusters and function, followed by a restoration of receptor function during recovery.[36] In vivo experiments have demonstrated that infusion of patients' antibodies into rat hippocampus tissue substantially reduced NMDAR density, which was similar to the decrease of these receptors found in the hippocampi of autopsy specimens.[35] The correlation between antibody titers and neurologic outcome and the reduction in number of postsynaptic NMDAR caused by the antibodies suggest that they play a role in the pathogenesis of the disease. Removing antibodies from the cultures increases the density of postsynaptic NMDAR and explains the potential reversibility of symptoms.[3,33–35] Postmortem analysis of the hippocampi of 2 patients who died of this disorder showed a significant decrease in NMDAR density.[35] The role of the immune response is further supported by the correlation between antibody titers and symptoms, and the frequent clinical response to immunotherapy.[34] The reversibility of the disorder suggests immune-mediated neuronal dysfunction rather than irreversible degeneration.

Synaptic plasticity is thought to be an important mechanism for memory, learning, and cognition. These neurologic processes require glutaminergic synaptic localization and trafficking via NMDA and AMPA receptors. A suggested model of the disorder is that a decrease of NMDARs in inhibitory GABA neurons and glutamate synapses causes multiple effects, including disinhibition of excitatory pathways and increased extracellular glutamate. The clinical syndrome disinhibits the frontostriatal network, leading to symptoms of psychosis, catatonia, rigidity, dystonia, and mutism. The brainstem central-pattern generator is disinhibited, causing complex movement disorders, and the brainstem respiratory network is disinhibited, resulting in respiratory dysfunction.[36]

The immunopathology, CSF pleocytosis, oligoclonal bands, and intrathecal synthesis of NMDAR antibodies suggests that the humoral immune also response plays an important role in the pathogenesis of this disorder.[33] The tumor immunopathology suggests that the tumor may assist in triggering the anti-NMDAR immune response, likely contributing to the breaking of immune tolerance. However, this disorder can also present as a nonparaneoplastic, autoimmune syndrome.[33] After initial systemic immune activation there is an expansion of the CNS immune response. Synaptic autoantibodies in the CNS may be the result of peripherally synthesized antibodies passively crossing a disrupted blood-brain barrier and intrathecal antibody synthesis by plasma cells.[34]

The prodromal illness may cause transient disruption of the blood-brain barrier. After systemic immune activation by an NMDAR -expressing tumor or unknown factors, memory B cells are restimulated. These cells undergo antigen-driven affinity maturation, clonal expansion, and differentiation to become NMDAR antibody-secreting plasma cells.[34] Cross-reactivity of antibodies against other antigens can occur if the epitopes are sufficiently similar. Symptoms of a viral prodrome occurred in 48% of children; however, a common virus was not found to suggest a postinfectious autoimmune process in patients without teratoma. A few patients had positive serology or direct demonstration of a systemic infection, preceding the symptoms of anti-NMDAR encephalitis. One out of 4 patients with neurologic complications, attributed to influenza H1N1, had NMDAR antibodies. This patient showed characteristic symptoms of anti-NMDAR encephalitis.[37] A few patients with

anti-NMDAR encephalitis had positive mycoplasma serology with negative CSF polymerase chain reaction.[4] A child was reported with anti-NMDAR encephalitis after a booster vaccination against tetanus, diphtheria, pertussis, and poliomyelitis.[38] These infections may act as an adjuvant, boosting the immune response. It is possible that a genetic predisposition in addition to a viral or neoplastic trigger may be necessary to initiate the disease. A 3-year-old child with anti-NMDAR encephalitis had a microdeletion of chromosome 6p that involved the human leukocyte antigen cluster, which suggested a predisposition to autoimmunity.[39] A genetic predisposition to autoimmunity has been suggested in children, with antinuclear or thyroid peroxidase antibodies in addition to NMDAR antibodies.[4]

Immunopathology

Postmortem examination of 2 adult patients who died of anti-NMDAR encephalitis showed microgliosis and IgG deposition in the hippocampus, forebrain, basal ganglia, and spinal cord. Anti-NMDAR antibodies were predominantly IgG1, and included IgG2 and IgG3 subtypes. No complement deposits were observed in the examined areas of the CNS. B cells (CD20) and plasma cells (CD79a) were predominant in the perivascular spaces. Cells expressing cytotoxic T-cell markers were rare or absent in the areas examined.[33] In 14 patients with anti-NMDAR encephalitis, a brain biopsy was normal or nonspecific. Histology included perivascular lymphocytic cuffing with predominantly B cells or microglial activation, and sparse parenchymal T-cell infiltrates. Neuronophagic nodules were absent and viral assays were negative.[3] The ovarian tumors of 2 patients who underwent postmortem examination and of 9 other patients with ovarian tumors who survived expressed neuronal antigens, and contained neurons that expressed NMDAR and reacted with patients' antibodies.[33] Nervous tissue was demonstrated by cell morphology and the presence of dendritic neuronal processes, using microtubule associated protein 2 (MAP-2) antibody.[33] All tumors from patients with NMDAR antibodies had extensive T-lymphocyte infiltrates, macrophages or monocytes, B lymphocytes, and plasma cells.[33]

DIFFERENTIAL DIAGNOSIS

The differential diagnosis of anti-NMDAR encephalitis is broad, and typically includes subacute and chronic diffuse inflammatory disorders of the brain. When all the clinical features are present, the diagnosis can be entertained on a clinical basis, although confirmation by serum and CSF anti-NMDAR antibodies is essential. The differential diagnosis widens in the absence of all clinical features and the presence of atypical signs and symptoms. It is clear that with an expanding phenotype and accruing literature, certain specific features may become more helpful in the clinical suspicion of this condition.

Because some cases present with status epilepticus, acute infectious causes such as bacterial and viral infections of the brain need to be considered at presentation. Herpes simplex virus type 1 (HSV-1), human herpesvirus type 6, enterovirus, and mycoplasma are among the multitude of viruses that are possible.[5] Subacute and chronic autoimmune-associated encephalitis, including pediatric autoimmune neuropsychiatric disorders associated with streptococcal infections, Sydenham chorea, autoimmune synaptic receptor encephalitides including neuronal antibodies to GABA, AMPA, and LGI1 receptors, Hashimoto encephalopathy, Rasmussen encephalitis, and encephalitis lethargica, are some of the other conditions that may need consideration based on the clinical features.[9–12,22] CNS vasculitis, either primary (primary CNS angiitis) or secondary (due to chronic infection, inflammatory processes),

also must be considered in the differential diagnosis at presentation. A presentation similar to anti-NMDAR encephalitis has been reported in seronegative neuromyelitis optica.[28] There are additional poorly understood conditions such as acute encephalitis with refractory repetitive partial seizures (AERRPS)[40] and febrile infection–related epilepsy syndrome (FIRES)[41] that may have overlapping clinical features. Primary psychiatric disorders need consideration if the clinical features are solely of psychiatric nature.

Finally, medication overuse and abuse are rare considerations such that ketamine, phencyclidine, and neuroleptics causing neuroleptic malignant syndrome might have to be considered in individual cases (Table 1).

TREATMENT

Management of anti-NMDAR encephalitis should focus on immunotherapy and teratoma detection and removal.[25] There is evidence that early immunotherapy may lead to more rapid recovery and reduced morbidity. Tumor detection and removal within 4 months of onset lead to a better recovery than for those patients without a tumor.[3,4,15,42]

Table 1
Differential diagnosis

Bacterial and viral infections of the brain	Herpes simplex virus type 1 Human herpes virus type 6 Enterovirus Mycoplasma
Autoimmune-associated encephalitis	PANDAS Sydenham chorea Hashimoto encephalopathy Rasmussen encephalitis Encephalitis lethargica
Autoimmune synaptic receptor encephalitides	Neuronal antibodies to GABA, AMPA, and LGI1receptors
CNS vasculitis	Primary CNS angiitis Secondary (due to chronic infection, inflammatory processes)
Demyelinating disorders	Acute disseminated encephalomyelitis Neuromyelitis optica
Poorly understood conditions	Acute encephalitis with refractory repetitive partial seizures[40] Febrile infection–related epilepsy syndrome[41]
Primary psychiatric disorders	
Medication overuse	Ketamine Phencyclidine
Neuroleptic malignant syndrome	Neuroleptics

Abbreviations: AMPA, 2-amino-3-(3-hydroxy-5-methyl-isoxazol-4-yl)propanoic acid; CNS, central nervous system; GABA, γ-aminobutyric acid; LGI1, leucine-rich, glioma-B inactivated 1; PANDAS, pediatric autoimmune neuropsychiatric disorders associated with streptococcal infections.

Current immunotherapy includes corticosteroids, immune plasmapheresis, intravenous immunoglobulins, and rituximab.[43]

In a case series of 31 children, 30 (97%) had immunotherapy with a combination of corticosteroids, intravenous immunoglobulin, or plasma exchange. Seven unresponsive patients received rituximab or cyclophosphamide, or both.[4] These treatments were well tolerated, and 4 patients started to improve shortly afterward (1 with cyclophosphamide, 3 with cyclophosphamide and rituximab). The other 3 had slow progressive improvement not clearly related to the treatment.[4] A case report of a child treated with methylprednisone, oral steroids, and intravenous immunoglobulin documented a good outcome.[42] A case report of a child with anti-NMDAR encephalitis showed no initial clinical response to high-dose prednisolone. After plasmapheresis there was a rapid reduction in antibody titers, and recovery occurred within a few weeks. Anti-NMDAR encephalitis was suspected early, and plasma exchange was followed by excellent recovery.[44] A case report of a male adolescent who presented with anti-NMDAR encephalitis noted that he responded well to pharmacologic immunotherapy but had residual cognitive deficits.[31]

Occasionally serum and CSF antibody titers remain elevated, and additional courses of intravenous immunoglobulin, methylprednisolone, or plasmapheresis may be beneficial.

Usually antibody serum titers are reduced or undetectable, whereas CSF titers remain elevated. Medications that have been shown to improve penetrance of the blood-brain barrier may be more effective.

Patients without a tumor, delayed diagnosis, or with severe refractory disease require additional treatment with second-line immunotherapy agents including rituximab, cyclophosphamide, or both.[4] A case report of a child with anti-NMDAR encephalitis noted minimal response to intravenous immunoglobulin and prednisone. The prednisone was replaced by a 5-day course of methylprednisolone, rituximab once a week for 4 weeks, and intravenous immunoglobulin once every other week. A substantial improvement in clinical symptoms occurred over the next 3 months.[15] A case report of a child without a primary tumor noted a response to treatment with corticosteroids, intravenous immunoglobulin, and rituximab.[26]

OUTCOME

Prognosis depends on early diagnosis, treatment with appropriate immunomodulatory therapy, and early tumor removal in paraneoplastic cases.[43]

The outcome in 31 children with anti-NMDAR encephalitis showed 9 patients (29%) with a full recovery; 14 (45%) with substantial improvement and mild deficits; and 8 (26%) with limited improvement, severe deficits, and slow recovery.[4] The median time from symptom onset to initial improvement was 6 weeks (range, 2–28 weeks). The median follow-up time was 4.5 months (range, 2–14.5 months).[4] Recovery from anti-NMDAR encephalitis takes place in multiple stages that occur in the reverse order of symptom presentation.[25] Despite severe symptoms and prolonged hospitalizations, the outcome is often positive. Symptoms usually stabilize over weeks to months.[18] During the acute stage of the disease, many patients need to be treated in hospital for 3 to 4 months, followed by a further several months of rehabilitation.[25] Residual symptoms usually reflect frontal and limbic dysfunction, including poor executive function. Long-term follow-up shows that in many patients these symptoms continue to improve, as do behavioral and language problems.[18] Signs of brain atrophy on MR imaging may improve with long-term follow-up. The positive outcomes are consistent with the proposed mechanism of NMDAR hypofunction. Despite the reduction of NMDAR cluster density, the structural integrity of the excitatory neurons and their synapses is not affected.[35]

Iizuka and colleagues[45] described 4 adult women with NMDAR antibodies in serum and CSF, and provided the best natural history of this illness at present. Despite an absence of immunotherapy or tumor removal, all patients had a gradual recovery. Anti-NMDAR encephalitis can recur in children. Eight patients (25%) had a history of one or several episodes of similar encephalitis 1 to 96 months before the diagnosis of anti-NMDAR encephalitis. None presented with an underlying tumor initially or at relapse.[4] Four patients relapsed while tapering corticosteroids or after immunotherapy was completed. The other 4 relapsed 1 year after full recovery or partial recovery from the previous episode of encephalitis.[4] The frequency of teratoma in children with anti-NMDAR encephalitis is low in comparison with adults; however, serial screening for ovarian teratoma with ultrasonography and MR imaging of the abdomen and pelvis for 2 years or longer is recommended.[4] In males the role of screening imaging remains unclear. A case series of 100 adults and children showed that 2 of 9 male patients had tumors (bilateral testicular teratoma, seminoma, and small-cell lung cancer), but none of 12 patients subsequently diagnosed had tumors.[3] Counseling families about long-term prognosis should be done with caution.[25]

Anti-NMDAR Encephalitis During Pregnancy

Three women were diagnosed with anti-NMDAR encephalitis while pregnant, of whom 2 had ovarian teratomas. Two patients completed their pregnancy to term and delivered healthy babies. One baby was negative for serum, cord blood, and CSF antibodies, while the mother had antibodies detectable in the CSF. This finding may have explained the lack of transfer to the fetus. In one mother who presented with bilateral, recurrent teratomas, the pregnancy was terminated. All patients were safely treated with methylprednisolone and intravenous immunoglobulin, and recovered following delivery or termination of the pregnancy. Recovery appeared to be assisted by delivery or termination of the pregnancy.[46] Concern for the fetus and neonate is appropriate, as the antibody subtypes IgG1 and IgG3 are involved in autoimmune newborn illnesses.[46]

Milder or Incomplete Forms of the Disorder

Patients may develop predominant or isolated psychiatric symptoms, seizures, or dystonia without developing the full spectrum of the disorder. Purely monosymptomatic syndromes are uncommon, occurring in fewer than 5% of patients.[3]

Mortality and Cause of Death

Despite a favorable outcome for most patients with anti-NMDAR encephalitis, this disorder is severe and may result in death. In the California Encephalitis Project, 10% of anti-NMDAR positive patients died. The mortality was higher than for enterovirus (6%), and lower than for HSV-1 (19%) and rabies (100%).[5] The estimated mortality for anti-NMDAR encephalitis is 4% from the information of 360 patients followed for at least 6 months.[25] Disease onset until death was a median time of 3·5 months (ranging from 1 to 8 months). Cause of death included sepsis, sudden cardiac arrest, acute respiratory distress, refractory status epilepticus, tumor progression, withdrawal of medical support, and unknown causes.[25]

PEARLS, PITFALLS, AND VARIANTS
Pearls

1. Anti-NMDAR encephalitis may present to a variety of physicians responsible for the care of children, including general and developmental pediatricians, pediatric neurologists, movement disorder specialists, and rheumatologists, and it is important that they be familiar with this disorder.

2. Acute infectious causes need to be considered in the differential diagnosis, and empiric antibiotic and antiviral medication may need to be implemented while awaiting the results of confirmatory tests.
3. In the initial stages of the disease the patient may present with psychiatric symptoms and receive treatment with neuroleptic medication. This scenario may lead to consideration of a differential diagnosis of neuroleptic malignant syndrome. The patient's response to withdrawal of neuroleptics may help determine the underlying etiology.

Pitfalls

The association of NMDAR encephalitis as a paraneoplastic syndrome appears to be less common in children and adult males; however, screening for ovarian teratoma in females and testicular carcinoma or small-cell lung carcinoma in males is recommended.

Variants

Recurrent optic neuritis with transient cerebral lesions, extensive longitudinal myelitis and optic neuritis mimicking neuromyelitis optica,[28] and unexplained new-onset epilepsy may be part of a spectrum of anti-NMDAR encephalitis.

WHAT THE REFERRING PHYSICIAN NEEDS TO KNOW

Clinical recovery usually corresponds to a reduction in CSF and serum antibody titers. Patients that do not respond to initial immunotherapy with intravenous immunoglobulin, corticosteroids, or plasma exchange may require repeat CSF and serum NMDAR antibody testing, and further second-line immunotherapy with rituximab or cyclophosphamide; this may require subspecialist referral.

SUMMARY

Anti-NMDAR encephalitis should be included in the differential diagnosis of children who present with acute changes of behavior, seizures, dystonia or dyskinesia, moderate CSF lymphocytosis, or oligoclonal bands. The EEG shows infrequent epileptiform activity, with slow, disorganized background activity that does not correlate with abnormal movements. The brain MR imaging is often normal, or shows transient T2 FLAIR hyperintense or contrast-enhancing cortical or subcortical abnormalities. Confirmatory testing of CSF or serum for antibodies to NR1 subunits of the NMDAR is required to confirm the diagnosis.[4]

Patients should be treated with immunotherapy and be examined for the presence of a tumor. Recovery takes months, and requires a multidisciplinary team including physical rehabilitation, occupational therapy, speech and language therapy, and psychiatric management.[4] Further research is needed to determine appropriate first-line treatment, the timeline for escalating therapy, and treatment selection according to the stage of the immune response within the CNS. The effectiveness of long-term immunosuppression should be also assessed.[4]

REFERENCES

1. Vitaliani R, Mason W, Ances B, et al. Paraneoplastic encephalitis, psychiatric symptoms, and hypoventilation in ovarian teratoma. Ann Neurol 2005;58:594–604.

2. Dalmau J, Tuzun E, Wu HY, et al. Paraneoplastic anti-N-methyl-D-aspartate receptor encephalitis associated with ovarian teratoma. Ann Neurol 2007;61:25–36.

3. Dalmau J, Gleichman AJ, Hughes EG, et al. Anti-NMDA-receptor encephalitis: case series and analysis of the effects of antibodies. Lancet Neurol 2008;7:1091–8.

4. Florance NR, Davis RL, Lam C, et al. Anti-N-methyl-D-aspartate receptor (NMDAR) encephalitis in children and adolescents. Ann Neurol 2009;66:11–8.

5. Gable MS, Gavali S, Radner A, et al. Anti-NMDA receptor encephalitis: report of ten cases and comparison with viral encephalitis. Eur J Clin Microbiol Infect Dis 2009;28:1421–9.

6. Sebire G, Devictor D, Huault G, et al. Coma associated with intense bursts of abnormal movements and long-lasting cognitive disturbances: an acute encephalopathy of obscure origin. J Pediatr 1992;121:845–51.

7. DeLong GR, Bean SC, Brown FR III. Acquired reversible autistic syndrome in acute encephalopathic illness in children. Arch Neurol 1981;38:191–4.

8. Hartley LM, Ng SY, Dale RC, et al. Immune mediated chorea encephalopathy syndrome in childhood. Dev Med Child Neurol 2002;44:273–7.

9. Dale RC, Irani SR, Brilot F, et al. N-methyl-D-aspartate receptor antibodies in pediatric dyskinetic encephalitis lethargica. Ann Neurol 2009;66:704–9.

10. Lai M, Hughes EG, Peng X, et al. AMPA receptor antibodies in limbic encephalitis alter synaptic receptor location. Ann Neurol 2009;65:424–34.

11. Lancaster E, Lai M, Peng X, et al. Antibodies to the GABA(B) receptor in limbic encephalitis with seizures: case series and characterisation of the antigen. Lancet Neurol 2010;9:67–76.

12. Lai M, Huijbers MG, Lancaster E, et al. Investigation of LGI1 as the antigen in limbic encephalitis previously attributed to potassium channels: a case series. Lancet Neurol 2010;9:776–85.

13. Pruss H, Dalmau J, Harms L, et al. Retrospective analysis of NMDA receptor antibodies in encephalitis of unknown origin. Neurology 2010;75:1735–9.

14. Granerod J, Ambrose HE, Davies NW, et al. Causes of encephalitis and differences in their clinical presentations in England: a multicentre, population-based prospective study. Lancet Infect Dis 2010;10:835–44.

15. Wong-Kisiel LC, Ji T, Renaud DL, et al. Response to immunotherapy in a 20-month-old boy with anti-NMDA receptor encephalitis. Neurology 2010;74:1550–1.

16. Luca N, Daengsuwan T, Dalmau J, et al. Anti-Nmethyl- D-aspartate receptor encephalitis: a newly recognized inflammatory brain disease in children. Arthritis Rheum 2011;63:2516–22.

17. Consoli A, Ronen K, An-Gourfinkel I, et al. Malignant catatonia due to anti-NMDA-receptor encephalitis in a 17-year-old girl: case report. Child Adolesc Psychiatry Ment Health 2011;5:15.

18. Florance-Ryan N, Dalmau J. Update on anti-N-methyl-D-aspartate receptor encephalitis in children and adolescents. Curr Opin Pediatr 2010;22:739–44.

19. Kleinig TJ, Thompson PD, Matar W, et al. The distinctive movement disorder of ovarian teratoma-associated encephalitis. Mov Disord 2008;23:1256–61.

20. Kurian M, Lalive PH, Dalmau JO, et al. Opsoclonus-myoclonus syndrome in anti-N-methyl-D-aspartate receptor encephalitis. Arch Neurol 2010;67:118–21.

21. Bayreuther C, Bourg V, Dellamonica J, et al. Complex partial status epilepticus revealing anti-NMDA receptor encephalitis. Epileptic Disord 2009;11:261–5.

22. Greiner H, Leach JL, Lee KH, et al. Anti-NMDA receptor encephalitis presenting with imaging findings and clinical features mimicking Rasmussen syndrome. Seizure 2011;20:266–70.

23. Niehusmann P, Dalmau J, Rudlowski C, et al. Diagnostic value of N-methyl-D-aspartate receptor antibodies in women with new-onset epilepsy. Arch Neurol 2009;66:458–64.

24. Sansing LH, Tuzun E, Ko MW, et al. A patient with encephalitis associated with NMDA receptor antibodies. Nat Clin Pract Neurol 2007;3:291–6.

25. Dalmau J, Lancaster E, Martinez-Hernandez E, et al. Clinical experience and laboratory investigations in patients with anti-NMDAR encephalitis. Lancet Neurol 2011;10:63–74.

26. Lebas A, Husson B, Didelot A, et al. Expanding spectrum of encephalitis with NMDA receptor antibodies in young children. J Child Neurol 2010;25:742–5.

27. Ishikawa N, Tajima G, Hyodo S, et al. Detection of autoantibodies against NMDA-type glutamate receptor in a patient with recurrent optic neuritis and transient cerebral lesions. Neuropediatrics 2007;38:257–60.

28. Kruer MC, Koch TK, Bourdette DN, et al. NMDA receptor encephalitis mimicking seronegative neuromyelitis optica. Neurology 2010;74:1473–5.

29. Pillai SC, Gill D, Webster R, et al. Cortical hypometabolism demonstrated by PET in relapsing NMDA receptor encephalitis. Pediatr Neurol 2010;43:217–20.

30. Llorens V, Gabilondo I, Gomez-Esteban JC, et al. Abnormal multifocal cerebral blood flow on Tc-99m HMPAO SPECT in a patient with anti-NMDA-receptor encephalitis. J Neurol 2010;257:1568–9.

31. McCoy B, Akiyama T, Widjaja E, et al. Autoimmune limbic encephalitis as an emerging pediatric condition: case report and review of the literature. J Child Neurol 2011;26:218–22.

32. Seki M, Suzuki S, Iizuka T, et al. Neurological response to early removal of ovarian teratoma in anti-NMDAR encephalitis. J Neurol Neurosurg Psychiatry 2008;79:324–6.

33. Tuzun E, Zhou L, Baehring JM, et al. Evidence for antibody-mediated pathogenesis in anti-NMDAR encephalitis associated with ovarian teratoma. Acta Neuropathol 2009;118:737–43.

34. Moscato EH, Jain A, Peng X, et al. Mechanisms underlying autoimmune synaptic encephalitis leading to disorders of memory, behavior and cognition: insights from molecular, cellular and synaptic studies. Eur J Neurosci 2010;32:298–309.

35. Hughes EG, Peng X, Gleichman AJ, et al. Cellular and synaptic mechanisms of anti-NMDA receptor encephalitis. J Neurosci 2010;30:5866–75.

36. Lancaster E, Martinez-Hernandez E, Dalmau J. Encephalitis and antibodies to synaptic and neuronal cell surface proteins. Neurology 2011;77:179–89.

37. Baltagi SA, Shoykhet M, Felmet K, et al. Neurological sequelae of 2009 influenza A (H1N1) in children: a case series observed during a pandemic. Pediatr Crit Care Med 2010;11:179–84.

38. Hofmann C, Baur MO, Schroten H. Anti-NMDA receptor encephalitis after TdaP-IPV booster vaccination: cause or coincidence? J Neurol 2011;258: 500–1.

39. Verhelst H, Verloo P, Dhondt K, et al. Anti-NMDA-receptor encephalitis in a 3 year old patient with chromosome 6p21.32 microdeletion including the HLA cluster. Eur J Paediatr Neurol 2011;15:163–6.

40. Sakuma H, Awaya Y, Shiomi M, et al. Acute encephalitis with refractory, repetitive partial seizures (AERRPS): a peculiar form of childhood encephalitis. Acta Neurol Scand 2010;121:251–6.

41. van Baalen A, Hausler M, Boor R, et al. Febrile infection-related epilepsy syndrome (FIRES): a non-encephalitic encephalopathy in childhood. Epilepsia 2010;51:1323–8.

42. Breese EH, Dalmau J, Lennon VA, et al. Anti-N-methyl-D-aspartate receptor encephalitis: early treatment is beneficial. Pediatr Neurol 2010;42: 213–4.

43. Wandinger KP, Saschenbrecker S, Stoecker W, et al. Anti-NMDA-receptor encephalitis: a severe, multistage, treatable disorder presenting with psychosis. J Neuroimmunol 2011;231:86–91.

44. Schimmel M, Bien CG, Vincent A, et al. Successful treatment of anti-N-methyl-D-aspartate receptor encephalitis presenting with catatonia. Arch Dis Child 2009;94:314–6.

45. Iizuka T, Sakai F, Ide T, et al. Anti-NMDA receptor encephalitis in Japan: long-term outcome without tumor removal. Neurology 2008;70:504–11.

46. Kumar MA, Jain A, Dechant VE, et al. Anti-N-methyl-D-aspartate receptor encephalitis during pregnancy. Arch Neurol 2010;67:884–7.

Mimics and Rare Presentations of Pediatric Demyelination

Julia O'Mahony, BSc[a], Manohar Shroff, MD, DABR, FRCPC[b,*],
Brenda Banwell, MD, FRCPC[c]

KEYWORDS

- Multiple sclerosis • Optic neuritis • Transverse myelitis • Acute disseminated encephalomyelitis
- Spinal cord infarct • Griscelli type 2 syndrome

KEY POINTS

- Demyelination of the optic nerves, spine, and brain may occur as a monophasic or transiently multiphasic illness without chronic relapsing demyelination typical of multiple sclerosis (MS). To date, no biomarker or magnetic resonance (MR) imaging pattern reliably identifies such individuals.
- Asymptomatic brain lesions outside of the optic nerve or spinal cord strongly favor MS.
- Anterior horn cell involvement can be prominent in both vascular and demyelinating disorders of the spinal cord.
- Diffusion restriction can be detected in the spinal cord but it is not pathognomonic for infarction in this region; diffusion restriction within the cord has been reported in transverse myelitis.
- Ring enhancement differentials include infections, granulomatous disease and neoplasms, but can be seen in patients with demyelination. Open-ring enhancement is more typical of demyelinating lesions. When open-ring sign is present in the brain, demyelination is much more likely than neoplasm or infection.

INTRODUCTION

Acquired demyelinating syndromes (ADS) of the central nervous system (CNS) are characterized by acute neurologic deficits, magnetic resonance (MR) imaging findings of focal or multifocal areas of abnormal signal on T2-weighted images in the brain, optic nerves, or spinal cord, and a response to corticosteroids. The clinical features of ADS relate to the localization of areas of inflammation. Common ADS presentations include optic neuritis (ON), transverse myelitis (TM), brainstem syndromes, polyfocal neurologic deficits, and polyfocal deficits accompanied by encephalopathy (termed acute disseminated encephalomyelitis

Disclosures: None (J.O'M., M.S.). B.B. has received Speaker's Honoraria from Biogen-Idec, Novartis, and Merk-Serono, and serves as an advisor for pediatric trials. None of these activities relate to the present work.
Funding: This article is on behalf of the Canadian Pediatric Demyelinating Disease Network, funding for which came from the Canadian Multiple Sclerosis Scientific Research Foundation.
[a] Divison of Neurology, Department of Pediatrics, Research Institute, The Hospital for Sick Children, 555 University Avenue, Room 6D33, Toronto, Ontario M5G 1X8, Canada; [b] Division of Neuroradiology, Department of Diagnostic Imaging, The Hospital for Sick Children, University of Toronto, 555 University Avenue, Toronto, Ontario M5G 1X8, Canada; [c] Divison of Neurology, Department of Pediatrics, Research Institute, The Hospital for Sick Children, University of Toronto, 555 University Avenue, Toronto, Ontario M5G 1X8, Canada
* Corresponding author.
E-mail address: manohar.shroff@sickkids.ca

Neuroimag Clin N Am 23 (2013) 321–336
http://dx.doi.org/10.1016/j.nic.2012.12.010

[ADEM]). For some patients, ADS occurs as a monophasic illness, whereas for others it represents the first clinical manifestation of multiple sclerosis (MS). **Table 1** provides a diagnostic evaluation for children suspected of having an acquired demyelinating syndrome or MS.

Although well characterized clinically and radiologically, the clinical features of acute

Table 1
Diagnostic evaluation for children evaluated for suspected acquired demyelinating syndromes and multiple sclerosis

The following investigations should be performed, as clinically indicated:

MR imaging	Brain MR imaging in all children
	Spine MR imaging in all children with clinical spine involvement
	Orbital MR imaging for children with visual loss
	The following MR imaging sequences are suggested:
	FLAIR or T2-weighted sequences in at least 2 planes
	Pre- and postgadolinium T1-weighted images
	Diffusion-weighted sequences
Evoked potentials	VEPs
	SSEPs
Laboratory screening for NMO and MAS	Serum NMO IgG
	CSF NMO IgG (if serum negative)
	Ferritin
	Triglycerides
Infection screening	CBC + differential
	Serum viral serologies (EBV, mycoplasma, HSV serology)
	VDRL
	Lyme disease (seasonal)
	Cysticercosis (based on travel to endemic areas only)
	HTLV (based on travel to endemic areas only)
Endocrine	TSH, T4, anti-TPO antibodies if Hashimoto encephalopathy is a consideration
Mitochondrial lactate serum + CSF	Pyruvate; if higher than normal lactate, calculate lactate to pyruvate ratio
	DNA studies, skin and muscle biopsy if mitochondrial disease strongly suspected
Rheumatologic disease	ESR, CRP
	ANA, dsDNA
	Anticardiolipin and antiphospholipid antibodies
	Angiotensin-converting enzyme
	CXR (if sarcoidosis is strongly suspected)
Nutritional	Vitamin B12 (serum)
	25-hydroxyvitamin D (25(OH)D)
CSF studies	Glucose
	Lactate
	Protein
	Cell count
	Culture and sensitivity, Gram stain when appropriate
	Oligoclonal bands (compared with concurrently obtained serum)[a]
	CSF viral cultures + PCR herpesviruses
	Cytology (if indicated)

Abbreviations: ANA, antinuclear antibody; CBC, complete blood count; CRP, C-reactive protein; CSF, cerebrospinal fluid; CT, computed tomography; CXR, chest radiograph; DNA, deoxyribonucleic acid; dsDNA, double-stranded deoxyribonucleic acid; EBV, Epstein-Barr virus; ESR, erythrocyte sedimentation rate; FLAIR, fluid-attenuated inversion recovery; HSV, herpes simplex virus; HTLV, human T-lymphotropic virus; IgG, immunoglobulin G; MAS, macrophage activation syndrome; NMO, neuromyelitis optica; PCR, polymerase chain reaction; SSEP, somatosensory evoked potential; T4, thyroxine test; TPO, Thyroid peroxidase; TSH, thyroid-stimulating hormone; VDRL, venereal disease research laboratory; VEP, visual evoked potential.

[a] The accuracy of oligoclonal band measurement depends on the diagnostic test used and on the experience of the laboratory performing the test. Isoelectric focusing has the highest sensitivity.

demyelination are not specific. Clinicians must be alert to other neurologic disorders with similar signs. The diagnosis of monophasic ADS and MS requires exclusion of other diagnoses. **Table 2** highlights some of the MR imaging features that should prompt clinicians to consider diagnoses other than ADS and MS. This article reviews the features that should prompt consideration of diseases that mimic ADS and MS, using vignettes to highlight unusual clinical and radiologic features.

TYPICAL FEATURES OF PEDIATRIC DEMYELINATION ON MR IMAGING

As detailed in the article elsewhere in this issue by Verhey and colleagues, MR imaging plays an increasingly important role in the diagnosis of monophasic ADS and MS. The MR imaging appearance of childhood MS is characterized by multiple white matter lesions, which are of increased signal on T2-weighted and fluid-attenuated inversion recovery (FLAIR)-weighted

images. Lesions may enhance with administration of gadolinium. However, enhancement may be absent even in acute lesions. Areas of hypointensity on T1-weighted images may reflect acute lesions or areas of long-standing regional tissue loss. Younger children often exhibit larger and more diffuse, bilateral white matter lesions with ill-defined borders that are frequently confluent at disease onset. Despite the important role played by MR imaging in the diagnosis of ADS and MS, it must be used in conjunction with clinical features.

DISTINGUISHING ACUTE DEMYELINATION FROM ACUTE VASCULAR INSULT IN THE SPINAL CORD

Acute neurologic deficits prompt consideration of vascular occlusion and cerebral or spinal cord infarction, key differentials of ADS. In patients with infarction, the rapid development over minutes to hours of maximal deficit favors vascular occlusion. However, acute deficits can occur in

---

Table 2
MR imaging red flags for the diagnosis of children with acquired demyelinating syndromes

MR imaging	Leptomeningeal enhancement	SVcPACNS Infection Tumor HLH	Leptomeningeal enhancement is not a feature of MS in adults, and emerged as a red flag for vasculitic or malignant processes in the pediatric cohort
	Lesion expansion	Tumor Lymphoma PML Sarcoidosis	Increased size of T2 lesions on serial imaging is well recognized in MS, although this should always prompt consideration of malignancy. Increasing size of a white matter–predominant lesion without lesion enhancement in a patient treated with immunosuppressant therapy (or a patient with known HIV) should prompt consideration of PML. PML is a risk for MS patients exposed to more intense immunosuppressive therapies
	Hemorrhage	ANE Stroke Cerebellitis AHLE Large-vessel CNS vasculitis SVcPACNS	Although susceptibility-weighted imaging reveals tiny microfoci of hemosiderin in MS patients, hemorrhage large enough to be visible on conventional MR imaging sequences is not a feature of ADS or MS, and should prompt consideration of disorders in which the cerebral vasculature is specifically involved

Abbreviations: ADS, acquired demyelinating syndrome; AHLE, acute hemorrhagic leukoencephalitis; CNS, central nervous system; HIV, human immunodeficiency virus; HLH, hemophagocytic lymphohistiocytosis; MS, multiple sclerosis; PML, progressive multifocal leukoencephalopathy; SVcPACNS, small-vessel childhood primary angiitis of the central nervous system.

CLINICAL VIGNETTE

An 11-year-old girl presented with acute onset of back pain, shooting pain down her legs, loss of bowel and bladder control, and 4-limb weakness that developed over 1 to 2 hours. Weakness then worsened progressively to complete paralysis over the next 5 days with concomitant respiratory failure. MR imaging of the spine on day of onset revealed a focal hyperintensity on T2-weighted images in the anterior aspect of the cervical cord, more prominently involving the anterior horn cells, extending from the C3 level to the T2/T3 level with no diffusion restriction (Fig. 1A, B). Repeat MR imaging on day 5 showed expansion of the cord from C3 to T2. MR imaging of the brain was normal. Spinal fluid analysis revealed a normal protein and cell count. Serum coagulation profile was normal.

The prominent back pain and initial rapid progression prompted consideration of spinal cord infarct, whereas the subsequent progressive worsening and delayed spinal cord expansion favored a demyelinating process. The extensive lesion length led to serologic evaluation for aquaporin-4 antibodies (results were negative), as longitudinally extensive TM is a core feature of neuromyelitis optica (NMO). Treatment with corticosteroids did not lead to neurologic improvement. Plasma exchange (PLEX) was initiated, and within 48 hours she was able to breathe independently. A course of 5 exchanges was completed. After 5 weeks in the intensive care unit (ICU), she was discharged to a rehabilitation hospital where she continued inpatient treatment for 4 months. Eighteen months after onset, she has moderate hand weakness and minor bladder-control issues, but has regained all lower extremity and proximal upper limb strength. Follow-up MR imaging reveals residual intramedullary T2 hyperintensity with associated volume loss of the upper cervical cord (Fig. 1C). Recovery and symptoms were ultimately deemed to be consistent with severe TM.

CLINICAL VIGNETTE

A 14-year-old girl developed acute-onset bilateral lower extremity weakness, numbness, and bladder incontinence that progressed to maximal initial deficit over the course of 2 hours. Her history was remarkable for a mild back injury that occurred 5 months prior during training for competitive gymnastics. At presentation to hospital, examination was remarkable for flaccid tone and absent reflexes in the lower extremities, bilateral lower limb weakness, and a sensory level at T4/5. MR imaging of the spine demonstrated spinal cord swelling in the distal lumbar to sacral segments with abnormal intramedullary signal (Fig. 2A) and diffusion restriction (Fig. 2B, C). In addition, a disc herniation was noted at T12-L1 level (see Fig. 2A). Spinal fluid analysis was unremarkable. The focal disc protrusion and diffusion restriction imaged on MR raised the possibility of fibrocartilaginous disc embolism. Treatment included low molecular weight heparin for possible anterior spinal artery stroke and a 5-day course of intravenous methylprednisolone to address a possible inflammatory component. Three days after onset, when performing a Valsalva maneuver in the context of constipation, she developed acute worsening of her lower limb weakness, leading to complete paraplegia. MR imaging demonstrated extension longitudinally of abnormal T2 signal hyperintensity from T11 to the mid L1 level (Fig. 2D), and extension transversely to involve the anterior horn cells (Fig. 2E). The diffusion-weighted images again showed some restriction of diffusion. The patient was discharged to a rehabilitation hospital for 4 months of inpatient treatment, has experienced minimal improvement, and remains wheelchair dependent. The very rapid progression to maximal deficit, prior history of back pain, MR imaging evidence of disc herniation, and poor recovery favor a diagnosis of fibrocartilaginous embolic spinal cord infarct.

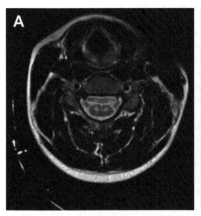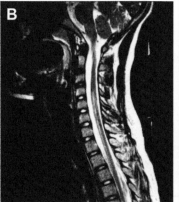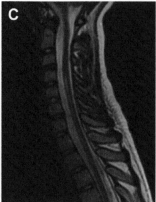

Fig. 1. Axial T2 image (A) on day of onset of symptoms shows focal hyperintensity in the anterior horn cells bilaterally. There was no diffusion restriction (not shown). Sagittal T2 image (B) on the same day shows the longitudinal extent of the abnormal signal in the anterior portion of the cord. Sagittal T2 image 18 months after onset (C) show residual hyperintensity with associated volume loss in the upper spinal cord.

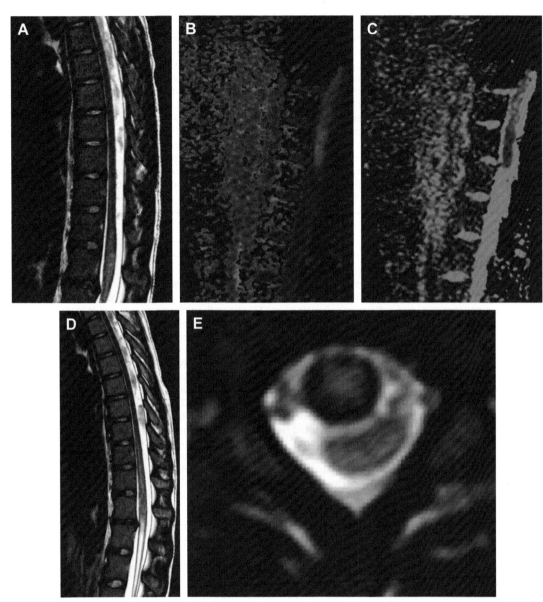

Fig. 2. Sagittal T2 image (*A*) shows swelling and abnormal increased signal in the distal lumbar segments and the conus medullaris, with evidence of increased signal on the trace diffusion image (*B*) and decreased signal on the apparent diffusion coefficient (ADC) map (*C*), in keeping with diffusion restriction. Note the abnormal hypointense signal at the T12-L1 disc with posterior herniation (*A*). Follow-up sagittal (*D*) and axial (*E*) T2 images show extension of abnormal signal longitudinally and transversely.

patients with ADS, particularly those with TM. MR imaging lesions that conform to specific vascular distributions in the brain or anterior spinal artery of the spinal cord would support vascular causes. As emphasized by the following 2 vignettes, distinguishing vascular from demyelinating disease can be difficult.

DISTINGUISHING ACUTE DEMYELINATION FROM ACUTE VASCULAR INSULT IN THE BRAIN

The diagnosis of isolated SVcPACNS necessitates brain biopsy, as angiographic studies and laboratory investigations are typically noninformative. Children with SVcPACNS may manifest with

A 7-year-old boy was admitted with a 3-day history of headache, fever, lethargy, and focal left-sided seizures. Spinal fluid investigations were normal. The patient commenced treatment with a broad spectrum of antibiotics and acyclovir. Initial examination was remarkable for a left hemiparesis involving the face, arm, and leg. Two days after onset, the patient became encephalopathic. An electroencephalogram (EEG) demonstrated slow electrical activity without ictal discharges. MR imaging of the brain showed increased T2 signal in multiple brain regions, including the basal ganglia (Fig. 3A). Diffusion restriction was detected in the right hemisphere (Fig. 3B, C)). MR angiogram was normal. Treatment with corticosteroids was associated with rapid improvement. At 3 weeks after onset the neurologic examination was normal. The patient remains well 6 years later, with neither residual deficits nor subsequent episodes. Polyfocal deficits and encephalopathy, MR imaging findings of diffuse white and deep gray matter involvement, and the prompt response to corticosteroids led to a diagnosis of ADEM. The diffusion restriction was hypothesized to be secondary to his initial seizures, rather than attributable to vascular etiology.

A previously healthy, developmentally normal 28-month-old boy presented with status epilepticus associated with fever. Treatment included lorazepam, fosphenytoin, phenobarbitone, intravenous acyclovir, vancomycin, and ceftriaxone. Continuous EEG showed no recurrence of seizures after initiation of phenobarbitone. Lumbar puncture revealed an opening pressure of 44 cm H_2O. Spinal fluid analyses were not suggestive of CNS infection. Head computed tomography (CT) and MR imaging of the brain on day 2 were normal. Following an initial improvement, the child became progressively encephalopathic with disorientation, loss of speech, and an inability to sit unsupported. On day 6 of illness, he experienced a second series of generalized seizures. MR imaging revealed multifocal white matter lesions involving cortical gray matter, yielding an initial diagnosis of ADEM. Diffusion restriction was notable in the frontal and temporal lobes bilaterally (Fig. 4). Treatment with corticosteroids led to improved alertness and resolution of ataxia, although the patient remained nonverbal with poor social interaction. Follow-up sedated sleep EEG was abnormal, with intermittent polymorphic slowing over the right anterior temporal region as well as multiple independent spike foci (Fig. 5). Fever-induced seizures followed by regression in cognitive skills led to a diagnosis of fever-induced refractory epileptic encephalopathy in school-aged children (FIRES). FIRES is a refractory epileptic encephalopathy, previously termed devastating epilepsy in school-aged children (DESC), which is characterized by fever-induced status epilepticus and severe cognitive impairment, mainly involving language.

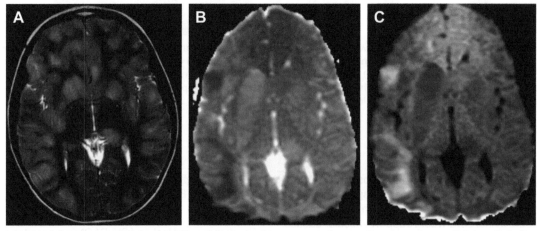

Fig. 3. Axial T2 image (A) shows diffuse bilateral white matter abnormality throughout all lobes including involvement of the subcortical white matter and basal ganglia, and moderate involvement of the brainstem. Multiple foci of decreased signal on the ADC map (B) and increased signal on the trace diffusion image (C) were confined to the right cerebral hemisphere.

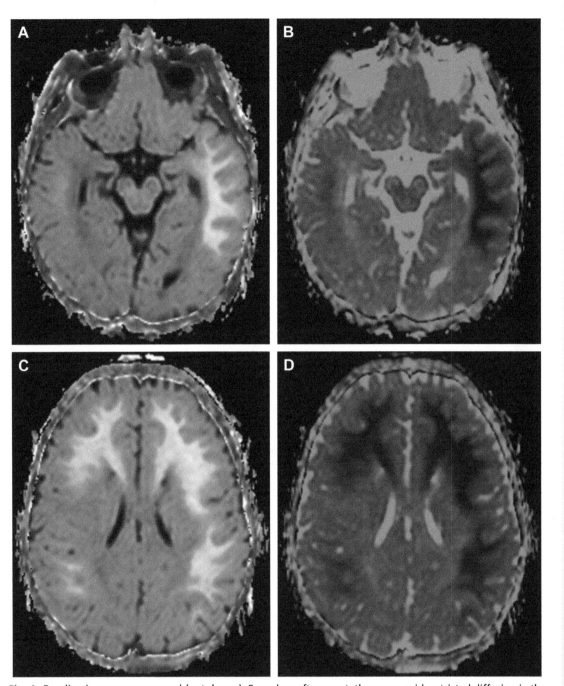

Fig. 4. Baseline images were normal (not shown). Four days after onset, there was avid restricted diffusion in the subcortical and deep white matter of the bilateral frontal, parietal, and left greater than right temporal lobes (*A–D*).

CLINICAL VIGNETTE

A previously healthy 15-year-old girl presented with a 2-day history of painful paresthesias in all 4 limbs, generalized fatigue, transient aphasia, right-sided weakness, right visual loss, vomiting, and headache. She experienced generalized tonic-clonic seizures. Her family history included a maternal grandmother with 3 sisters who had MS and an older sister with ankylosing spondylitis. CSF was normal and negative for oligoclonal bands (OCBs). Antinuclear antibody (ANA), antineutrophil cytoplasmic antibodies (ANCA), and anti–double-stranded deoxyribonucleic acid (anti-dsDNA) were negative. MR imaging of the brain revealed right optic nerve enhancement (Fig. 6) as well as bifrontal leptomeningeal enhancement (Fig. 7). MR imaging of the spinal cord revealed abnormal intramedullary signal at C4/5 and C6 levels (Fig. 8). Treatment with corticosteroids led to resolution of visual loss and focal deficits. One month later she presented with headache, photophobia, generalized fatigue, and malaise. Examination revealed bilateral conjunctival injection with painful eye movement as well as papillary edema. Formal cerebral angiogram revealed no evidence of intracranial vasculitis in the large, middle, or small vessels. Persistent unrelenting headaches provoked a brain biopsy that revealed evidence of isolated small-vessel childhood primary angiitis of the central nervous system (SVcPACNS) vasculitis (Fig. 9). Treatment with oral prednisone, monthly immune globulin, and mycophenolate mofetil has led to clinical remission over the last 6 years.

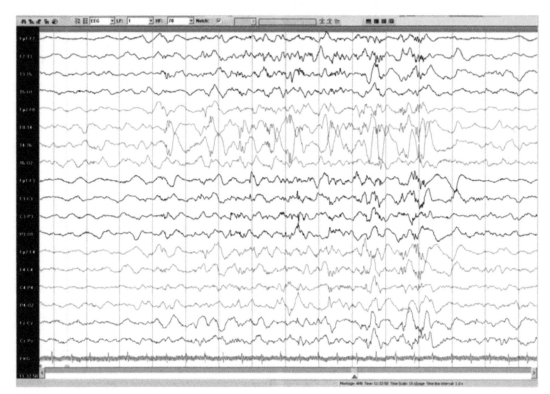

Fig. 5. Sedated electroencephalogram shows frequent generalized or diffuse polyspikes/spikes and slow-wave discharges with slight predominance over the right frontal temporal regions.

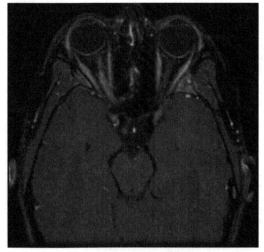

Fig. 6. Axial T1 + C image shows thickening, high T2 signal, and enhancement of the right optic nerve beginning at the globe and extending to the chiasm.

features of ON, spinal cord inflammation, or encephalopathy (ADEM-like), rendering distinction from demyelination difficult. Persistent headache, rarely observed in MS or in children with transient demyelination, has been reported as a key feature of other CNS vasculitis cohorts. Leptomeningeal enhancement, when present, argues against MS and favors vasculitis, neurosarcoidosis, or CNS infection.

DISTINGUISHING GENETIC AND ACQUIRED CNS INFLAMMATORY DISEASE

Griscelli syndrome type 2 (GS2) is a rare autosomal recessive disorder that is characterized by hypomelanosis, immunologic abnormalities including HLH, and often neurologic impairment. GS2 is caused by biallelic mutations in the *RAB27A* gene.

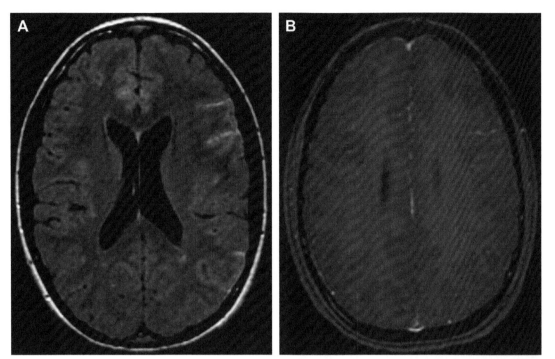

Fig. 7. Axial T2 fluid-attenuated inversion recovery (FLAIR) (*A*) and axial T1 (*B*) images following the administration of gadolinium show abnormal leptomeningeal enhancement in several sulci over the left frontal lobe near the vertex.

CLINICAL VIGNETTE

A 17-year-old boy presented with a 3-week history of headache, weight loss, and severe fatigue, a 2-week history of low-grade fever, bowel and bladder dysfunction, and visual impairment, and a 1-day history of numbness of the right hand and slurred speech. Neurologic examination revealed reduced visual acuity bilaterally, mild encephalopathy, limb and truncal ataxia, and diffuse hyperreflexia. Brain MR imaging revealed multiple small white matter hyperintensities on FLAIR images, with leptomeningeal enhancement in the cerebellar folia (Fig. 10). MR imaging of the spine revealed several ill-defined small areas of T2 hyperintensity in the cervical and thoracic cord without cord expansion or enhancement (Fig. 11). Medical history was remarkable for a diagnosis in infancy of hemophagocytic lymphohistiocytosis (HLH). Treatment from age 5 months to 2 years with etoposide, corticosteroids, and cyclosporine led to complete clinical resolution, and the patient was well from age 2 to 17 years without medication. A 5-day course of intravenous methylprednisolone led to marked improvement. The diagnosis of recurrent HLH with CNS involvement was supported by his silver-colored hair, progressive elevation in serum ferritin, bone marrow aspirate demonstrating hemophagocytosis, and genetic studies that confirmed a mutation in RAB27A. Allogeneic bone marrow transplant is planned.

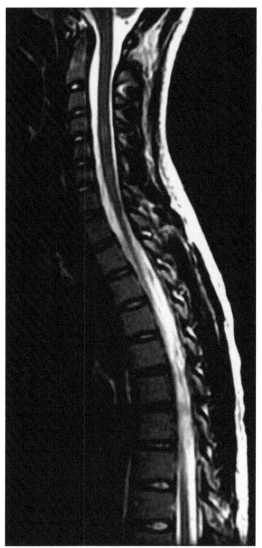

Fig. 8. Sagittal T2 image shows abnormal intramedullary signal seen in the cervical cord at the C4-5 and C6 levels.

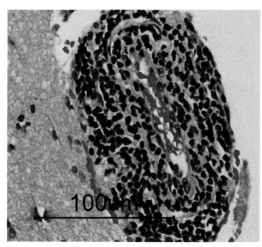

Fig. 9. Hematoxylin-eosin stain demonstrating perivascular inflammatory cell infiltrate, with hyalinization of the vessel wall and crenated red blood cells in the vessel lumen.

DISTINGUISHING INFLAMMATORY DEMYELINATION FROM CNS INFECTION

Acute CNS infection should be considered in all children with acute CNS deficits; spinal fluid analysis for infection is a standard component of initial investigation. CSF lymphocytosis is seen in ADS, whereas neutrophils in the CSF should prompt concern for infection, necrosis, HLH, NMO, and rare cases of ADEM. The MR imaging features of CNS infection must also be considered.

CLINICAL VIGNETTE

A young patient presented with a 3-day history of tingling and numbness in both lower limbs. Clinical concerns were raised for a demyelinating disease, Guillain-Barré syndrome, and infection. CSF showed slightly increased eosinophils and was otherwise not specific. MR imaging of the spine was performed with gadolinium contrast enhancement (Fig. 12A–C). There was a small cystic lesion in the conus medullaris with an intramural nodule. There was minimal contrast enhancement at this site, with mildly increased contrast enhancement in nerve roots of the cauda equina. The presence of a cystic lesion with an intramural eccentric nodule as seen on the sagittal T2 image (see Fig. 12A) strongly suggested the diagnosis of cysticercosis. Although spinal cord cysticercosis is rare, the patient's background and travel history was in keeping with areas where cysticercosis is endemic (South East Asia and South America). Treatment was initiated with albendazole, and a follow-up MR imaging obtained at 6 months showed a decrease in the size of this cystic lesion (Fig. 12D–F).

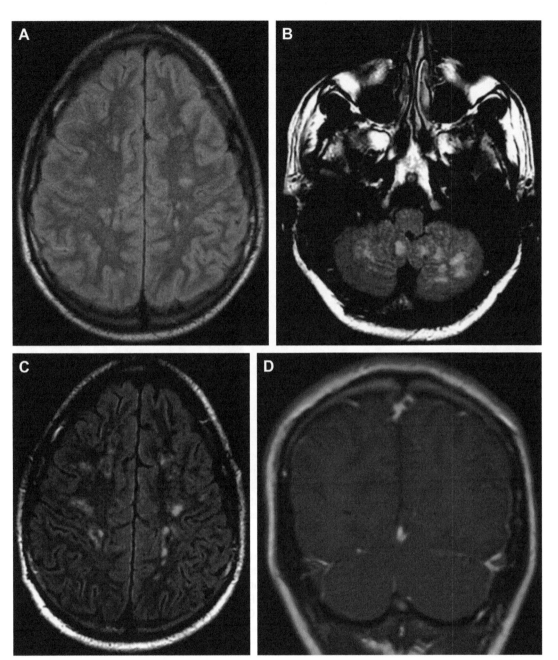

Fig. 10. Axial FLAIR images (*A–C*) show areas of hyperintense signal involving the deep white matter of the cerebral and cerebellar hemispheres, more on the left side (*B*). Coronal T1 + C (*D*) Shows subtle leptomeningeal enhancement at the level of the cerebellar folia.

CLINICAL VIGNETTE

A previously healthy 12-year-old girl presented with a 2-week history of progressive difficulty with gait. MR imaging of the spine revealed intramedullary T2 signal abnormality from T7 to T9 and ring enhancement (Fig. 13A). MR imaging of the brain was remarkable for nonenhancing lesions in the anterior limb of the right internal capsule, left centrum semiovale, and along the subcortical location of the right inferior frontal lobe (Fig. 13B, C). Neurologic examination was remarkable for severe lower limb weakness and increased deep tendon reflexes in both her upper and lower extremities. CSF investigations were normal. Treatment with corticosteroids led to complete clinical recovery. The diagnosis of TM was made.

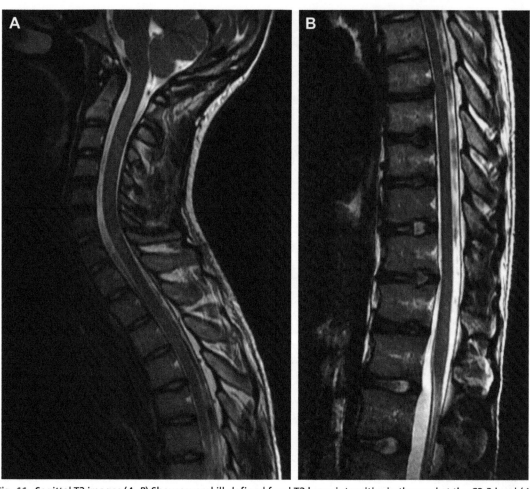

Fig. 11. Sagittal T2 images (*A, B*) Show several ill-defined focal T2 hyperintensities in the cord at the C2-3 level (*A*) and in the thoracic cord at the T3-4 and T8 levels (*B*). There was no evidence of cord expansion, syrinx, or abnormal enhancement.

DISTINGUISHING DIFFERENT TYPES OF RELAPSING DEMYELINATING DISORDERS

Of key interest to clinicians, patients, and parents is the ability to predict future risk of MS when patients present at the time of a first clinical attack of demyelination. However, even children who experience more than 1 episode of demyelination are not necessarily destined for a diagnosis of MS. Forms of recurrent demyelination that do not yield a diagnosis of MS include recurrent and multiphasic ADEM, NMO, NMO spectrum disorders, relapsing TM without features of NMO, and chronic relapsing inflammatory optic neuropathy (CRION).

CRION is a recurrent, frequently bilateral, steroid-dependent ON, without evidence of any additional neurologic deficits, sarcoidosis, or systemic autoimmune disease. The latency between episodes varies from days to decades. Patients with CRION have normal brain MR imaging and absent spinal fluid oligoclonal bands.

CLINICAL VIGNETTE

A 10-year-old girl was admitted to hospital with a 5-day history of progressive bilateral visual loss and pain with eye movement. On examination, visual acuity was finger counting on the right and 20/800 on the left. Examination revealed bilateral optic disc swelling. Neurologic examination was otherwise unremarkable. MR imaging of the brain and orbits showed enhancement and abnormal signal of the optic nerves bilaterally (Fig. 14). Treatment with corticosteroids led to resolution of eye pain and marked improvement in vision to 20/40 on the right and 20/50 on the left. Nineteen months after the initial episode, she experienced recurrent pain with eye movement and reduced vision in the left eye. Visual acuity was 20/25 in the right eye, with light perception only in the left eye. MR imaging of the orbits showed enhancement and thickening of the optic nerves bilaterally. Testing for NMO immunoglobulin G (IgG) was negative. Five years after her initial episode, the patient remains well without further evidence of clinical or MR imaging disease activity.

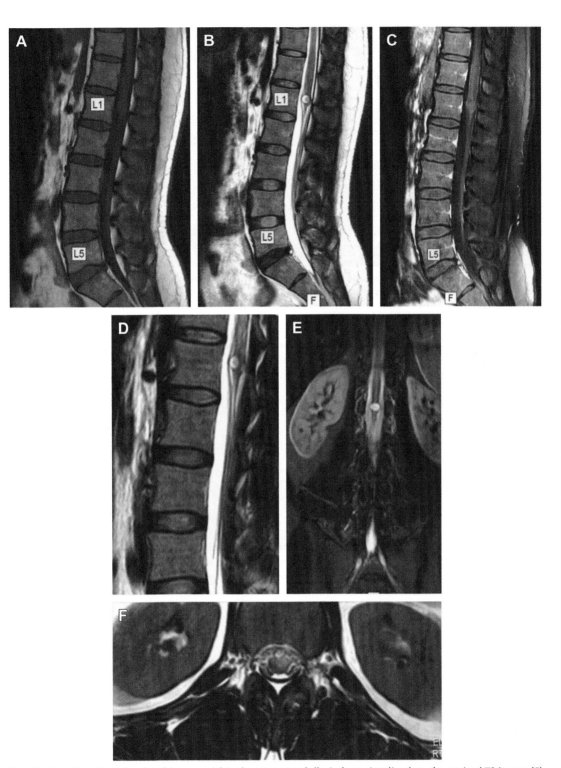

Fig. 12. A small cystic lesion (*A–C*) is seen within the conus medullaris, best visualized on the sagittal T2 image (*B*). The small intramural nodule within the cyst is highly suggestive of cysticercosis. Postcontrast images showed mild enhancement of the cauda equina. Follow-up images (*D–F*) 6 months after treatment with albendazole show decrease in the size of the lesion. (*Courtesy of* Dr Ashish Atre, MD, Pune, India.)

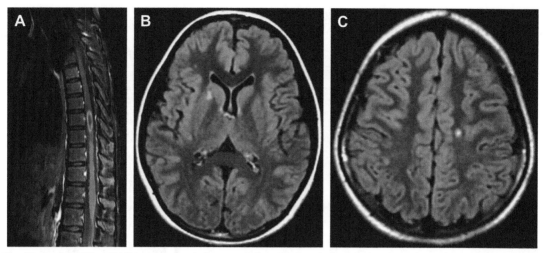

Fig. 13. Sagittal T1 + C (*A*) image reveals intramedullary T2 signal abnormality for T7-9 and ring enhancement. Axial T2 FLAIR of the brain (*B, C*) is remarkable for nonenhancing lesions.

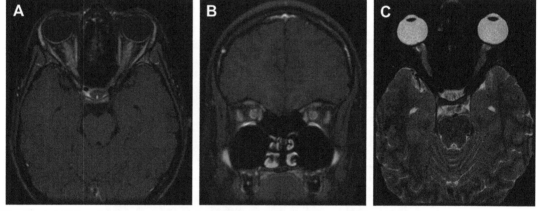

Fig. 14. Axial T1 + C (*A*), coronal T1 + C (*B*), and axial T2 with fat saturation (*C*) show prominent optic nerve sheaths bilaterally. The optic nerves within the optic nerve sheaths are abnormal in signal and show abnormal enhancement.

DISTINGUISHING VITAMIN B12 DEFICIENCY FROM ACQUIRED DEMYELINATION

CLINICAL VIGNETTE

A 13-year-old boy with a recent episode of pneumonia presented with a 3-month history of abdominal pain, weakness, difficulty with short-term memory, fatigue, and vomiting. Physical examination was remarkable for diffusely tender abdomen, jaundice, bilateral leg weakness, tremor, abnormal gait, diminished reflexes, and sensory loss at L4. Laboratory investigations showed elevated liver enzymes and substantially low ceruloplasmin. Extensive workup for Wilson disease was negative. MR imaging of the brain was normal. Over the following few weeks, serial laboratory evaluations indicated elevated bilirubin, hemoglobin of 76 g/L, and B12 deficiency. MR imaging of the spine revealed extensive cord signal abnormality within the dorsal columns (Fig. 15). A diagnosis of vitamin B12 deficiency due to pernicious anemia (intrinsic factor positive) was conferred. He improved dramatically on initiation of B12 supplementation; however, 4 years later he continues to experience difficulty with fine motor movements.

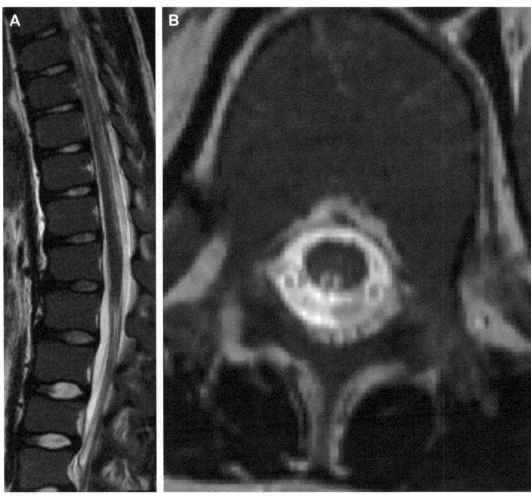

Fig. 15. Sagittal T2 (A) and axial T2 (B) images through the thoracic cord show increased signal within the dorsal columns in this child with vitamin B12 deficiency.

DISTINGUISHING MALIGNANCY FROM ACQUIRED DEMYELINATION

Tumefactive lesions share many commonalities with CNS malignancy, making it difficult to distinguish between the two even with MR imaging. Although rare in children, metastatic malignancy should be considered, and all patients with tumefactive demyelination should be followed with frequent MR imaging to avoid brain biopsy.

CLINICAL VIGNETTE

An 8-year-old girl presented with a 1-month history of a sixth-nerve palsy. Deficits on examination were confined to a left sixth-nerve palsy, nystagmus on right gaze, and slightly brisk reflexes at the knees bilaterally. MR imaging revealed an inferior pontine lesion and periventricular white matter lesions (Fig. 16A–C). Cytology, cell count, protein, and glucose in CSF were all normal. A diagnosis of monofocal brainstem demyelination was conferred with appreciation for close follow-up in the context of suspicion of malignancy. There was neither clinical nor radiologic improvement after treatment with oral prednisone, pulse methylprednisolone, and intravenous immunoglobulin.

Five months after symptom onset, the patient's clinical symptoms progressed to left-sided facial weakness. Follow-up imaging at that time revealed an increase in size of the pontine lesion and progression of the periventricular abnormalities (Fig. 16D–F). Brain biopsy from the septum pellucidum revealed infiltrative astrocytoma. Treatment with chemotherapy and radiation was commenced.

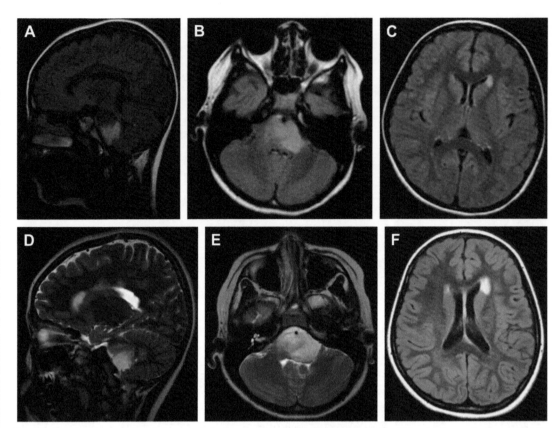

Fig. 16. Baseline images (*A–C*) show an inferior pontine lesion extending to the left middle cerebellar peduncle, which shows increased T2 and low T1 (not shown) signal. Also noted are periventricular white matter lesions (*C*). Follow-up imaging (*D–F*) 5 months after onset reveal progression of the brainstem tumor, with an increase in mass effect of the posterior aspect of the pons and the fourth ventricle. Axial T2 image (*E*) shows increased encasement of the basilar artery by the mass and the left distal vertebral artery, and (*F*) progression of the periventricular white matter signal abnormalities surrounding the frontal horns with thickening and increased signal of the septum pellucidum (*F*). Biopsy from the septum pellucidum showed this to be an infiltrative astrocytoma.

- White matter lesions with the accompaniment of discrete tumefactive lesions favor a diagnosis of demyelination. However, as illustrated by this patient, follow-up imaging is essential, as an occasional muticentric neoplasm can mimic demyelinating white matter lesions.
- Polyfocal neurologic deficits on examination, acute worsening of clinical symptoms, detection of an infectious agent, and resolution of lesions on MR imaging with corticosteroid therapy all support a diagnosis of tumefactive demyelination over malignancy.

SUMMARY

ADS and MS are important diseases that require prompt identification and early treatment. However, even with thorough clinical, laboratory, and imaging evaluation, their diagnoses remain challenging. As illustrated by the patients presented in this article, diagnosis of MS or ADS often requires time for the evolution of clinical symptoms and changes on MR imaging. The identification of serum or CSF biological markers that reliably distinguish patients with MS and ADS from other demyelinating disorders is needed. The potential for advanced MR imaging techniques to visualize underlying features of myelin integrity and repair provides exciting possibilities for future research.

ACKNOWLEDGMENTS

The authors wish to acknowledge the help of Stephanie Khan, Dr Tina Go, and Dr William Halliday.

Advanced Magnetic Resonance Imaging in Pediatric Multiple Sclerosis

Leonard H. Verhey, PhD[a,b], John G. Sled, PhD[c,d],*

KEYWORDS

- Multiple sclerosis • Pediatric • Magnetic resonance imaging • Advanced imaging techniques

KEY POINTS

- Advanced MR imaging techniques are more specific than conventional sequences to the heterogenous features of MS disease and permit quantification of tissue damage in normal appearing brain tissue.
- Recent volumetric studies have revealed that global brain volume and head size are reduced in children with MS compared to matched healthy children. These findings suggest that pediatric MS may affect primary brain and skull growth.
- Thalamic volume and diffusion tensor indices such as fractional anisotropy and mean diffusivity are associated with cognitive impairment in children with MS.
- Studies applying techniques such as focussed cortical imaging, magnetization transfer and functional MR imaging, and MR spectroscopy are limited, and should represent key areas of MR imaging research in pediatric-onset MS to aid in understanding the some of the earliest signatures of MS disease.

INTRODUCTION

The sensitivity of conventional magnetic resonance (MR) imaging (ie, proton density, T2-weighted, fluid-attenuated inversion recovery (FLAIR), and T1-weighted sequences) to detect subclinical disease activity has led to its incorporation into diagnostic criteria for individuals suspected of having multiple sclerosis (MS), and to its use in providing prognostic information for patients in the earliest disease stages. However, the strength of association between conventional MR imaging findings and clinical parameters in patients with established MS is only modest. This association may

be explained by the lack of specificity of conventional MR imaging for the heterogeneous features of MS disease as well as its inability to quantitatively characterize damage to normal-appearing white matter (NAWM) and normal-appearing gray matter (NAGM). Over the past 2 decades, advanced MR imaging techniques have been developed with the objective to identify in vivo quantitative pathologic substrates of clinical disability and provide more specific or sensitive end points for treatment trials. These techniques are not routinely available for clinical use, because they require standardized acquisition, rigorous

[a] Pediatric Demyelinating Disease Program, Program in Neuroscience and Mental Health, The Hospital for Sick Children, Room 11-105, Elm Wing, 555 University Avenue, Toronto, Ontario M5G 1X8, Canada; [b] Institute of Medical Science, University of Toronto, Medical Science Building, 1 King's College Circle, Room 2374, Toronto, Ontario M5S 1A8, Canada; [c] Department of Medical Biophysics, University of Toronto, Ontario Cancer Institute, Princess Margaret Hospital, 610 University Avenue, Room 7-411, Toronto, Ontario M5G 2M9, Canada; [d] Program in Physiology and Experimental Medicine, The Hospital for Sick Children, Toronto Centre for Phenogenomics, Mouse Imaging Centre, 25 Orde Street, Toronto, Ontario M5T 3H7, Canada
* Corresponding author. Mouse Imaging Centre, Toronto Centre for Phenogenomics, 25 Orde Street, Toronto, Ontario M5T 3H7, Canada.
E-mail address: jgsled@phenogenomics.ca

Neuroimag Clin N Am 23 (2013) 337–354
http://dx.doi.org/10.1016/j.nic.2012.12.011
1052-5149/13/$ – see front matter © 2013 Elsevier Inc. All rights reserved.

image analysis pipelines, MR imaging scanner quality-control monitoring, and control or reference data. Multicenter studies on the sensitivity of these techniques to natural history of disease and treatment response are required before their implementation into clinical imaging protocols.

This review summarizes results from studies that have applied advanced MR imaging techniques to patients with pediatric-onset MS, and includes a discussion of cortical imaging techniques, volumetry, magnetization transfer (MT) and diffusion tensor (DT) imaging, proton magnetic resonance spectroscopy (^{1}H-MRS), and functional MR imaging (fMR imaging). The application of advanced MR imaging techniques to pediatric MS is still in its infancy, and therefore, for several techniques, the literature available for review is limited.

CORTICAL IMAGING
Background

Several histopathologic studies have shown that a substantial proportion of the focal cerebral lesion load in adult patients with MS is located within the cortex or at the junction between the cortex and subcortical white matter[1-3] and that cortical lesions are actively inflammatory and appear early on in the MS disease course.[4] Postmortem studies of adult patients have shown that cortical lesions can be classified according to 4 subtypes: (1) lesions involving the cortical gray matter and adjacent subcortical white matter, termed leukocortical lesions; (2) intracortical lesions located solely within the cortex and not involving the subpial cortex or subcortical white matter; (3) lesions beginning in the subpial cortex but that do not reach the boundary between gray and white matter; and (4) lesions involving the entire width of the cerebral cortex, from subpial cortex to the border between gray and white matter.[5,6] These lesions are not typically resolved on conventional MR imaging sequences because of their small size, their poor contrast against normal-appearing cortical gray matter, and the effects of partial voluming from the surrounding cerebrospinal fluid.

The ability to detect and quantify the level of cortical involvement has important implications, because quantitative MR imaging studies in adults with MS have shown evidence of cortical gray matter damage in the earliest clinical stages of the disease,[7-9] and cortical gray matter volume loss occurs at a faster rate than that of the white matter.[10] In addition, MR imaging measures of cortical gray matter damage, specifically accumulation of intracortical lesions, have shown stronger correlations with clinical measures of physical and cognitive impairment[11-14] and with co-occurring

epilepsy,[15] compared with measures of white matter lesion burden. Guidelines for the scoring of cortical lesions have recently been proposed.[16] The presence of at least 1 cortical lesion independently predicts MS diagnosis in adults with a first attack of central nervous system (CNS) demyelination.[17] Disease-modifying therapy in adults with MS has also been shown to decrease the number of new cortical lesions and slow the rate of cortical atrophy when compared with untreated patients.[18]

Cortical Imaging Techniques

Several pulse sequences have been shown to substantially improve detection of cortical lesions. Compared with two-dimensional T2-weighted spin-echo imaging, the three-dimensional (3D) fast FLAIR sequence, which allows acquisition of thinner slices, has an increased sensitivity for cortical lesions.[19-21] However, delineation of cortical lesions on T2-weighted and FLAIR imaging remains a challenge because of poor gray matter–white matter contrast, which makes complicates classification of lesions as intracortical, leukocortical, or juxtacortical.[22] Limited blood-brain barrier permeability and low inflammatory cell infiltration in cortical lesions,[3,23] as well as low myelin density in the upper layers of the neocortex,[24] decrease T2 contrast.

Introduction of the double inversion recovery (DIR) sequence has substantially increased the in vivo detection of cortical lesions.[25] By selecting inversion times that can simultaneously achieve T1-based suppression of the signals from both white matter and cerebrospinal fluid, the DIR sequence yields images in which T2 variations within gray matter are more easily detected. The result is superior delineation of the gray matter and the boundary between the cortex and subcortical white matter, with lesions appearing hyperintense. Using DIR imaging, intracortical lesion detection rates per patient increase by 152% compared with FLAIR imaging, and by 538% when compared with T2-weighted imaging.[22,26] DIR imaging at 3 T results in a 192% increase in cortical lesion detection compared with 1.5-T DIR images.[27] A study of the probabilistic distribution and frequency of cortical lesions in adults with MS confirmed earlier histopathologic studies, showing that more than 80% of lesions were found in the frontotemporal cortex, with a predilection for the motor cortex in approximately 35% of patients and anterior cingulate gyrus in 10%.[28] There are likely still many cortical lesions not resolved by DIR, because only about 10% to 20% of cortical lesions identified through postmortem immunohistochemistry are detected on DIR imaging.[1]

Given that DIR imaging is limited by a low cortical lesion detection rate compared with histopathologic studies, poor delineation of lesion borders, artifacts caused by cerebrospinal fluid flow and pulsation, and an intrinsically low signal-to-noise ratio, combining DIR imaging with other sequences may improve cortical lesion detection and reliability of cortical lesion classification. Using a combination of phase-sensitive inversion recovery (PSIR) and DIR techniques yields a 337% increase in total number of cortical lesions detected when compared with FLAIR; intracortical lesion detection was increased by 417%, mixed gray-white matter lesions by 396%, and juxtacortical lesions by 130%.[29]

3D spoiled gradient-recalled (SPGR) echo imaging provides high spatial resolution and high signal-to-noise ratio images within a clinically acceptable acquisition time. The superior contrast between gray matter and white matter achievable with SPGR permits increased classification accuracy for cortical lesions.[30,31] One study reported that 30 of the 119 cortical lesions (11 patients) initially identified on DIR and PSIR images were reclassified after reviewing the 3D-SPGR images, with most reclassified from mixed gray-white matter lesions to purely intracortical.[30]

Cortical Lesion Detection in Pediatric MS

Only 1 study has evaluated the presence, frequency, and type of cortical lesions in individuals with pediatric-onset MS compared with adult patients.[32] Only 8% of the pediatric patients had cortical lesions, compared with 66% of adults with MS. Although the number and volume of white matter lesions did not differ between pediatric and adult patients with MS, mean cortical lesion count in pediatric patients was only 0.08, compared with 1.99 cortical lesions per adult patient. Median cortical lesion volume was also lower in pediatric versus adult patients. All cortical lesions in the pediatric patients were located at the gray matter–white matter boundary, which is where proliferation of myelin into the peripheral cortical neuropil occurs during childhood and adolescence.[33]

These data suggest that cortical lesion formation is rare in patients with pediatric MS. Whether the formation of cortical lesions is rare in the early stages of MS cannot be determined from this study because the median disease duration was 2 years longer for adult-onset compared with pediatric-onset patients. It is possible that the degree of gray matter maturation in pediatric versus adult patients may explain why children with MS have fewer cortical lesions. Quantification of cortical volume by measuring cortical thickness

has been conducted in adults with MS.[34–37] Studies to assess whether cortical thinning is more prominent than cortical lesion accrual seen in children with MS have not yet been performed. Additional studies in children with MS are required to identify optimal MR imaging techniques for cortical lesion detection, and to better understand the frequency and localization of cortical lesions and their correlation with clinical parameters such as cognitive impairment.

VOLUMETRY
Background

MR imaging measurement of volume loss in MS is appealing because it is believed to reflect a sensitive but nonspecific measure of irreversible axonal loss and the neurodegenerative aspect of MS pathobiology.[38] Longitudinal studies in adults with MS have shown that volume loss is evident in the earliest stages of the disease and predicts clinical progression[9,39] and that patients with the highest rate of volume loss early in the disease reach higher levels of disability than those with a slower rate of volume loss.[39–41] Gray matter volume loss specifically develops at a faster rate than does white matter volume loss[42,43] and shows stronger correlations with clinical disability than white matter loss and conventional T2 lesion measures.[44–46]

Methodology for Measuring Brain Volume

From a technical point of view, measurement of brain volume is appealing, because it can be achieved using a conventional T1-weighted MR imaging pulse sequence. However, because the typical rate of brain volume loss in adults with relapsing-remitting MS is only between 0.5% and 1% per year,[38] detection of these subtle volume changes requires quantitative techniques that rely on careful and consistent image acquisition, the use of image analysis algorithms that are not typically available or too intensive to run on MR imaging consoles, as well as the oversight of a trained operator. The technical demands of performing volumetric measurements have prevented their use outside the research setting.

The available methods for estimating brain volume differ depending on whether the intent is to measure volume change from serial images or to measure absolute or normalized volume from individual scans. When measuring absolute brain volume, 2 broad strategies apply. One is to classify each of the voxel elements of the image as either brain parenchyma or nonbrain.[47–50] This classification can be based on image intensity, perhaps with the aid of spatial maps of prior probability, or by evolving a deformable model to find the brain surface. The brain volume is then directly computed by summing the volumes of the constituent voxels. A second strategy is to use image registration to warp the shape of a reference brain image onto the given image.[51,52] Volume is then computed using the spatial transformation and the brain boundary defined on the reference image.

A challenge to estimating absolute brain volume is that the MR imaging scanner may not have sufficient geometric accuracy to correctly report the differences on the order of 1% that are anticipated.[38] This limitation can be overcome by careful geometric calibration of the MR imaging scanner with a specialized phantom or by normalizing the brain volume to another structure. Normalization of brain volume to intracranial volume is a common strategy for analyzing cross-sectional data.[53,54]

Deformation-based and voxel-based morphometry are 2 methods that allow estimation of brain volume change from serial images. In the case of deformation-based morphometry, images from the time series are warped to align with each other using image registration, and the brain boundary is estimated once for the entire series.[55] Compared with estimating brain volume from individual scans, this approach has the advantage that the alignment between consecutive scans after warping tends to be more accurate than the alignment between a given image and the generic reference image. Voxel-based morphometry takes a similar approach, except that only linear or coarse scale nonlinear alignment is applied.[56–59] The changes between consecutive images are then detected as small changes in gray level intensity that correspond to shifts in the position of the boundary that are smaller than the dimensions of the voxel. These brain shifts can be integrated across cortical regions or averaged across individuals to obtain estimates of volume change. Both deformation-based and voxel-based morphometry are generic methods that apply equally well to analyzing subregions of the brain or to boundaries other than the cortical surface.

Unique Methodological Issues in Brain Volume Measurement in Children

In healthy individuals, brain volume is nearly constant between the ages of 20 and 55 years,[60] but in children and adolescents, the brain is still growing with age, and the rate of growth varies between individuals. Thus, choosing appropriate metrics to compare brain volumes among children is challenging. Methods of brain volume measurement that rely on normalization to the inner surface of the skull are inaccurate in children, especially between the ages of 10 and 12 years, because the skull and brain show a differential rate of brain growth. To overcome this challenge, a recent study that compared brain volume loss in children with MS with healthy controls[61] proposed a novel approach of using a z score at each location in the brain to represent whether the local volume at each given location was larger or smaller than that for a database of age-matched controls (**Fig. 1**). The z scores were computed by warping the given brain image to a reference image and computing the Jacobian determinant of this transformation. These Jacobian determinants can then be compared with those found for the age-matched reference population to compute the number of standard deviations by which the given individual deviates from the mean for that location. A positive Jacobian determinant value indicates a local volume increase relative to the template, and a negative determinant value indicates a local decrease in brain volume.

Volumetry in Pediatric MS

Several cross-sectional studies have been conducted to assess brain volume change in children with MS compared with healthy individuals and correlate these changes with clinical measures of disability and cognitive impairment. One study used a segmentation technique to calculate the brain parenchymal fraction, which normalizes parenchymal volume to the volume bounded by the inner skull surface; similarly, normalized gray and white matter fractions were also computed.[62] Three key findings can be noted from this study. First, compared with adults with MS matched for disease duration, pediatric patients showed a higher brain parenchymal fraction and gray matter fraction. Second, when comparing adults with pediatric-onset MS with adult-onset patients matched for disease duration to assess the long-term impact of pediatric disease, no differences were found between groups for brain parenchymal fraction or white matter fraction, but adult patients trended toward greater gray matter volume loss compared with pediatric-onset adult patients. To assess age at onset-related differences in brain volume, a comparison between adults with pediatric-onset MS and adult-onset patients of similar age showed lower brain parenchymal and gray matter fractions in the adult pediatric-onset adult group compared with the adult-onset patients.

Another study used voxel-based morphometry to evaluate the pattern of gray matter loss in pediatric patients with MS compared with a control group matched for age and sex.[63] No differences were detected in normalized brain and gray matter

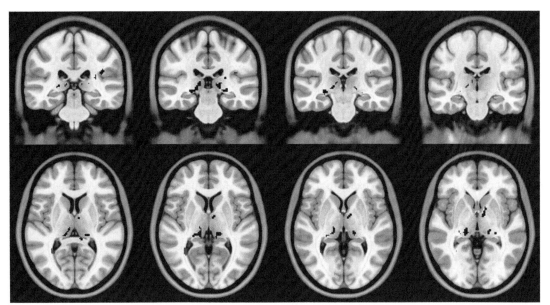

Fig. 1. Clusters of significant tissue loss (*blue*) and expansion (*red*) in children with MS compared with age-matched and sex-matched healthy controls (*P*<.05, corrected for multiple comparisons). (*Courtesy of* Collins DL, PhD, Aubert-Broche B, PhD, McConnell Brain Imaging Center, Montreal Neurological Institute, McGill University, Montreal, Canada.)

volume or intracranial volume between healthy individuals and children with MS, but patients showed locally reduced gray matter volume in the right and left thalami compared with controls. Although T2 lesion load was significantly negatively correlated with both left and right thalamic volume, no correlations were found with disability or disease duration. Children included in this study had a mean disease duration of only 3 years, and the accrual of disability in patients with pediatric-onset MS typically occurs 15 to 20 years after onset.[64,65] The association between T2 lesion load and thalamic volume suggests that focal white matter lesions may cause retrograde or anterograde transynaptic degeneration of the afferent and efferent neuronal connections that relay through the thalamus. Evidence for this hypothesis is further given by a study that used deformation-based morphometry to evaluate the spatial distribution of brain volume loss in children with MS in a cross-sectional manner (see Fig. 1).[61] Significant volume reductions were seen in the pulvinar and anterior nuclei of the left and right thalami as well as in the splenium of the corpus callosum and globus pallidus in pediatric patients compared with age-matched and sex-matched controls. T2 lesion load was negatively correlated with volume loss in the splenium of the corpus callosum, supporting the notion of Wallerian degeneration of the crossing nerve fiber tracts caused by axonal transection within hemispheric white matter focal lesions.[66] Loss of volume within the

optic tract (from the chiasm to the lateral geniculate bodies, and the anterior portion of the optic radiations) was associated with disease duration but not T2 lesion volume; however, post hoc analyses did not show any correlation between history of optic neuritis and optic pathway volume loss.

Using a region-of-interest method to analyze brain volume in children and adolescents with MS compared with healthy individuals, a significant reduction in global brain volume was detected in patients with MS.[67] After correction for global brain volume, an even greater reduction in thalamic volume was observed in patients with MS compared with control individuals. Reduced normalized brain volume correlated moderately with increased T1 and T2 lesion volumes, suggesting an important contribution of focal MR imaging-visible lesions to the neurodegenerative process of MS. The investigators also observed a reduction in head size of the patients with pediatric-onset MS compared with matched healthy control individuals. Given that skull size is largely determined by brain growth during the first 10 years after birth,[68] these findings suggest that pediatric-onset MS may affect primary brain and skull growth.[67]

In a study of MR imaging correlates of cognitive impairment in children with MS, thalamic volume and corpus callosal area were positively correlated with an index of global intellectual function, mental processing speed, and confrontation naming.[69] These findings support the notion that the neurodegenerative aspect of MS pathobiology is operative in the earliest stages of the disease and that immune-mediated damage of immature neural networks may have significant deleterious consequences on cognitive function. Longitudinal studies are needed to determine whether resiliency of developing neural networks is able to protect children with MS from long-term cognitive deficits.

MT IMAGING
Background

MR imaging studies have been pivotal in showing that pathologic changes are present not only within lesions but also in the normal-appearing brain matter (NABM) of patients with MS. MT imaging is a technique that can be used to quantify the level of microstructural damage within T2 visible lesions as well as NAWM and NAGM.[70–73]

On MT ratio (MTR) maps, demyelinating lesions (T2 visible lesions) appear as hypointense (**Fig. 2**). Postmortem studies of patients with MS have shown the relationship between low MTR and neuroaxonal damage and myelin loss both within lesions as well as in NABM.[74–78] Remyelinated lesions have a higher MTR than demyelinated lesions,[76] suggesting the potential role of MT imaging in monitoring remyelination.

Physics of MT Imaging

Conventional MR imaging pulse sequences exploit the properties (ie, T1 and T2 relaxation behavior as well as spin density) of free-water protons to produce tissue contrast. There is a pool of nonaqueous protons associated with proteins and macromolecules, such as myelin, which may permit quantification of myelin integrity in the context of MS. However, because of the short transverse (T2) relaxation times of these bound proton spins, signal decays too rapidly and prohibits acquisition of an MR imaging signal. Another challenge to imaging bound protons is that the frequency of the signal from aqueous protons is near that of the signal from the nonaqueous proton pool.

Using MT imaging, the protons bound to macromolecules can be probed via their exchange or transfer of magnetization with free-water protons.[79,80] To achieve this goal, a selective radiofrequency pulse that is off the water resonance is applied to excite primarily the bound proton pool, thereby partially saturating its magnetization. Magnetization exchange between the partially saturated bound proton pool and the more mobile pool of spins causes a reduction in the signal measured by MR imaging. The MTR represents

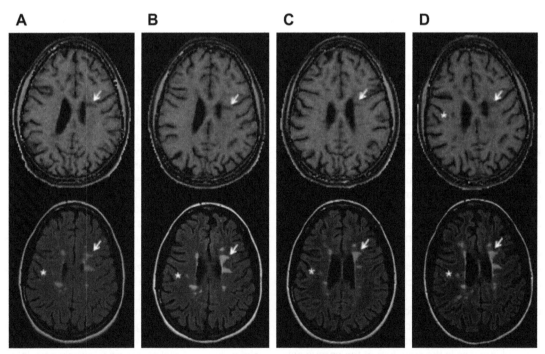

Fig. 2. Axial MTR maps (*top row*) and corresponding axial FLAIR images (*bottom row*) of a girl who presented with a first attack of MS at 11 years of age. Scans were acquired at 5 years (*A*), 6 years (*B*), 7 years (*C*), and 8 years (*D*) after onset. A subset of the T2 lesions is visible on the corresponding MTR maps. The periventricular T2 lesion denoted by the arrow on FLAIR images shows decreased MTR on corresponding MT images across all time points. The T2 lesion demarcated by an asterisk on all serial FLAIR images shows a decreased MTR at the 8-year follow-up scan.

the efficiency of this magnetization exchange, and is calculated as a difference in signal between the images acquired with and without the off-resonance radiofrequency pulse. MTR maps are computed at a voxel level according to the following equation:

$$MTR = (1 - MT_{on}/MT_{off}) \times 100\%$$

where MT_{on} refers to the signal intensity with the off-resonance radiofrequency pulse and MT_{off} refers to the intensity without the off-resonance pulse.

Methods to Analyze MT Imaging Data

Several methods exist for analyzing MTR maps. These methods include computing average MTR within regions of interest such the NAWM or NAGM or within lesions; computing histograms of MTR for the whole brain; or voxel-by-voxel analysis. Voxel-by-voxel analysis is more technically demanding because image registration is required to identify corresponding voxels in multiple scans from a time series or across scans of different individuals.

MT Imaging in Pediatric MS

Only 3 studies[62,81,82] have evaluated microstructural tissue abnormalities in children with MS using MT imaging. A preliminary study evaluated the average MTR and histogram peak height (ie, the most frequently occurring MTR value) in both the NABM and cervical spinal cord of 13 children with MS compared with age-matched and sex-matched healthy controls. However, no significant differences were found.[81] In a follow-up study of 23 children with MS and 16 age-matched and sex-matched healthy controls, average MTR and histogram peak height in both the NAWM and NAGM were similar.[82] In a study comparing 33 adults with pediatric-onset MS with 381 adults with adult-onset disease, MTR values tended to be lower within T2 lesions, NAWM, and NAGM,[62] suggesting a greater degree of microstructural abnormality in pediatric-onset adult patients than adult-onset patients, perhaps explained by a longer disease duration. Further studies using voxel-based methods and longitudinal MTR analyses are required to determine the extent and time course for neuroaxonal and myelin injury in children and whether children show enhanced reparative capacity.

DT IMAGING
Background

Diffusion imaging is a powerful and sensitive technique used to noninvasively measure restriction of water diffusion in vivo within an image voxel, thereby providing information on the structural organization of the brain and spinal cord, as well as pathologic changes not visualized on conventional MR imaging scans. In diffusion imaging, the displacement (on the order of 10–15 μm[83]) of thermally driven, randomly moving (ie, Brownian motion) water molecules is measured. This distance is sufficient for restriction caused by subcellular and cellular structure to affect the measured signal; however, establishing which aspects of cellular structure account for observed changes is difficult. In white matter, the axonal membrane, intra-axonal structures such as neurofilaments, as well as the ensheathing layers of myelin, are all believed to affect the diffusion signal observed by MR imaging.[83]

Physics of DT Imaging

The addition of a pair of strong gradient pulses to a spin-echo sequence is the most common strategy to create a diffusion-weighted imaging sequence, and is typically combined with an echo planar imaging readout for rapid acquisition. The amplitude, duration, and interval between the gradient pulses determine the diffusion weighting of the sequences and can be summarized by a single variable termed the b value. The exponential rate of signal loss with increasing b values is used to define the apparent diffusion coefficient (ADC) for a tissue and reflects both the diffusivity of water as well as the restrictions on water motion imposed by cellular structures. For the modest b values that are obtainable using clinical MR imaging systems, ADC shows little variation with b.

A limitation of reporting ADC alone is that for tissue with oriented structure, such as white matter tracts, the coefficient varies with the direction of the diffusion weighting gradients. A useful way to represent this directional dependence is to imagine an ellipsoidal region that describes where a given water molecule is likely to be found a short time later. Although this ellipsoidal confidence region needs to grow with time to allow for larger displacements of the water molecule, its shape remains the same. The ellipsoidal region can be represented mathematically by a 3-by-3 tensor, in which the eigenvectors of the tensor describe the axes of the ellipsoid and the eigenvalues the diffusivity along each axis. A minimum of 6 different diffusion-weighting directions is needed to estimate the DT for a given tissue.

Where water freely diffuses in all directions, such as in cerebrospinal fluid, this confidence region is spherical, representing isotropic diffusion. In tissue, where there are obstacles to water diffusion in certain directions, the confidence could be ellipsoidal, representing anisotropic diffusion. In myelinated tracts of the brain, for example, diffusion within each voxel occurs principally parallel to the axons, with relatively little diffusion perpendicular to the axon, possibly because of the hydrophobic nature of myelin.[84] The principal eigenvector (λ_1) represents the diffusion direction of greatest magnitude within the voxel and is parallel to the white matter fibers. The secondary (λ_2) and tertiary (λ_3) eigenvectors are perpendicular to λ_1 and transverse to white matter fiber tracts.

Four diffusion parameters derived from the DT are typically reported in DT imaging studies: (1) mean diffusivity (MD) is the arithmetic average of the 3 diffusivities; (2) fractional anisotropy (FA) is a measure of the eccentricity of the ellipsoidal confidence region[85]; (3) parallel (axial) diffusivity ($\lambda_\parallel$) is the same as λ_1; and (4) transverse (radial) diffusivity ($\lambda_\perp$) is the average of λ_2 and λ_3 (**Fig. 3**).

DT Imaging Analysis Methodology

Several DT imaging techniques have been developed to selectively localize white matter tracts and evaluate their diffusion-related changes in individuals with MS. Using a voxel-wise comparisons method, several studies have shown correlations between FA and clinical parameters such as physical disability and cognitive impairment.[56,86,87] Voxel-wise methods rely on rigorous spatial registration and spatial smoothing, both of which can affect the consistency of results and the influence of partial volume.[88,89]

A relatively new technique that permits whole-brain evaluation without a priori knowledge of location of white matter tract damage, known as tract-based spatial statistics (TBSS), eliminates the requirements for spatial smoothing and robust nonlinear image registration.[90] When conducting TBSS, an initial approximate nonlinear FA image registration is first performed and images are then projected onto a group mean, white matter tract FA skeleton, permitting coregistration between individuals or patient groups. Voxel-wise statistics can then be computed across individuals on the data projected to the FA skeleton.

Another DT imaging analysis technique is to characterize white matter pathways through fiber tracking.[91–93] Fiber-tracking techniques can be summarized as deterministic or probabilistic. Deterministic methods involve propagation of a line from a seed point to another coordinate in the brain by interpolating DTs or following orientations of primary eigenvectors.[93] Applying this technique in patients with MS has some limitations because decreased FA values within lesions lead to uncertainty about orientation of the primary eigenvector or deterministic tracts may terminate altogether within a lesion.[94] An alternative method, probabilistic fiber tracking, is to consider multiple tract trajectories emanating from a given voxel and weight these by the probability density function for water diffusion at that location.[95]

DT Imaging in Pediatric MS

The earliest DT imaging studies conducted in children with MS[81,82] report histogram analyses of lesions, NAWM, and NAGM. In patients with pediatric-onset MS, the NABM average MD is lower compared with healthy controls.[81] More specifically, the microstructural abnormalities seen in the NABM of children with MS may be specific to the NAWM, given the increased average MD and decreased MD histogram peak height observed in the NAWM group when compared with controls.[82] The NAWM group also shows lower average FA and higher peak height, compared with healthy children.[82,96] Increased MD and decreased FA in the NAWM of children with MS suggests the presence of white matter tract disorganization and may support the

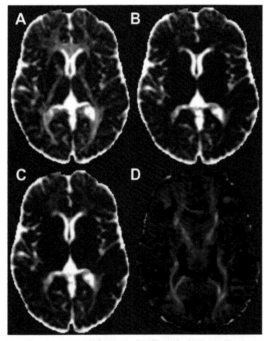

Fig. 3. Axial diffusivity (A), radial diffusivity (B), MD (C), and FA (D) maps of a child with MS. In (D), fibers oriented right-left are in red, fibers oriented superior-inferior are in blue, and fibers oriented anteroposterior are in green.

hypothesis of glial proliferation because glial cells do not have the same anisotropic morphology as myelinated fibers.[82] When compared with adults with a first attack of CNS demyelination, the FA and MD of NAWM, NAGM, or lesions was not different for children with acute demyelination.[96] However, adult patients with relapsing-remitting MS had higher average MD values both within lesions and within the NAGM compared with pediatric patients with relapsing-remitting MS.[96] Average lesion FA and MD as well as FA and MD of NAWM correlate with T2 lesion volume,[82,96] suggesting that NAWM damage may be a phenomenon of Wallerian degeneration of axons that pass through visible T2 lesions.

One study has used a tract-based approach to characterize diffusion abnormalities of the callosal, projection, and association pathways in children with MS.[97] In lesional white matter, mean ADC values within corpus callosal, posterior limb of the internal capsule, and long association fiber regions of interest are higher in children with MS compared with healthy individuals and FA values are lower. When considering only NAWM, higher ADC and lower FA values are observed.[97] Tract-based measures of NAWM fibers show higher ADC and lower FA values in children with MS compared with healthy controls.[97]

Recently, a study was conducted to assess the functional consequence of loss of microstructural integrity in children with MS using DT imaging and cognitive measures of processing speed.[98] In a cohort of 36 children with MS and 30 age-matched and sex-matched healthy controls, children with MS showed lower FA values in the NAWM of both the genu and splenium of the corpus callosum as well as in the NAWM of the bilateral temporal, parietal, and occipital lobes, compared with controls.[98] FA and MD values of the averaged right-left thalami did not differ between patients and controls. For children with MS, T2 lesion volume was associated with corpus callosal FA, specifically the genu and splenium, and NAWM hemispheric FA, but not with thalamic FA. In children with MS, processing speed, measured with the Symbol Digit Modalities Test (SDMT) and the Visual Matching subtest of the Woodcock-Johnson III Test of Cognitive Abilities, was faster in children with higher FA values within the lobar NAWM, particularly in the right hemisphere. Faster processing speed on the SDMT was correlated with higher FA in the genu of the corpus callosum, whereas faster performance on the Visual Matching subtest was associated with higher FA in all corpus callosal regions. Lower MD values in the corpus callosum were correlated with faster processing speed on both tests. FA of the thalamus in children with MS was positively correlated with performance on the SDMT but not the Visual Matching subtest.

These studies together suggest that disruption of normal white matter structure occurs early in the disease, that the white matter integrity disruption is widespread, and that this early damage to the NAWM has functional consequences.

¹H-MRS
Background and Summary of the Technique

¹H-MRS is similar in technique to MR imaging, but instead of using the signal from water protons to provide structural information, ¹H-MRS acquires information from hydrogen nuclei of molecules or metabolites present in tissues, and this metabolic information has pathologic specificity not obtainable from water proton signals.[99] Magnetic resonance spectra are identified by their resonance frequency and expressed as a shift in frequency in parts-per-million (ppm) relative to a reference standard. Two major factors determine whether metabolite resonances can be usefully studied by ¹H-MRS: (1) only freely mobile molecules yield well-defined, discrete resonances, and (2) only those molecules with high concentrations (ie, on the order of millimoles per liter) produce sufficient signal-to-noise.[100]

The concentration of water in brain tissue is greater than that of metabolites, and therefore produces a greater signal compared with the signals produced by metabolite protons. Therefore, ¹H-MRS studies use MR imaging sequences that suppress the signal from water protons. The echo time in a water-suppressed ¹H-MRS study determines the number of observed spectral peaks as well as their amplitude. Four major metabolite resonances are revealed in the brain at long echo times (eg, TE = 144 milliseconds): (1) the methyl resonance of tetramethylamines, especially the choline-containing phospholipids at 3.2 ppm, which include choline, phosphocholine, glycerophosphocholine, and betaine; (2) methyl resonance of creatine and phosphocreatine at 3.0 ppm; (3) methyl resonance of N-acetyl (NA)-containing compounds, especially N-acetylaspartate (NAA) at 2.0 ppm; and (4) methyl resonance of lactate as a doublet at 1.3 ppm, which is normally difficult to visualize above baseline noise and mobile lipids and other macromolecules.[101] At shorter echo times, signals from molecules with short T2 relaxation times can be obtained. These metabolite resonances include amino acids such as γ-aminobutyric acid and glutamate, and sugars such as myoinositol. Short-echo time ¹H-MRS measurements can be complicated by gradient-induced distortions and a poorly defined baseline.

Obtaining estimates of absolute metabolite concentrations from ^{1}H-MRS is challenging, because the spectral peak area depends on acquisition parameters as well as the T1 of the metabolite. Although reference phantoms can aid in calibrating such studies,[102] many studies use another endogenous metabolite as a reference and report a metabolite ratio. The source of metabolite signals collected is spatially localized to a given brain region by using either a single-voxel (^{1}H-MRS) or multivoxel (^{1}H-MR spectroscopic imaging) technique. Single-voxel techniques often use larger volume elements (eg, 2–3 cm^3) than multivoxel techniques (eg, 0.5–1 cm^3 per voxel) and obtain a proportionately higher signal-to-noise ratio.[101]

Description of the ^{1}H-MRS Resonances

To understand in vivo measures of chemical pathology associated with impairments in axonal metabolic and structural integrity, the normal physiology of metabolite resonances commonly studied in MS are briefly reviewed.

The methyl resonance from NA groups

The NA resonance represents NAA primarily and *N*-acetylaspartylglutamate (NAAG) to a lesser degree. NAA is synthesized by neuronal mitochondria and localizes almost exclusively in neurons and neuronal processes. It is important in myelin lipid synthesis, water pump function in myelinated neurons, and as a precursor for NAAG.[103,104] Decreases in NAA can result from any of the following intravoxel changes: (1) decrease in axonal density secondary to axonal loss or atrophy, (2) mitochondrial metabolic dysfunction within neurons and axons, or (3) dilution of NAA secondary to edema or non-NAA-containing cells. NAA as a specific marker of axonal integrity in patients with MS has been shown by strong correlations between in vivo ^{1}H-MRS measurements of NAA resonance and immunohistochemical analyses of brain biopsy specimens.[105]

The creatine resonance

The resonance of creatine (Cr) reflects the presence of Cr and phosphocreatine, which play roles in energy metabolism and homeostasis. Although present in neurons and glial cells, the concentration of Cr is highest in astrocytes and oligodendrocytes.[106] Cr is often used as an intravoxel standard for other metabolites because of its constant concentration and resistance to change throughout the brain. In the study of patients with MS, the intravoxel NAA/Cr ratio is commonly used as an

The glutamate resonance

Glutamate, produced from glutamine in neurons, is the primary excitatory neurotransmitter in the CNS. The glutamate resonance is of interest in ^{1}H-MRS studies of patients with MS because glutamate excitotoxicity is associated with neurodegeneration.[110] Glutamate is also produced by lymphocytes and microglia,[111,112] and, in excess, is associated with axonal and oligodendrocyte damage.[111] Oligodendrocyte-mediated clearance of glutamate in the extrasynaptic white matter of the CNS in adult patients with MS is impaired, and therefore glutamate levels are increased in acute lesions and NAWM, but not in chronic lesions.[113–115]

Evidence for the NA Resonance as a Marker of Axonal Injury in MS

Because of its prominence in the ^{1}H-MR spectrum and its localization within neurons, decreases in NAA are often used as indicators of MS disease and disease progression.[101,108,116] The presence of low NAA, measured both as an absolute concentration and as a ratio of NAA/Cr, has been confirmed within lesional white matter, NAWM, and normal-appearing cortical gray matter of adult patients with MS relative to healthy controls.[105,109,117–124] Decreases in NAA resonance intensity of up to 50% can be observed in the NAWM of adult patients[125] and of up to 80% in white matter regions of T2 hyperintensity.[126] The loss in neuronal integrity measured by decreased NAA/Cr ratios follows a gradient around T2 lesions, with greater injury proximal to the lesion relative to the more distal NAWM.[119] Based on brain biopsy and postmortem spinal cord analyses of adults with MS, decreases in NAA resonance intensities are associated with decreases in axonal density.[105,127,128] Loss of neuronal integrity as measured by MRS has been shown even in the earliest stages of disease.[129,130] The NAA/Cr ratio in adult patients with relapsing-remitting MS shows a strong negative correlation with measures of clinical disability,[131–133] a negative correlation with cerebral atrophy measures,[134] and a positive correlation with functional measures of adaptive reorganization.[135] In a study evaluating multiple MR imaging techniques, cerebral NAA/Cr values were most strongly associated with clinical disability measures.[131]

^{1}H-MRS in Pediatric MS

Fig. 4 shows single-voxel ^{1}H-MRS spectra from the NAWM of a child with MS and healthy control. The application of ^{1}H-MRS to children with MS has been limited to 3 studies. The first study[136]

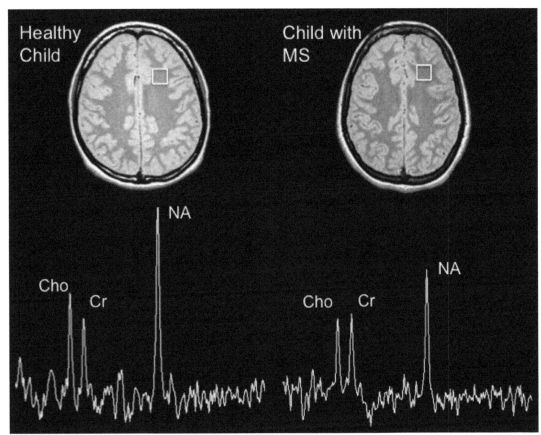

Fig. 4. ^{1}H-MRS resonances showing a reduced NA/Cr ratio in the left frontal NAWM of a child with MS compared with a healthy child. The NA peak includes methyl resonances from NA groups of NAA and NAAG. The Cr resonance includes Cr and phosphocreatine. The choline peak includes methyl resonances of all choline-containing compounds (choline, phosphocholine, glycerophosphocholine, and betaine). (*Courtesy of* Narayanan S, PhD, McConnell Brain Imaging Center, Montreal Neurological Institute, McGill University, Montreal, Canada.)

included 8 individuals with pediatric-onset MS and the findings mimic that seen in patients with adult-onset disease, showing decreased NAA and Cr resonances and increased resonances of choline and myoinositol within lesions relative to healthy age-matched controls. In contrast to observations in adults, 2 studies[136,137] have shown that the ^{1}H-MR spectra of the NAWM of pediatric patients are not different from white matter of healthy controls. However, according to unpublished work by the authors of this article, a decreased NAA/Cr can be observed in the NAWM of children with MS compared with healthy controls (see **Fig. 4**).

A second study evaluated the resonance of citrulline in the brains of 27 children with MS compared with 23 control individuals.[137] Citrullination is a posttranslational modification of myelin basic protein (MBP), the only essential structural proteolipid protein for myelin formation, by which arginine is converted to citrulline via deamination. Increased citrullination of MBP diminishes its

ability to organize lipid bilayers into compact multilayers, resulting in myelin instability.[138,139] Increased levels of citrullinated MBP have been shown in brain specimens from patients with MS,[140] suggesting that citrullination may predispose the white matter to demyelination. This hypothesis was tested in children with MS with ^{1}H-MRS using spectral narrowing to search for the citrulline resonance.[137] A total of 44% of children with MS showed a citrulline peak compared with only 13% of control individuals who were imaged for headache or syncope. A citrulline peak was observed in both NAWM and T2 hyperintense lesions, and conforms with histopathologic evidence of increased citrullinated MBP in the white matter of patients with MS.[141] The NAA/Cr and choline/Cr ratios were not different between pediatric-onset patients and controls, raising the possibility of better metabolic neuroaxonal recovery in children. However, mean myoinositol/Cr ratio was significantly higher within lesions than NAWM of patients and the white matter of controls, suggesting significant glial proliferation, as suggested by other studies.[142]

The third study[143] included 7 children with acute disseminated encephalomyelitis (ADEM) with the goal of identifying an MRS signature of monophasic ADEM that is distinct from that reported in MS. ADEM represents a monophasic inflammatory disorder characterized by large edematous lesions within the CNS. The investigators reported a substantial reduction in the myoinositol/Cr ratio in children with ADEM,[143] which contrasts with the increased intralesional myoinositol/Cr ratio reported in patients with MS.[144] Myoinositol is an osmolyte and a precursor of myelin phosphatidyl inositol found in astrocytes and is considered a glial marker.[145] Functioning as an osmolyte, decreases in myoinositol could indicate decreases in regulatory volume necessary to reduce cell swelling and normalize edema.[146] Reduced myoinositol resonance in children with ADEM could therefore be explained as a compensatory mechanism to counteract edema.

FMR IMAGING
Background and Summary of the Technique

The concept that regional cerebral blood flow reflects neuronal activity is the basis for fMR imaging. A focal increase in neuronal synaptic and electrical activity triggers a local increase in cerebral blood flow, cerebral blood volume, cerebral metabolic rate of oxygen use, and cerebral metabolic rate of glucose rate consumption. Increased neuronal activity leads to a local increase in blood flow, which exceeds the heightened demand for oxygen, thereby causing a net increase in blood oxygenation in that region. Because deoxyhemoglobin is paramagnetic, the reduction in the deoxyhemoglobin concentration that occurs with increased blood flow results in a reduction in T2* and a local increase in the signal observed in T2*-weighted MR imaging scans. This blood oxygenation-dependent contrast (BOLD) effect is the basis of most fMR imaging studies. The BOLD response is closely coupled with neuronal firing rate,[147] and functional localization derived from fMR imaging agrees with the localization obtained in electrophysiologic studies.[148]

Methods of fMR Imaging Acquisition and Analysis

Several experimental designs are used when acquiring fMR imaging data. Task-dependent paradigms can be used to address several questions of interest in MS related to visual or motor function, cognition, fatigue, and depression. Another paradigm, resting-state fMR imaging, is unique in that it does not require a stimulus presentation. The objective of this paradigm is to detect signal fluctuations (up to 3%) that are correlated between different parts of the brain. These fluctuating patterns are analyzed to determine network connectivity.

Several factors can confound the detection of activation patterns in patients with MS. For example, the disease-modifying therapy interferon β-1a increases basal ganglia blood flow,[149] and benzodiazepines and baclofen, which are used to relieve hypertonia, reduce cerebral metabolism.[150] The BOLD signal can also be affected by caffeine intake,[151] circadian rhythm,[152] and menstrual cycle.[153] These potential confounders must be mitigated against in the design of fMR imaging studies.

fMR Imaging in Pediatric MS

Two studies have evaluated cortical activation patterns and functional connectivity using fMR imaging in children with MS.[154,155] Natural history studies have shown that time to reach physical disability in children with MS is on average 10 years longer than that seen in adults.[64,156–158] One plausible explanation for this finding is the enhanced capacity for brain network reorganization in pediatric-onset versus adult-onset patients. To test this hypothesis, the first study evaluated the movement-associated pattern of cortical activations and motor network connectivity in 17 children with MS compared with 9 age-matched and sex-matched healthy controls.[154] Increased activation was observed in the contralateral sensorimotor cortex compared with controls, which was correlated with T2 lesion volume. The investigators suggested that the increased contralateral activation represents an adaptation to the presence of tissue disruption. In a functional connectivity analysis, the investigators found reduced connectivity between the left primary sensorimotor cortex and left thalamus, left insula and left secondary sensorimotor cortex, supplementary motor area and the left secondary sensorimotor cortex, left thalamus and left insula, and the left thalamus and left secondary somatosensory cortex, when compared with controls. The investigators speculated that this connectivity downregulation could be compensatory, representing a functional reservoir that may be upregulated when irreversible structural damage accumulates.

The investigators expanded on these findings in a second study by evaluating effective connectivity changes within the motor network in children with MS compared with adult-onset patients, and considered the influence of structural damage to the corpus callosum and corticospinal tracts on connectivity.[155] No changes in effective connectivity were detected between pediatric MS patients and age-matched and sex-matched healthy controls, suggesting that the adaptive properties or plasticity of the cortex may be preserved in children. The effective intrahemispheric and interhemispheric motor network connectivity was increased in adults with a first attack of CNS demyelination, and more markedly so in adults with MS compared with children with MS. These connectivity changes were associated with microstructural changes within the corpus callosum and corticospinal tracts as measured by MD and FA. Taken together, the incremental recruitment of networks in adult-onset compared with pediatric-onset MS and the association between this recruitment and structural damage suggests that the propensity for brain plasticity or the functional reservoir may deplete over time, and manifest as accrual of physical disability.

SUMMARY

The application of advanced MR imaging techniques to MS undoubtedly enhances understanding of disease pathophysiology and holds promise in its ability to resolve the discrepancy between conventional MR imaging findings and clinical disability, a necessary step to identifying imaging markers of prognosis and therapeutic response. Although application of these modern techniques to pediatric MS is still in its infancy, several challenges unique to the pediatric population are being resolved, such as optimization of brain atrophy measurement in individuals in whom brain and skull growth is ongoing, and standardization of MR imaging acquisition and image analysis to permit multicentered studies necessary for obtaining sufficient sample sizes to address unique questions. Several techniques have not yet been applied to pediatric MS or at most have only been piloted, including multicomponent T2 (myelin water content) imaging, MT imaging, susceptibility-weighted imaging, cortical imaging, fMR imaging, high-resolution imaging of the optic nerve and spinal cord, and imaging at very high field strengths (>3 T). Children with MS represent a unique cohort in which these techniques can be applied to aid in elucidating the earliest signatures of MS disease, given the short window of time between potential inciting exposures and disease onset. Further work is required to determine whether these advanced techniques can be used in treatment trials. Implementation and optimization of multicentered standardized protocols for advanced imaging techniques is timely, given that pediatric trials of MS-related therapies are soon to be launched.

REFERENCES

1. Geurts JJ, Bo L, Pouwels PJ, et al. Cortical lesions in multiple sclerosis: combined postmortem MR imaging and histopathology. AJNR Am J Neuroradiol 2005;26:572–7.
2. Peterson JW, Bo L, Mork S, et al. Transected neurites, apoptotic neurons, and reduced inflammation in cortical multiple sclerosis lesions. Ann Neurol 2001;50:389–400.
3. Kidd D, Barkhof F, McConnell R, et al. Cortical lesions in multiple sclerosis. Brain 1999;122(Pt 1):17–26.
4. Lucchinetti CF, Popescu BF, Bunyan RF, et al. Inflammatory cortical demyelination in early multiple sclerosis. N Engl J Med 2011;365:2188–97.
5. Bo L, Vedeler CA, Nyland HI, et al. Subpial demyelination in the cerebral cortex of multiple sclerosis patients. J Neuropathol Exp Neurol 2003;62:723–32.
6. Bo L, Vedeler CA, Nyland H, et al. Intracortical multiple sclerosis lesions are not associated with increased lymphocyte infiltration. Mult Scler 2003; 9:323–31.
7. Chard DT, Griffin CM, McLean MA, et al. Brain metabolite changes in cortical grey and normal-appearing white matter in clinically early relapsing-remitting multiple sclerosis. Brain 2002;125: 2342–52.
8. De SN, Matthews PM, Filippi M, et al. Evidence of early cortical atrophy in MS: relevance to white matter changes and disability. Neurology 2003; 60:1157–62.
9. Dalton CM, Chard DT, Davies GR, et al. Early development of multiple sclerosis is associated with progressive grey matter atrophy in patients presenting with clinically isolated syndromes. Brain 2004;127:1101–7.
10. Chard DT, Griffin CM, Rashid W, et al. Progressive grey matter atrophy in clinically early relapsing-remitting multiple sclerosis. Mult Scler 2004;10: 387–91.
11. Nelson F, Datta S, Garcia N, et al. Intracortical lesions by 3T magnetic resonance imaging and correlation with cognitive impairment in multiple sclerosis. Mult Scler 2011;17:1122–9.
12. Roosendaal SD, Moraal B, Pouwels PJ, et al. Accumulation of cortical lesions in MS: relation with cognitive impairment. Mult Scler 2009;15: 708–14.
13. Sanfilipo MP, Benedict RH, Weinstock-Guttman B, et al. Gray and white matter brain atrophy and neuropsychological impairment in multiple sclerosis. Neurology 2006;66:685–92.

14. Amato MP, Bartolozzi ML, Zipoli V, et al. Neocortical volume decrease in relapsing-remitting MS patients with mild cognitive impairment. Neurology 2004;63:89–93.

15. Calabrese M, De SN, Atzori M, et al. Extensive cortical inflammation is associated with epilepsy in multiple sclerosis. J Neurol 2008;255:581–6.

16. Geurts JJ, Roosendaal SD, Calabrese M, et al. Consensus recommendations for MS cortical lesion scoring using double inversion recovery MRI. Neurology 2011;76:418–24.

17. Filippi M, Rocca MA, Calabrese M, et al. Intracortical lesions: relevance for new MRI diagnostic criteria for multiple sclerosis. Neurology 2010;75:1988–94.

18. Calabrese M, Bernardi V, Atzori M, et al. Effect of disease-modifying drugs on cortical lesions and atrophy in relapsing-remitting multiple sclerosis. Mult Scler 2011;18(4):418–24.

19. Tan IL, Pouwels PJ, van Schijndel RA, et al. Isotropic 3D fast FLAIR imaging of the brain in multiple sclerosis patients: initial experience. Eur Radiol 2002;12:559–67.

20. Bakshi R, Ariyaratana S, Benedict RH, et al. Fluid-attenuated inversion recovery magnetic resonance imaging detects cortical and juxtacortical multiple sclerosis lesions. Arch Neurol 2001;58:742–8.

21. Tubridy N, Barker GJ, MacManus DG, et al. Three-dimensional fast fluid attenuated inversion recovery (3D fast FLAIR): a new MRI sequence which increases the detectable cerebral lesion load in multiple sclerosis. Br J Radiol 1998;71:840–5.

22. Geurts JJ, Pouwels PJ, Uitdehaag BM, et al. Intracortical lesions in multiple sclerosis: improved detection with 3D double inversion-recovery MR imaging. Radiology 2005;236:254–60.

23. van HJ, Brink BP, de Vries HE, et al. The blood-brain barrier in cortical multiple sclerosis lesions. J Neuropathol Exp Neurol 2007;66:321–8.

24. Calabrese M, Filippi M, Gallo P. Cortical lesions in multiple sclerosis. Nat Rev Neurol 2010;6:438–44.

25. Bedell BJ, Narayana PA. Implementation and evaluation of a new pulse sequence for rapid acquisition of double inversion recovery images for simultaneous suppression of white matter and CSF. J Magn Reson Imaging 1998;8:544–7.

26. Calabrese M, De SN, Atzori M, et al. Detection of cortical inflammatory lesions by double inversion recovery magnetic resonance imaging in patients with multiple sclerosis. Arch Neurol 2007;64:1416–22.

27. Simon B, Schmidt S, Lukas C, et al. Improved in vivo detection of cortical lesions in multiple sclerosis using double inversion recovery MR imaging at 3 Tesla. Eur Radiol 2010;20:1675–83.

28. Calabrese M, Battaglini M, Giorgio A, et al. Imaging distribution and frequency of cortical lesions in patients with multiple sclerosis. Neurology 2010;75:1234–40.

29. Nelson F, Poonawalla AH, Hou P, et al. Improved identification of intracortical lesions in multiple sclerosis with phase-sensitive inversion recovery in combination with fast double inversion recovery MR imaging. AJNR Am J Neuroradiol 2007;28:1645–9.

30. Nelson F, Poonawalla A, Hou P, et al. 3D MPRAGE improves classification of cortical lesions in multiple sclerosis. Mult Scler 2008;14:1214–9.

31. Bagnato F, Butman JA, Gupta S, et al. In vivo detection of cortical plaques by MR imaging in patients with multiple sclerosis. AJNR Am J Neuroradiol 2006;27:2161–7.

32. Absinta M, Rocca MA, Moiola L, et al. Cortical lesions in children with multiple sclerosis. Neurology 2011;76:910–3.

33. Gogtay N, Thompson PM. Mapping gray matter development: implications for typical development and vulnerability to psychopathology. Brain Cogn 2010;72:6–15.

34. Nakamura K, Fox R, Fisher E. CLADA: cortical longitudinal atrophy detection algorithm. Neuroimage 2011;54:278–89.

35. Derakhshan M, Caramanos Z, Giacomini PS, et al. Evaluation of automated techniques for the quantification of grey matter atrophy in patients with multiple sclerosis. Neuroimage 2010;52:1261–7.

36. Chen JT, Narayanan S, Collins DL, et al. Relating neocortical pathology to disability progression in multiple sclerosis using MRI. Neuroimage 2004;23:1168–75.

37. Sailer M, Fischl B, Salat D, et al. Focal thinning of the cerebral cortex in multiple sclerosis. Brain 2003;126:1734–44.

38. Miller DH, Barkhof F, Frank JA, et al. Measurement of atrophy in multiple sclerosis: pathological basis, methodological aspects and clinical relevance. Brain 2002;125:1676–95.

39. Kalkers NF, Ameziane N, Bot JC, et al. Longitudinal brain volume measurement in multiple sclerosis: rate of brain atrophy is independent of the disease subtype. Arch Neurol 2002;59:1572–6.

40. Fisher E, Rudick RA, Cutter G, et al. Relationship between brain atrophy and disability: an 8-year follow-up study of multiple sclerosis patients. Mult Scler 2000;6:373–7.

41. Minneboo A, Jasperse B, Barkhof F, et al. Predicting short-term disability progression in early multiple sclerosis: added value of MRI parameters. J Neurol Neurosurg Psychiatry 2008;79:917–23.

42. Valsasina P, Benedetti B, Rovaris M, et al. Evidence for progressive gray matter loss in patients with relapsing-remitting MS. Neurology 2005;65:1126–8.

43. Chard D, Miller D. Grey matter pathology in clinically early multiple sclerosis: evidence from magnetic resonance imaging. J Neurol Sci 2009; 282:5–11.

44. Tedeschi G, Lavorgna L, Russo P, et al. Brain atrophy and lesion load in a large population of patients with multiple sclerosis. Neurology 2005; 65:280–5.

45. Rudick RA, Lee JC, Nakamura K, et al. Gray matter atrophy correlates with MS disability progression measured with MSFC but not EDSS. J Neurol Sci 2009;282:106–11.

46. Khaleeli Z, Cercignani M, Audoin B, et al. Localized grey matter damage in early primary progressive multiple sclerosis contributes to disability. Neuroimage 2007;37:253–61.

47. Chard DT, Parker GJ, Griffin CM, et al. The reproducibility and sensitivity of brain tissue volume measurements derived from an SPM-based segmentation methodology. J Magn Reson Imaging 2002;15:259–67.

48. Korteweg T, Rovaris M, Neacsu V, et al. Can rate of brain atrophy in multiple sclerosis be explained by clinical and MRI characteristics? Mult Scler 2009; 15:465–71.

49. Bedell BJ, Narayana PA. Automatic removal of extrameningeal tissues from MR images of human brain. J Magn Reson Imaging 1996;6:939–43.

50. Goldszal AF, Davatzikos C, Pham DL, et al. An image-processing system for qualitative and quantitative volumetric analysis of brain images. J Comput Assist Tomogr 1998;22:827–37.

51. Fox NC, Jenkins R, Leary SM, et al. Progressive cerebral atrophy in MS: a serial study using registered, volumetric MRI. Neurology 2000;54: 807–12.

52. Smith SM, De SN, Jenkinson M, et al. Normalized accurate measurement of longitudinal brain change. J Comput Assist Tomogr 2001;25:466–75.

53. Rudick RA, Fisher E, Lee JC, et al. Use of the brain parenchymal fraction to measure whole brain atrophy in relapsing-remitting MS. Multiple Sclerosis Collaborative Research Group. Neurology 1999;53:1698–704.

54. Kalkers NF, Bergers E, Castelijns JA, et al. Optimizing the association between disability and biological markers in MS. Neurology 2001;57: 1253–8.

55. Tao G, Datta S, He R, et al. Deep gray matter atrophy in multiple sclerosis: a tensor based morphometry. J Neurol Sci 2009;282:39–46.

56. Ceccarelli A, Rocca MA, Pagani E, et al. The topographical distribution of tissue injury in benign MS: a 3T multiparametric MRI study. Neuroimage 2008; 39:1499–509.

57. Andreasen AK, Jakobsen J, Soerensen L, et al. Regional brain atrophy in primary fatigued patients with multiple sclerosis. Neuroimage 2010;50:608–15.

58. Audoin B, Zaaraoui W, Reuter F, et al. Atrophy mainly affects the limbic system and the deep grey matter at the first stage of multiple sclerosis. J Neurol Neurosurg Psychiatry 2010;81:690–5.

59. Ashburner J, Friston KJ. Voxel-based morphometry–the methods. Neuroimage 2000;11:805–21.

60. Pfefferbaum A, Mathalon DH, Sullivan EV, et al. A quantitative magnetic resonance imaging study of changes in brain morphology from infancy to late adulthood. Arch Neurol 1994;51:874–87.

61. Aubert-Broche B, Fonov V, Ghassemi R, et al. Regional brain atrophy in children with multiple sclerosis. Neuroimage 2011;58(2):409–15.

62. Yeh EA, Weinstock-Guttman B, Ramanathan M, et al. Magnetic resonance imaging characteristics of children and adults with paediatric-onset multiple sclerosis. Brain 2009;132:3392–400.

63. Mesaros S, Rocca MA, Absinta M, et al. Evidence of thalamic gray matter loss in pediatric multiple sclerosis. Neurology 2008;70:1107–12.

64. Banwell B, Ghezzi A, Bar-Or A, et al. Multiple sclerosis in children: clinical diagnosis, therapeutic strategies, and future directions. Lancet Neurol 2007;6:887–902.

65. Banwell BL, Sled JG. Starting early: MRI evidence of gray matter atrophy in children with multiple sclerosis. Neurology 2008;70:1065–6.

66. Evangelou N, Konz D, Esiri MM, et al. Regional axonal loss in the corpus callosum correlates with cerebral white matter lesion volume and distribution in multiple sclerosis. Brain 2000;123(Pt 9):1845–9.

67. Kerbrat A, Aubert-Broche B, Fonov V, et al. Reduced head and brain size for age and disproportionately smaller thalami in child-onset MS. Neurology 2012;78:194–201.

68. Giedd JN, Blumenthal J, Jeffries NO, et al. Brain development during childhood and adolescence: a longitudinal MRI study. Nat Neurosci 1999;2: 861–3.

69. Till C, Ghassemi R, Aubert-Broche B, et al. MRI correlates of cognitive impairment in childhood-onset multiple sclerosis. Neuropsychology 2011; 25:319–32.

70. Vrenken H, Geurts JJ, Knol DL, et al. Normal-appearing white matter changes vary with distance to lesions in multiple sclerosis. AJNR Am J Neuroradiol 2006;27:2005–11.

71. Laule C, Vavasour IM, Whittall KP, et al. Evolution of focal and diffuse magnetisation transfer abnormalities in multiple sclerosis. J Neurol 2003;250: 924–31.

72. Fazekas F, Ropele S, Enzinger C, et al. Quantitative magnetization transfer imaging of pre-lesional white-matter changes in multiple sclerosis. Mult Scler 2002;8:479–84.

73. Pike GB, De Stefano N, Narayanan S, et al. Multiple sclerosis: magnetization transfer MR imaging of white matter before lesion appearance on T2-weighted images. Radiology 2000;215:824–30.

74. Dousset V, Gayou A, Brochet B, et al. Early structural changes in acute MS lesions assessed by serial magnetization transfer studies. Neurology 1998;51:1150–5.

75. van Waesberghe JH, Kamphorst W, De Groot CJ, et al. Axonal loss in multiple sclerosis lesions: magnetic resonance imaging insights into substrates of disability. Ann Neurol 1999;46:747–54.

76. Schmierer K, Scaravilli F, Altmann DR, et al. Magnetization transfer ratio and myelin in post-mortem multiple sclerosis brain. Ann Neurol 2004; 56:407–15.

77. Giacomini PS, Levesque IR, Ribeiro L, et al. Measuring demyelination and remyelination in acute multiple sclerosis lesion voxels. Arch Neurol 2009;66:375–81.

78. Chen JT, Collins DL, Freedman MS, et al. Local magnetization transfer ratio signal inhomogeneity is related to subsequent change in MTR in lesions and normal-appearing white-matter of multiple sclerosis patients. Neuroimage 2005;25:1272–8.

79. Wolff SD, Balaban RS. Magnetization transfer imaging: practical aspects and clinical applications. Radiology 1994;192:593–9.

80. McGowan JC, Leigh JS Jr. Selective saturation in magnetization transfer experiments. Magn Reson Med 1994;32:517–22.

81. Mezzapesa DM, Rocca MA, Falini A, et al. A preliminary diffusion tensor and magnetization transfer magnetic resonance imaging study of early-onset multiple sclerosis. Arch Neurol 2004; 61:366–8.

82. Tortorella P, Rocca MA, Mezzapesa DM, et al. MRI quantification of gray and white matter damage in patients with early-onset multiple sclerosis. J Neurol 2006;253:903–7.

83. Le Bihan D, Mangin JF, Poupon C, et al. Diffusion tensor imaging: concepts and applications. J Magn Reson Imaging 2001;13:534–46.

84. Moseley ME, Cohen Y, Kucharczyk J, et al. Diffusion-weighted MR imaging of anisotropic water diffusion in cat central nervous system. Radiology 1990;176:439–45.

85. Pierpaoli C, Basser PJ. Toward a quantitative assessment of diffusion anisotropy. Magn Reson Med 1996;36:893–906.

86. Van HW, Nagels G, Leemans A, et al. Correlation of cognitive dysfunction and diffusion tensor MRI measures in patients with mild and moderate multiple sclerosis. J Magn Reson Imaging 2010;31:1492–8.

87. Bodini B, Khaleeli Z, Cercignani M, et al. Exploring the relationship between white matter and gray matter damage in early primary progressive multiple sclerosis: an in vivo study with TBSS and VBM. Hum Brain Mapp 2009;30:2852–61.

88. Jones DK, Symms MR, Cercignani M, et al. The effect of filter size on VBM analyses of DT-MRI data. Neuroimage 2005;26:546–54.

89. Jones DK, Cercignani M. Twenty-five pitfalls in the analysis of diffusion MRI data. NMR Biomed 2010;23:803–20.

90. Smith SM, Jenkinson M, Johansen-Berg H, et al. Tract-based spatial statistics: voxelwise analysis of multi-subject diffusion data. Neuroimage 2006; 31:1487–505.

91. Conturo TE, Lori NF, Cull TS, et al. Tracking neuronal fiber pathways in the living human brain. Proc Natl Acad Sci U S A 1999;96:10422–7.

92. Mori S, Crain BJ, Chacko VP, et al. Three-dimensional tracking of axonal projections in the brain by magnetic resonance imaging. Ann Neurol 1999;45:265–9.

93. Mori S, van Zijl PC. Fiber tracking: principles and strategies–a technical review. NMR Biomed 2002; 15:468–80.

94. Pagani E, Bammer R, Horsfield MA, et al. Diffusion MR imaging in multiple sclerosis: technical aspects and challenges. AJNR Am J Neuroradiol 2007;28: 411–20.

95. Lowe MJ, Beall EB, Sakaie KE, et al. Resting state sensorimotor functional connectivity in multiple sclerosis inversely correlates with transcallosal motor pathway transverse diffusivity. Hum Brain Mapp 2008;29:818–27.

96. Absinta M, Rocca MA, Moiola L, et al. Brain macro- and microscopic damage in patients with paediatric MS. J Neurol Neurosurg Psychiatry 2010;81(12): 1357–62.

97. Vishwas MS, Chitnis T, Pienaar R, et al. Tract-based analysis of callosal, projection, and association pathways in pediatric patients with multiple sclerosis: a preliminary study. AJNR Am J Neuroradiol 2010;31:121–8.

98. Bethune A, Tipu V, Sled JG, et al. Diffusion tensor imaging and cognitive speed in children with multiple sclerosis. J Neurol Sci 2011;309: 68–74.

99. Ross B, Bluml S. Magnetic resonance spectroscopy of the human brain. Anat Rec 2001;265:54–84.

100. Narayanan S, Caramanos Z, Matthews P, et al. Axonal pathology in patients with multiple sclerosis: evidence from in vivo proton magnetic resonance spectroscopy. In: Cohen JA, Rudick RA, editors. Multiple sclerosis therapeutics. 4th edition. New York: Cambridge University Press; 2011. p. 150–64.

101. De SN, Filippi M. MR spectroscopy in multiple sclerosis. J Neuroimaging 2007;17(Suppl 1):31S–5S.

102. Provencher SW. Automatic quantitation of localized in vivo 1H spectra with LCModel. NMR Biomed 2001;14:260–4.

103. Baslow MH. Evidence supporting a role for N-acetyl-L-aspartate as a molecular water pump in myelinated neurons in the central nervous system. An analytical review. Neurochem Int 2002; 40:295–300.

104. Simmons ML, Frondoza CG, Coyle JT. Immunocytochemical localization of N-acetyl-aspartate with monoclonal antibodies. Neuroscience 1991;45: 37–45.

105. Bitsch A, Bruhn H, Vougioukas V, et al. Inflammatory CNS demyelination: histopathologic correlation with in vivo quantitative proton MR spectroscopy. AJNR Am J Neuroradiol 1999;20:1619–27.

106. Urenjak J, Williams SR, Gadian DG, et al. Proton nuclear magnetic resonance spectroscopy unambiguously identifies different neural cell types. J Neurosci 1993;13:981–9.

107. Arnold DL, De SN, Narayanan S, et al. Proton MR spectroscopy in multiple sclerosis. Neuroimaging Clin North Am 2000;10:789–98.

108. Arnold DL, Wolinsky JS, Matthews PM, et al. The use of magnetic resonance spectroscopy in the evaluation of the natural history of multiple sclerosis. J Neurol Neurosurg Psychiatry 1998; 64(Suppl 1):S94–101.

109. Caramanos Z, Narayanan S, Arnold DL. 1H-MRS quantification of tNA and tCr in patients with multiple sclerosis: a meta-analytic review. Brain 2005;128:2483–506.

110. Doble A. The role of excitotoxicity in neurodegenerative disease: implications for therapy. Pharmacol Ther 1999;81:163–221.

111. Werner P, Pitt D, Raine CS. Multiple sclerosis: altered glutamate homeostasis in lesions correlates with oligodendrocyte and axonal damage. Ann Neurol 2001;50:169–80.

112. Centonze D, Muzio L, Rossi S, et al. The link between inflammation, synaptic transmission and neurodegeneration in multiple sclerosis. Cell Death Differ 2010;17:1083–91.

113. Pitt D, Nagelmeier IE, Wilson HC, et al. Glutamate uptake by oligodendrocytes: implications for excitotoxicity in multiple sclerosis. Neurology 2003;61: 1113–20.

114. Hurd R, Sailasuta N, Srinivasan R, et al. Measurement of brain glutamate using TE-averaged PRESS at 3T. Magn Reson Med 2004;51:435–40.

115. Srinivasan R, Sailasuta N, Hurd R, et al. Evidence of elevated glutamate in multiple sclerosis using magnetic resonance spectroscopy at 3 T. Brain 2005;128:1016–25.

116. De SN, Bartolozzi ML, Guidi L, et al. Magnetic resonance spectroscopy as a measure of brain damage in multiple sclerosis. J Neurol Sci 2005; 233:203–8.

117. Sarchielli P, Presciutti O, Pelliccioli GP, et al. Absolute quantification of brain metabolites by proton magnetic resonance spectroscopy in normal-appearing white matter of multiple sclerosis patients. Brain 1999;122(Pt 3):513–21.

118. Matthews PM, Francis G, Antel J, et al. Proton magnetic resonance spectroscopy for metabolic characterization of plaques in multiple sclerosis. Neurology 1991;41:1251–6.

119. Arnold DL, Matthews PM, Francis GS, et al. Proton magnetic resonance spectroscopic imaging for metabolic characterization of demyelinating plaques. Ann Neurol 1992;31:235–41.

120. Miller DH, Austin SJ, Connelly A, et al. Proton magnetic resonance spectroscopy of an acute and chronic lesion in multiple sclerosis. Lancet 1991;337:58–9.

121. Husted CA, Goodin DS, Hugg JW, et al. Biochemical alterations in multiple sclerosis lesions and normal-appearing white matter detected by in vivo 31P and 1H spectroscopic imaging. Ann Neurol 1994;36:157–65.

122. Van Hecke P, Marchal G, Johannik K, et al. Human brain proton localized NMR spectroscopy in multiple sclerosis. Magn Reson Med 1991;18:199–206.

123. Grossman RI, Lenkinski RE, Ramer KN, et al. MR proton spectroscopy in multiple sclerosis. AJNR Am J Neuroradiol 1992;13:1535–43.

124. Caramanos Z, DiMaio S, Narayanan S, et al. (1)H-MRSI evidence for cortical gray matter pathology that is independent of cerebral white matter lesion load in patients with secondary progressive multiple sclerosis. J Neurol Sci 2009;282:72–9.

125. Fu L, Matthews PM, De Stefano N, et al. Imaging axonal damage of normal-appearing white matter in multiple sclerosis. Brain 1998;121(Pt 1):103–13.

126. De SN, Matthews PM, Arnold DL. Reversible decreases in N-acetylaspartate after acute brain injury. Magn Reson Med 1995;34:721–7.

127. Bjartmar C, Kidd G, Mork S, et al. Neurological disability correlates with spinal cord axonal loss and reduced N-acetyl aspartate in chronic multiple sclerosis patients. Ann Neurol 2000;48:893–901.

128. Evangelou N, Esiri MM, Smith S, et al. Quantitative pathological evidence for axonal loss in normal appearing white matter in multiple sclerosis. Ann Neurol 2000;47:391–5.

129. Inglese M, Ge Y, Filippi M, et al. Indirect evidence for early widespread gray matter involvement in relapsing-remitting multiple sclerosis. Neuroimage 2004;21:1825–9.

130. Rocca MA, Mezzapesa DM, Falini A, et al. Evidence for axonal pathology and adaptive cortical reorganization in patients at presentation with clinically isolated syndromes suggestive of multiple sclerosis. Neuroimage 2003;18:847–55.

131. Mainero C, De Stefano N, Iannucci G, et al. Correlates of MS disability assessed in vivo using aggregates of MR quantities. Neurology 2001;56:1331–4.

132. Tartaglia MC, Narayanan S, Francis SJ, et al. The relationship between diffuse axonal damage and fatigue in multiple sclerosis. Arch Neurol 2004;61: 201–7.

133. De Stefano N, Narayanan S, Francis GS, et al. Evidence of axonal damage in the early stages of multiple sclerosis and its relevance to disability. Arch Neurol 2001;58:65–70.

134. De Stefano N, Iannucci G, Sormani MP, et al. MR correlates of cerebral atrophy in patients with multiple sclerosis. J Neurol 2002;249:1072–7.

135. Reddy H, Narayanan S, Arnoutelis R, et al. Evidence for adaptive functional changes in the cerebral cortex with axonal injury from multiple sclerosis. Brain 2000;123(Pt 11):2314–20.

136. Bruhn H, Frahm J, Merboldt KD, et al. Multiple sclerosis in children: cerebral metabolic alterations monitored by localized proton magnetic resonance spectroscopy in vivo. Ann Neurol 1992;32:140–50.

137. Oguz KK, Kurne A, Aksu AO, et al. Assessment of citrullinated myelin by 1H-MR spectroscopy in early-onset multiple sclerosis. AJNR Am J Neuroradiol 2009;30:716–21.

138. Pritzker LB, Joshi S, Harauz G, et al. Deimination of myelin basic protein. 2. Effect of methylation of MBP on its deimination by peptidylarginine deiminase. Biochemistry 2000;39:5382–8.

139. Pritzker LB, Joshi S, Gowan JJ, et al. Deimination of myelin basic protein. 1. Effect of deimination of arginyl residues of myelin basic protein on its structure and susceptibility to digestion by cathepsin D. Biochemistry 2000;39:5374–81.

140. Wood DD, Bilbao JM, O'Connors P, et al. Acute multiple sclerosis (Marburg type) is associated with developmentally immature myelin basic protein. Ann Neurol 1996;40:18–24.

141. Moscarello MA, Mastronardi FG, Wood DD. The role of citrullinated proteins suggests a novel mechanism in the pathogenesis of multiple sclerosis. Neurochem Res 2007;32:251–6.

142. Vrenken H, Barkhof F, Uitdehaag BM, et al. MR spectroscopic evidence for glial increase but not for neuro-axonal damage in MS normal-appearing white matter. Magn Reson Med 2005; 53:256–66.

143. Ben SL, Miller E, Artzi M, et al. 1H-MRS for the diagnosis of acute disseminated encephalomyelitis: insight into the acute-disease stage. Pediatr Radiol 2010;40:106–13.

144. Brex PA, Parker GJ, Leary SM, et al. Lesion heterogeneity in multiple sclerosis: a study of the relations between appearances on T1 weighted images, T1 relaxation times, and metabolite concentrations. J Neurol Neurosurg Psychiatry 2000;68:627–32.

145. Ashwal S, Holshouser B, Tong K, et al. Proton spectroscopy detected myoinositol in children with traumatic brain injury. Pediatr Res 2004;56:630–8.

146. Elberling TV, Danielsen ER, Rasmussen AK, et al. Reduced myo-inositol and total choline measured with cerebral MRS in acute thyrotoxic Graves' disease. Neurology 2003;60:142–5.

147. Mukamel R, Gelbard H, Arieli A, et al. Coupling between neuronal firing, field potentials, and FMRI in human auditory cortex. Science 2005; 309:951–4.

148. Logothetis NK, Pauls J, Augath M, et al. Neurophysiological investigation of the basis of the fMRI signal. Nature 2001;412:150–7.

149. Mackowiak PA, Siegel E, Wasserman SS, et al. Effects of IFN-beta on human cerebral blood flow distribution. J Interferon Cytokine Res 1998;18: 393–7.

150. de WH, Metz J, Wagner N, et al. Effects of diazepam on cerebral metabolism and mood in normal volunteers. Neuropsychopharmacology 1991;5:33–41.

151. Liu TT, Behzadi Y, Restom K, et al. Caffeine alters the temporal dynamics of the visual BOLD response. Neuroimage 2004;23:1402–13.

152. Buysse DJ, Nofzinger EA, Germain A, et al. Regional brain glucose metabolism during morning and evening wakefulness in humans: preliminary findings. Sleep 2004;27:1245–54.

153. Dietrich T, Krings T, Neulen J, et al. Effects of blood estrogen level on cortical activation patterns during cognitive activation as measured by functional MRI. Neuroimage 2001;13:425–32.

154. Rocca MA, Absinta M, Ghezzi A, et al. Is a preserved functional reserve a mechanism limiting clinical impairment in pediatric MS patients? Hum Brain Mapp 2009;30:2844–51.

155. Rocca MA, Absinta M, Moiola L, et al. Functional and structural connectivity of the motor network in pediatric and adult-onset relapsing-remitting multiple sclerosis. Radiology 2010;254:541–50.

156. Renoux C, Vukusic S, Mikaeloff Y, et al. Natural history of multiple sclerosis with childhood onset. N Engl J Med 2007;356:2603–13.

157. Confavreux C, Vukusic S, Adeleine P. Early clinical predictors and progression of irreversible disability in multiple sclerosis: an amnesic process. Brain 2003;126:770–82.

158. Simone IL, Carrara D, Tortorella C, et al. Course and prognosis in early-onset MS: comparison with adult-onset forms. Neurology 2002;59:1922–8.

Index

A

Anterior commissure, 210
Anti-NMDA receptor encephalitis. See *Encephalitis, anti-NMDA receptor.*
Arcuate fascicle, 205
Association fibers, 204–209

B

Brain, acute vascular insult in, and acute pediatric demyelination, differentiation of, 325–328
Brain volume, measurement in children, methodological issues in, 340, 341
   volumetry for measuring, methodology for, 339–340
Brainstem fibers, 212–215
Brainstem tracts, 212

C

Central nervous system, acquired inflammatory disease of, and genetic disease of, distinguishing of, 328–330
   malignancy of, and acquired demyelination, distinguishing of, 335–336
Central nervous system infection, and inflammatory pediatric demyelination, distinguishing of, 330–331, 333, 334
Central nervous system vasculitis, in childhood, **293–308**
   primary, 294–302
     angiography-negative SV-c, 300–302
     angiography-positive NP-c, 294–298
       clinical features of, 294
       laboratory tests in, 294–295
       neuroimaging features of, 295–296
     angiography-positive P-c, 298–300
     etiopathogenesis of, 296
     management of, 297–298
     outcome of, 298
   secondary, in rheumatic and systemic inflammatory diseases, 302–305
     in systemic diseases/exposures, 305
     infection-associated, 300
Cerebellar peduncle, inferior, 213–215
   superior, 213
Cerebrospinal venous insufficiency, chronic, in multiple sclerosis, 229

Children, central nervous system vasculitis in, **293–308**
   magnetic resonance imaging in, unique considerations in, 218
   multiple sclerosis in. See *Multiple sclerosis, pediatric.*
Cingulum, 210–211, 212
Commissural fibers, 209–210
Cord compression, extra-axial, 272
   in skeletal disorders, 275
Corpus callosum, 209–210, 214
Cortical imaging, in pediatric multiple sclerosis, 338–339
Cortical lesions, in pediatric multiple sclerosis, detection of, 339
Corticobulbar tracts, projection fibers in, 202
Corticopontine tracts, projection fibers in, 202
Corticospinal tract(s), 214
   projection fibers in, 198–201

D

Demyelinating disease, pediatric, acquired, and multiple sclerosis, diagnostic evaluation of, 322
   diagnosis of, MR imaging flags for, 323
   typical features of, on MR imaging, 323
   acute, and acute vascular insult in brain, differentiation of, 325–328
   and acute vascular spinal cord insult, differentiation of, 323–325
   clinical vinettes of, 324–325, 326–328
   inflammatory, and CNS infection, distinguishing of, 330–331, 333, 334
   magnetic resonance imaging reporting template for, 223
   mimics and rare presentations of, **321–336**
   standard lexicon magnetic resonance imaging in, 221–223
   standard protocol magnetic resonance imaging in, 218–221
Demyelinating disorders, relapsing, distinguishing different types of, 332–333
Demyelination, acquired, and central nervous system malignancy, distinguishing of, 335–336
   and vitamin B12 deficiency, distinguishing of, 334–335
Diffusion tensor imaging, 197–198
   in pediatric multiple sclerosis, 343–345

E

Encephalitis, anti-NMDA receptor, **309–320**
    autonomic dysfunction in, 311
    cerebrospinal fluid and serum assessment in,
        312–314
    clinical presentation of, 310–311
    cognitive problems in, 311
    differential diagnosis of, 315–316
    during pregnancy, 318
    electroencephalography in, 312
    epidemiology of, 310
    functional imaging in, 312
    immunopathology of, 315
    neuroimaging in, 311–312
    neurologic features of, 310–311
    outcome of, 317–318
    pathogenesis of, 314–315
    pearls, pitfalls, and variants of, 318
    physical examination in, 311
    prodromal features of, 310
    psychiatric features of, 310
    seizures in, 311
    treatment of, 316–317
    tumor association in, 314
  monophasic acute disseminated, computed
    tomography of brain in, 250
    differential diagnosis of, 256–259
    DT imaging in, 254
    DW imaging in, 253–254
    epidemiology and clinical presentation of,
        246–248
    immunogenesis of, 248–249
    in children, quantitative parameters of, 252
    inflammatory cascade theory of, 249
    International MS Study Group criteria for, 246
    laboratory findings in, 250
    magnetic resonance imaging appearance of,
        245–266
    magnetic resonance imaging of brain and
        spine in, 250–252
    molecular mimicry theory of, 249
    MR spectroscopy in, 254–255
    MT imaging in, 253
    neuroimaging in, 250–255
    neurologic features of, 248
    PET and SPECT in, 255
    prognosis in, 259–260
    treatment of, 256–259
    variants of, 260
Encephalomyelitis, monophasic acute disseminated,
    and relapsing-remitting multiple sclerosis,
    distinguishing of, 238

F

Fasciculus. See specific fasciculus.
Fibrocartilaginous embolization, 275–276

Fornix, 211
Functional magnetic resonance imaging, in pediatric
    multiple sclerosis, 348–349

G

Geniculocalcarine tract (optic radiation), projection
    fibers in, 203–204, 206

I

Internal capsule, projection fibers in, 202, 203

L

Limbic system fibers, 210–211
Longitudinal fasciculus, inferior, 206, 207, 208, 214
    middle, 206–207, 208
    superior, 204–205, 207, 208

M

Magnetic resonance imaging, diagnostic criteria, for
    multiple sclerosis diagnosis, 224
    in children, unique considerations in, 218
    of spinal cord and optic nerve, of children, 221
    standard lexicon, for pediatric demyelination,
        221–223
    standard protocol, for pediatric demyelination,
        218–221
    standardized reporting, in pediatric multiple
        sclerosis, 223
    standarized aquisition and reporting, of pediatric
        multiple sclerosis, **217–226**
Magnetization transfer imaging, in pediatric multiple
    sclerosis, 342–343
Medial lemniscus, 214, 215
Meyer loop, 203, 206
Multiple sclerosis, and acquired pediatric
    demyelinating disease, diagnostic evaluation of,
    322
    and neuromyelitis optica, features of, compared,
    280
    pediatric, **227–243**
        2010 McDonald criteria for, 235
        advanced magnetic resonance imaging in,
            337–354
        basal ganglia lesion in, 226(5)
        brainstem lesion in, 226(6)
        cerebral lesion in, 226(7)
        cerebral white matter lesion in, 226(2)
        children at risk for, MR imaging predictors and,
            235–238
        chronic cerebrospinal venous insufficiency in,
            229
        cortical imaging in, 338–339
        cortical lesions in, detection of, 339

demographic and clinical characteristics in, 229–230

diffusion tensor imaging in, 343–345

environmental risk factors for, 228

functional magnetic resonance imaging in, 348–349

genetic disposition to, 228

gyral projection in, 222, 226(1)

incidence of, 227

internal capsule lesion in, 226(5)

international pediatric consensus criteria for, 234

intracallosal lesion in, 226(3)–226(4)

juxtacortical lesion in, 226(3)

leptomeningeal contrast-enhancement in, 226(2)

lesion distribution in, 222, 226(1)

lesional contrast enhancement in, 222, 226(2)

magnetic resonance imaging diagnostic criteria for, 224

magnetization transfer imaging in, 342–343

MR imaging and diagnosis of, 233–235, 237

MR imaging features of, in very young children, 233

    spinal cord in, 233

    typical, 231–233, 234, 236

onset of, and adult-onset, MR imaging features of, compared, 238–239

    MR imaging diagnostic criteria developed for, 235–238

pathobiology of, 229

pediatric-specific MR criteria for diagnosis of, 235–238

periventricular lesion in, 226(2)

physical and cognitive outcome of, 231

proton magnetic resonance spectroscopy in, 346–348

relapsing-remitting, and neoplasic acute disseminated encephalitis, distinguishing of, 238

    MR imaging appearance of, 231–233

standardized, magnetic resonance imaging acquisition and reporting of, **217–226**

standardized reporting magnetic resonance imaging in, 223

T1 hypointensity in, 222, 226(1)

thalamic lesion in, 226(5)

treatment of, 230–231

volumetry in, 339–342

risk of, following transverse myelitis, 276

Myelin, function and structure of, 183

  MR imaging appearance of, 188–190

Myelination, normal, **183–195**

    imaging of, 185–192

    progression of, 184, 190–193

    terminal zones of, 193, 194

Myelitis, acute transverse, brain lesions in, 276

childhood transverse, mimics of, 272–276

    spinal cord lesions in, 270, 271

transverse, clinical and radiologic mimics of, 268

    follow-up MR imaging in, 276

    in neuromyelitis optica, MR imaging features of, 283–284

    radiologic features of, 270–271

    risk of multiple sclerosis following, 276

    trivial trauma and, 276

N

Neuromyelitis optica, and multiple sclerosis, features of, compared, 280

  brain MR imaging in, 284–285

  clinical course of, 280–281

  demographics and epidemiology of, 279–280

  diagnosis of, **279–291**

  diagnostic criteria for, 282

  immunopathogenesis of, 280

  laboratory investigations in, 285–286

  magnetic resonance imaging in, 282–285

  pathologic abnormalities in, 286–288

  spectrum disorders, 281

  symptomatic brain involvement in, 281–282

  systemic autoimmunity of, 282

  transverse myelitis in, MR imaging features of, 283–284

O

Occipitofrontal fasciculus, inferior, 207–208, 209, 214

  superior, 206, 207, 208, 214

P

Projection fibers, in corticobulbar tracts, 198–201

  in corticopontine tracts, 198–201

  in corticospinal tracts, 198–201

  in geniculocalarine tract (optic radiation), 203–204, 206

  in internal capsule, 202, 203

  in thalamic radiations, 202–203

Proton magnetic resonance spectroscopy, in pediatric multiple sclerosis, 346–348

S

Spinal cord, anatomy of, 267, 269

  disorders of, anatomic considerations in, 267–268

  imaging of, technical aspects of, 268–270

  inflammatory disorders surrounding, 275

  intramedullary disorders of, 275

  vascular disorders of, 275

Spinal cord and optic nerve, of children, magnetic resonance imaging of, 221

Spinal cord insult, acute vascular, and acute pediatric demyelination, differentiation of, 323–325

Stria terminalis, 211–212

T

Temporal stem, 210

Thalamic radiations, projection fibers in, 202–203

U

Uncinate fasciculous, 206, 208, 209, 214

V

Vasculitis, central nervous system. See *Central nervous system vasculitis.*

Vitamin B12 deficiency, and acquired demyelination, distinguishing of, 334–335

Volumetry, in pediatric multiple sclerosis, 339–342

W

White matter, anatomy of, **197–216**

White matter tracts, classification of, 198

  MR imaging of, 197

Moving?

Make sure your subscription moves with you!

To notify us of your new address, find your **Clinics Account Number** (located on your mailing label above your name), and contact customer service at:

Email: **journalscustomerservice-usa@elsevier.com**

800-654-2452 (subscribers in the U.S. & Canada)
314-447-8871 (subscribers outside of the U.S. & Canada)

Fax number: 314-447-8029

Elsevier Health Sciences Division
Subscription Customer Service
3251 Riverport Lane
Maryland Heights, MO 63043

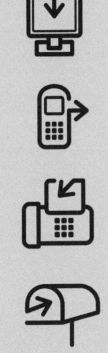